Gastrointestinal Radiology

THE REQUISITES
SECOND EDITION

SERIES EDITOR **James H. Thrall,** M.D.

Radiologist-in-Chief
Massachusetts General Hospital
Juan M. Taveras Professor of Radiology
Harvard Medical School
Boston, Massachusetts

Gastrointestinal Radiology

THE REQUISITES

SECOND EDITION

ROBERT D. HALPERT, M.D.
Chief of General Radiology
Residency Program Director
Henry Ford Hospital
Detroit, Michigan

PETER J. FECZKO, M.D.
Section Chief of Gastrointestinal Radiology
Henry Ford Hospital
Detroit, Michigan

*with **590** illustrations*

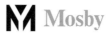 Mosby

St. Louis Baltimore Boston Carlsbad
Chicago Minneapolis New York Philadelphia Portland
London Milan Sydney Tokyo Toronto

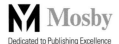

Dedicated to Publishing Excellence

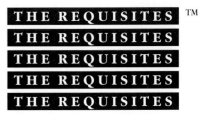

Developmental Editor: Mia Cariño
Project Manager: Patricia Tannian
Production Editor: Kevin Schofield/Richard Hund
Design Manager: Gail Morey Hudson
Manufacturing Supervisor: Don Carlisle

SECOND EDITION

Copyright © 1999 by Mosby, Inc.

Composition by Graphic World Inc.
Printing/binding by Maple Vail Book Mfg Group

Mosby, Inc.
11830 Westline Industrial Drive
St. Louis, MO 63146

Library of Congress Cataloging in Publication Data

Halpert, Robert D., M.D.
    Gastrointestinal radiology : the requisites / Robert D. Halpert,
Peter J. Feczko. — 2nd ed.
      p.   cm.
    Includes bibliographical references and index.
    ISBN 0-8151-4370-2
    1. Gastrointestinal system—Radiography. I. Feczko, Peter J.
II. Title.
    [DNLM: 1. Gastrointestinal System—radiography. 2. Diagnostic
Imaging. WI 141 H195g 1999]
RC804.R6H27 1999
616.3′307572—dc21
DNLM/DLC
for Library of Congress   99-10221
                                    CIP

99 00 01 02 03 / 9 8 7 6 5 4 3 2 1

To my wife
Sylvia
whose love, patience, and support make all things possible,
and to my children
Heather Anne, Stephenie, Janie, Emily, Maggie, *and* **Robbie**
who were willing, for a limited period of time,
to share their Dad with this venture

R.D.H.

To my father
Joseph
my wife
Claire
and my children
Matthew, Julia, *and* **Andrea**

P.J.F.

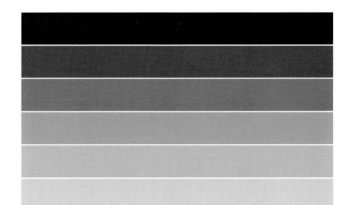

Foreword

Gastrointestinal Radiology was the first volume in THE REQUISITES™ in radiology series. The original book stood alone for quite some time but has turned out to be a harbinger of the success of the entire series. Drs. Robert D. Halpert and Philip Goodman captured and even helped define the central attribute of the series: authoritative information presented efficiently to the reader. The second edition retains this characteristic while updating factual and illustrative material.

The first edition of *Gastrointestinal Radiology: THE REQUISITES* was organized in a very logical way that Drs. Halpert and Peter J. Feczko have maintained in the second edition. Each chapter begins with a brief overview of examination techniques. These discussions include information on the reasons for using specialized maneuvers and different imaging modalities, as well as descriptions of how to perform the examinations. Thereafter, each chapter proceeds sensibly on the basis of radiological findings and their differential diagnosis. This approach defines a particular strength of *Gastrointestinal Radiology: THE REQUISITES*: the reader encounters the gastrointestinal tract and its diseases the way they are encountered by the radiologist in clinical practice. Appropriately performed examinations reveal patterns of abnormality that must first be recognized and categorized and then evaluated for etiology. Knowledge of the radiological differential diagnosis, coupled with clinical context, brings the observer to the most likely possibilities.

Each chapter in the second edition has been updated to reflect new knowledge and practice patterns. In particular, Drs. Halpert and Feczko have added a significant number of new illustrations. They have also added summary and review material in the form of tables and boxes. These have proven to be a particularly popular feature of THE REQUISITES™ series, since they allow the reader to review large amounts of material quickly while reading the complete text.

In the 6-year interval since the first edition, cross-sectional imaging techniques have markedly advanced in quality. New clinical applications have blossomed. In particular, spiral computed tomography (CT) has become available and is now the imaging standard for many abdominal applications. New material on CT, ultrasound, and magnetic resonance imaging is appropriately incorporated throughout the second edition of *Gastrointestinal Radiology: THE REQUISITES*. At the same time, the excellent presentations of conventional imaging methods employing barium are retained. The high quality and succinctness of this subject matter are especially important, since residents and fellows now receive less personal training in conventional barium techniques than in the past.

The philosophy of THE REQUISITES™ series is retained in the second edition. The goal of the series has always been to create a concise book providing core material in each important subspecialty of radiology. Since most radiology residencies are designed in a format of subspecialty-based rotations, THE REQUISITES™ series provides an efficient method by which residents go from a limited radiological knowledge of an area to a useful working knowledge in the short period of time embraced by the subspecialty rotation. At the same time, when residents are preparing for in-service and other examinations, the compact nature of the books in THE REQUISITES™ is a great advantage in covering substantial material in the inevitably limited time available.

I believe the resident in radiology will continue to find *Gastrointestinal Radiology: THE REQUISITES* a concise, useful introduction to the subject, especially with the enhancement of the second edition. Residents, fellows, and practicing radiologists should also find this a very manageable text for review of the subspecialty. We further hope that surgeons and internists and their resident and fellowship trainees interested in the gastrointestinal tract will also continue to find this a user-friendly book. Congratulations to Drs. Halpert and Feczko on their outstanding accomplishment.

James H. Thrall, MD

Radiologist-in-Chief
Massachusetts General Hospital
Professor of Radiology
Harvard Medical School
Boston, Massachusetts

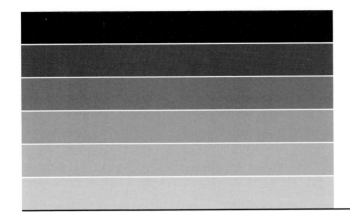

Preface

With the release of the second edition of this work, the reader will note that because of time constraints, Dr. Philip Goodman has not participated in this new edition. His role has been assumed capably by Dr. Peter Feczko, a gastrointestinal radiologist of considerable stature. However, it remains for me to acknowledge the substantial contribution that Dr. Goodman made to the first edition, much of which is carried into the second. His role in the birthing of this venture and its subsequent success is most gratefully appreciated, and I count it an honor to have worked with such a gentleman.

I would also like to acknowledge the privilege of being involved in a series like THE REQUISITES™ and especially of having co-authored the first volume in this unique series. To be involved in THE REQUISITES™ was a challenge in that it was a bold and innovative undertaking by the publisher, Mosby, Inc., and the series editor, Dr. Jim Thrall. The format common to many medical textbooks seldom results in interesting reading. To this author, the new series provided, for the first time in decades, the opportunity to become "part of the text." THE REQUISITES™ was a first in a new style of textbooks in which the personality and views of the authors are not largely bleached out by draconian editorial dogma. As a result, readers find that what is being discussed is well amplified and highlighted by personal insights and experiences of the author. The text returned a certain richness to medical/scientific writing that had been absent for several decades. For this, I must credit the publisher and Dr. Thrall for their determination to undertake something different.

Over the last several years, I have had the opportunity to discuss the text and the series with numerous people from around the world. I confess that I had some initial concerns as to how such a text style would be received. However, the very positive response from readers, both within the specialty of radiology and in other specialties, has been most encouraging and gratifying. In particular, I have been pleased to see how the book has been received by radiology residents.

In the launching of this new edition, I hope that we have not lost sight of those things that made the first edition of *Gastrointestinal Radiology: THE REQUISITES* so successful. Indeed, it is my hope that we have made gastrointestinal and abdominal radiology all the more interesting and inviting to our readers.

Robert D. Halpert, MD

1998

I greatly acknowledge those people whose efforts and contributions were instrumental in the completion of this project. I thank colleagues at the H. Lee Moffitt Cancer Center and Research Institute and the University of Texas Medical Branch at Galveston who so willingly contributed material to this book, as well as those at the Henry Ford Hospital who have shared cases with us or helped in the organization of this new edition. These include Dr. Dan Eurman and Dr. David L. Spizarny, Dr. Brigitte Ala, and Dr. Eric Ward.

R.D.H.

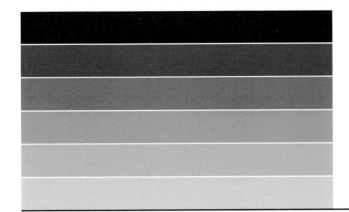

Preface to the First Edition

In August of 1879, while attending the Annual Meeting of the American Association for the Advancement of Science in Saratoga, New York, the renowned physician, Sir William Osler chanced to meet the inventor, Thomas Edison. Edison, having a passing interest in the medical applications of his inventions, suggested to Osler that it might be possible to "illumine the interior of the body by passing a small electric burner into the stomach." Sir William's response is not recorded, but his account of the encounter suggests some degree of amusement at the prospect of passing a tube with a light on the end into the stomach.

Nevertheless, Edison's words were prophetic and 114 years later, endoscopic direct visualization of the mucosal surface has established itself as the standard of gastrointestinal (GI) diagnosis, following several decades of virtual domination of this field by radiologists. However, the expected demise of radiological imaging of the gastrointestinal tract has not occurred. Instead, a collaborative, complementary relationship between endoscopy and radiological imaging of the gut has evolved, spurred on and encouraged by the profound effect of cost constraint and the increasing diagnostic sensitivity and relatively low cost of the radiological procedures.

Barium studies have decreased but not disappeared since the advent of widely available endoscopy. Moreover, the technical refinement of low-cost barium examinations may, in all likelihood, carve out a well-defined niche as a screening examination for many patients.

In addition, the development of other imaging methods has tremendously enhanced the role of imaging in GI diagnosis. Without doubt, the use of helical computer-assisted tomography, real-time ultrasound, and to an increasing extent, magnetic resonance imaging has greatly impacted gastrointestinal imaging. Indeed, modern cross-sectional multiplanar imaging has opened the abdomen for radiological inspection in a way that had been hitherto unattainable. Enhanced liver diagnosis and evaluation of the spleen, pancreas, lymphatics, and the structures surrounding the gut are now possible and signal the beginning of yet a new era in abdominal imaging and diagnosis.

In recent decades, our clinical colleagues have developed what they refer to as the *problem-oriented approach* to patient care and patient records. This refers to an orderly approach to patient diagnosis and management wherein the problems of greatest concern are appropriately weighted, while diagnoses of lesser importance are not lost sight of or neglected in the process. The goal is to establish a global perspective of patient care. Moreover, it should also facilitate a more readable and organized medical record.

In a similar fashion, we have tried to view the "radiological terrain" through the eyes of a first-year resident, a resident preparing for boards, or possibly a radiologist desiring to acquire a concise and abbreviated review of the specialty of gastrointestinal imaging. It would seem appropriate, from our view, to develop a problem-oriented approach to radiology to best address all of these demands and to attempt to present radiological problem solving (diagnosis) in an organized prioritized fashion.

This is generally referred to in radiology as the pattern approach. However, in keeping with a patient-orientated perspective on the practice of radiology, I would prefer to call these radiological patterns of disease, "problems." The irregular thickened gastric fold, from the referring physician's point of view (and especially the patient's perspective) is not a pattern, but a problem! For the attending radiologist, the issue is one of problem solving. Although some may see this as nothing more than hair splitting and semantics (and they may be correct), it is, nevertheless, an accurate reflection of a philosophical perspective on the practice of radiology, no doubt left over from my days as a family practitioner.

The advantage of this approach, as opposed to the disease-oriented method, is to allow a closer paralleling of the real day-to-day world of radiology, and as a result, be of more practical value. The disadvantage is in the complexities of presenting material. In terms of writing a textbook, it is easier to describe a disease and all its radiological presentations, than to start with the radiological problem and work backward toward a reasonable differential diagnosis. The former is the organizational basis of almost all reference texts, while the latter is the daily experience of most radiologists. However, in the problem-oriented clinical management of a patient, problems often overlap, or the same disease may result in several very different problems. In the same way, a disease may have several radiological presentations. Gastric carcinoma, for example, may present as a problem of gastric folds, gastric mass, or ulceration. Hence, the inherent weakness in such a presentation of material.

Accordingly, we have tried to avoid undue redundancy while at the same time overlapping wherever necessary. Usually, the more in depth discussion will be reserved for the most common radiological problem posed by the disease entity.

Robert D. Halpert, MD

1993

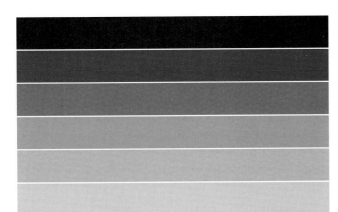

Contents

Gastrointestinal Radiology

THE REQUISITES

SECOND EDITION

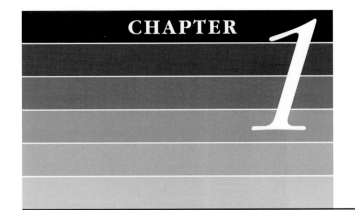

CHAPTER 1

Esophagus and Gastroesophageal Junction

EXAMINATION TECHNIQUES

Radiographic examination of the esophagus encompasses both conventional fluoroscopic studies and various cross-sectional imaging methods. Esophagram or barium swallow is most often performed as a biphasic examination in which both double- and single-contrast techniques are employed (Box 1-1). In the upright position, the patient ingests an effervescent agent followed by a cup of high-density barium. Films obtained during this time demonstrate the esophageal lumen distended with gas and the mucosal surface coated with barium (Fig. 1-1). This double-contrast phase of the examination is especially useful for showing fine mucosal detail, such as superficial nodules or ulcerations. When pooling of barium prevents visualization of the distal esophagus, a tube esophagram can be performed by injecting air directly into the esophageal lumen through a tube placed in the esophagus. This technique, how-

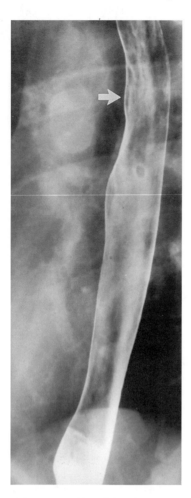

Fig. 1-1 Double-contrast film of the thoracic esophagus. Note mild marginal nodularity *(arrow)* at the impression of the left main bronchus. This is a normal finding and should not be confused with disease.

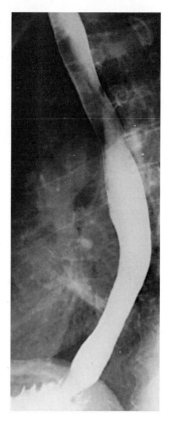

Fig. 1-2 Single-contrast film of the thoracic esophagus.

Box 1-1   Components of the Esophagram

Oral pharyngeal function
Morphology of the esophageal tube
Esophageal motility
Esophageal mucosal surface
Appearance of the gastroesophageal junction
Presence or absence of spontaneous gastroesophageal
    reflux and efficiency of secondary wave clearance

---

ever, is not frequently used and is associated with considerable patient discomfort. However, it is a highly effective method of demonstrating subtle strictures in patients with a dysphagia history. Fluoroscopically following the course of a 12.5-mm barium tablet taken with water is also an effective and less traumatic alternative to demonstrate the presence of a subtle stricture.

If the esophagram is performed as part of an upper gastrointestinal (UGI) series, double-contrast films of the stomach and duodenum are obtained following double-contrast films of the esophagus. Single-contrast examination of the esophagus is usually performed with the patient in the right anterior oblique prone position. Esophageal peristalsis is observed fluoroscopically after the patient has taken a single swallow of low-density barium. Films are then obtained as the patient continues to drink the cup of low-density barium (Fig. 1-2). This single-contrast phase of the examination is especially useful for evaluating esophageal motility and distensibility and for detecting certain abnormalities of the distal esophagus, including sliding hiatal hernia and mucosal ring (B-ring).

Spontaneous gastroesophageal reflux may also be observed fluoroscopically during the single-contrast phase of the examination. Provocative maneuvers to increase intraabdominal pressure and thereby elicit reflux are sometimes performed, but the significance of reflux induced by these maneuvers remains controversial. Mucosal-relief views of the collapsed esophagus show the longitudinal fold pattern and may be useful for demonstrating esophageal varices. Although esophagram is usually performed as part of a complete UGI series, it is sometimes requested as an isolated examination in patients with dysphagia or other complaints localized to the esophagus. However, all esophagrams should include evaluation of the proximal stomach because proximal stomach lesions may cause dysphagia, chest pain, or other symptoms suggesting esophageal disease.

Detailed examination of the pharynx and cervical esophagus may be incorporated into the routine esophagram in patients with cervical dysphagia or other symptoms localized to the neck. This is performed during the double-contrast phase with the patient in an upright position. Rapid-sequence films (three exposures per second) or a video recording is obtained in frontal and lateral projections while the patient drinks high-density barium. This allows dynamic evaluation of swallowing function and detection of physiological abnormalities, such as incomplete cricopharyngeal relaxation. Frontal and lateral spot films are then obtained while the patient phonates to distend the hypopharynx. The distention and mucosal coating seen on these spot films provide detailed anatomical information that might be obscured by barium on rapid-sequence or videotape recording.

In cases of suspected esophageal perforation, water-soluble contrast material is recommended because leakage of barium into the mediastinum may induce mediastinitis. If water-soluble contrast material does not demonstrate an esophageal perforation, the study may be repeated using barium because a small leak of water-soluble contrast material can be difficult to visualize. Water-soluble contrast material is hyperosmolar; therefore it can induce pulmonary edema when introduced into the respiratory tract, either by aspiration from the hypopharynx or by extension through an esophagorespiratory fistula. However, low-osmolality, water-soluble contrast material does not cause pulmonary edema and can be used safely in patients with suspected esophageal perforation who are at risk of aspirating or who are known to have an esophagorespiratory fistula. Nevertheless, its palatability leaves much to be desired.

Computed tomography (CT) is the most commonly used cross-sectional technique for evaluating the esophagus. CT is most helpful for demonstrating the extraluminal component of esophageal disease. This includes staging of esophageal carcinoma (wall thickening, invasion of adjacent structures, and distant metastases) and evaluation of esophageal trauma (extension to mediastinum or pleural cavity). Magnetic resonance imaging (MRI) offers cross-sectional evaluation with the advantages of multiplanar capabilities and lack of ionizing radiation. Although MRI has been of limited usefulness because of motion artifact, image quality is improving with the use of cardiorespiratory gating techniques. Endoscopic ultrasound, in which a transducer is endoscopically placed into the esophageal lumen, can differentiate the individual layers of the esophageal wall and

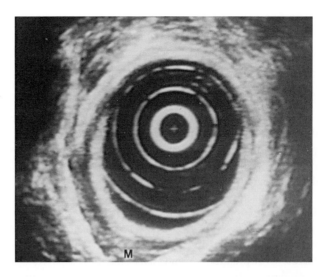

Fig. 1-3 Endoscopic ultrasound shows a hypoechoic mural mass *(M)*, representing esophageal carcinoma.

has been especially useful in evaluating the depth of esophageal tumors (Fig. 1-3).

SOLITARY MUCOSAL MASSES

Nonneoplastic

Inflammatory esophagogastric polyp/fold

Inflammatory esophagogastric polyp/fold is a prominent fold extending from the gastric cardia into the distal esophagus. This fold often has a protuberant tip that may simulate an esophageal polyp (Fig. 1-4). This polyp/fold complex (sometimes referred to as a sentinel polyp) is usually associated with gastroesophageal reflux. If the polypoid tip is larger than 2.5 cm in diameter or appears irregular, a biopsy is indicated to exclude adenocarcinoma of the gastroesophageal junction.

Neoplastic

Carcinomas

Primary squamous cell carcinoma of the hypopharynx or esophagus can present as a solitary mucosal mass, either small and plaquelike or large and polypoid (Figs. 1-5 and 1-6). Ulceration of the mass can occur in both small and large lesions.

Squamous cell carcinoma represents up to 95% of esophageal carcinomas. The most common risk factors (Box 1-2) for development of squamous cell carcinoma of the esophagus are cigarette smoking and alcohol ingestion. Other risk factors include the following:
- Chronic food stasis (achalasia)
- Chronic inflammation and scarring (lye stricture or radiation)
- Tylosis (a rare genetic disease of the skin characterized by palmar and plantar hyperkeratosis)

- Plummer-Vinson syndrome (association of cervical esophageal webs, iron-deficiency anemia, and dysphagia)
- Sprue
- Certain skin disorders such as pemphigoid and epidermolysis bullosa

Squamous cell carcinomas of the head and neck are also associated with an increased incidence of subsequent squamous cell carcinoma of the esophagus, resulting from either common risk factors (e.g., cigarettes and alcohol) or radiation used to treat the original tumor.

Adenocarcinoma of the esophagus accounts for fewer than 5% of esophageal carcinomas. Most cases represent either superior extension of gastric adenocarcinoma or malignant transformation of gastric-type epithelium in Barrett's esophagus. Adenocarcinoma develops in approximately 10% of patients with Barrett's esophagus, suggesting the need for regular surveillance of this condition.

Spindle-cell carcinoma represents an uncommon variant of squamous cell carcinoma that has undergone focal mesenchymal metaplasia. This typically appears as a bulky, polypoid intraluminal mass. Carcinosarcoma, oat cell carcinoma, and primary malignant melanoma of the esophagus are rare epithelial malignancies that appear morphologically similar to spindle-cell carcinoma.

Adenomas and papillomas

Adenomas and papillomas are uncommon, benign tumors of the esophagus that arise from columnar and squamous epithelium, respectively.

MULTIPLE MUCOSAL MASSES

Nonneoplastic

Candida esophagitis

Fungal esophagitis caused by *Candida albicans* is most commonly seen in patients with acquired immuno-deficiency syndrome (AIDS) or patients with other immunocompromising diseases. This fungus causes whitish, slightly raised plaques that may also involve the pharynx or tongue (oral thrush). In the esophagus, these plaques resemble small mucosal nodules that often occur in longitudinal columns (Figs. 1-7 and 1-8). Patients with esophageal stasis, such as those with achalasia or scleroderma, are also at risk for developing *Candida* esophagitis.

Reflux esophagitis

Reflux esophagitis may occur in patients with gastroesophageal reflux as a result of sensitivity of the esophageal mucosa to the acidic gastric fluid. Because reflux usually does not extend beyond the distal esophagus, esophagitis is most commonly confined to this area. Abnormal esophageal motility and mucosal edema are early signs of reflux esophagitis, with erosions, ulcerations, and stricture formation occurring with prolonged or severe reflux.

Glycogenic acanthosis

Glycogenic acanthosis is a benign degenerative condition of the esophagus seen in middle-aged and elderly people. Focal deposits of glycogen form discrete plaques that appear as mucosal nodules on contrast studies (Fig. 1-9). This does not cause dysphagia and is usually an incidental finding.

Crohn's disease

Filiform polyps are a rare manifestation of Crohn's disease of the esophagus. These thin, tubular or branching mucosal polyps resemble those seen in the colon or ileum in the healing stage of inflammatory bowel disease.

Pemphigoid and epidermolysis bullosa

Subepidermal bullae or blebs in the esophagus may be associated with cutaneous lesions in both benign mucous membrane pemphigoid and epidermolysis bullosa.

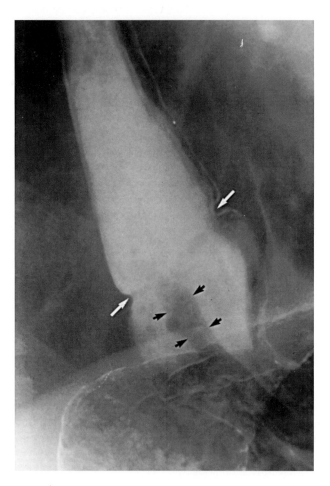

Fig. 1-4 Inflammatory esophagogastric polyp/fold *(black arrows)* in a small hiatal hernia. A nonobstructing B-ring *(white arrows)* is also present.

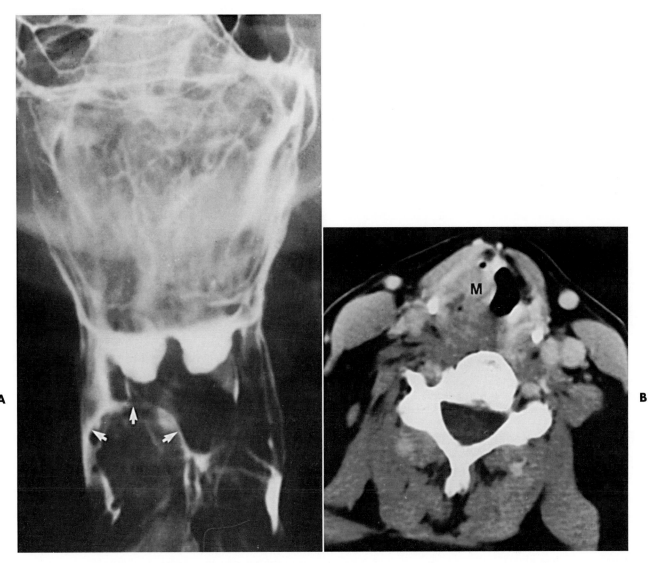

Fig. 1-5   **A,** Frontal film of the pharynx shows a large mass in the right pyriform sinus *(arrows)* representing squamous cell carcinoma. **B,** CT shows the soft tissue mass *(M)* obliterating the right pyriform sinus.

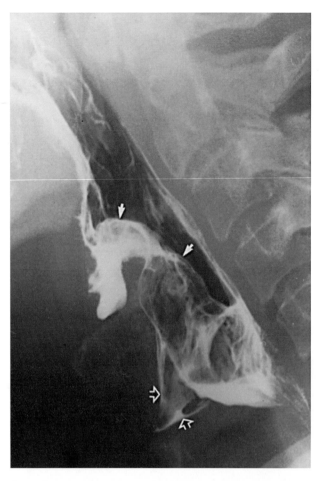

Fig. 1-6   Lateral film of the hypopharynx reveals a large mass involving the epiglottis and aryepiglottic fold *(arrows)*, representing squamous cell carcinoma. Barium is also seen in the larynx and supraglottic portion of the airway *(open arrows)*.

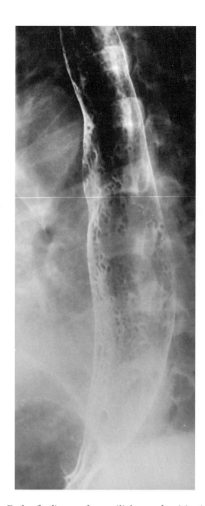

Fig. 1-7   Early findings of monilial esophagitis (colonization stage). Note the well-developed rounded plaques without ulceration.

Box 1-2   Risk Factors for Esophageal Cancer

Tobacco
Alcohol
Achalasia
Lye stricture
Plummer-Vinson syndrome
Head and neck cancers
Plantar and palmar hyperkeratosis
Sprue
Chronic reflux/Barrett's metaplasia

These appear initially as small mucosal nodules but subsequently undergo inflammation, ulceration, and fibrosis with stricture formation.

"Hairy" esophagus
Following pharyngoesophageal reconstructive surgery, hair follicles from the skin graft may appear as multiple small mucosal masses ("hairy" or hirsute esophagus).

Neoplastic

Papillomatosis
Papillomatosis is a rare condition characterized by multiple esophageal papillomas. These benign epithelial growths are usually solitary, but they can be multiple in squamous papillomatosis, an unusual genetic disease, or in acanthosis nigricans, a disease in which esophageal papillomas occur in association with focal thickening and hyperpigmentation of the skin.

Superficial spreading carcinoma
Superficial spreading carcinoma is an unusual form of squamous cell carcinoma characterized by small mucosal nodules. These tumors are limited to the mucosal and submucosal layers of the esophagus, but metastasis to adjacent lymph nodes may be present.

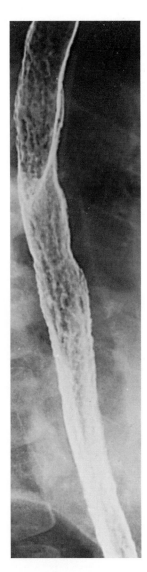

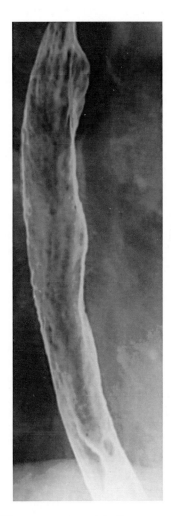

Fig. 1-8   Diffuse mucosal nodularity and ulceration represents advanced esophageal candidiasis in a patient with AIDS.

Fig. 1-9   Diffuse mucosal nodularity represents glycogenic acanthosis.

Cowden's syndrome

Cowden's syndrome is a rare genetic disease in which tiny hamartomas may cause diffuse mucosal nodularity of the gastrointestinal (GI) tract, including the esophagus. This disorder is often associated with various tumors of the skin, breast, and thyroid gland.

Leukoplakia

Leukoplakia represents small, whitish plaques resulting from hyperplasia of squamous epithelium. This rare cause of esophageal nodularity has an uncertain malignant potential, although it appears histologically identical to the more common premalignant leukoplakia of the oropharynx.

SUBMUCOSAL MASSES

Nonneoplastic

Varices

Esophageal varices represent dilated veins in the submucosal layer of the esophageal wall (Box 1-3). The more common uphill varices involve the distal esophagus and result from elevated portal venous pressure, usually secondary to cirrhosis of the liver. This causes increased blood flow through the coronary (left gastric) vein into the distal esophageal venous plexus, which then empties through the azygous system into the superior vena cava. Gastric fundal varices are sometimes associated with distal esophageal varices.

The less common downhill varices involve the proximal thoracic esophagus and result from obstruction of the superior vena cava. Collateral blood flow bypasses the obstruction and enters the superior vena cava through the azygous system, thereby sparing the distal esophageal veins (Fig. 1-10). However, an obstruction involving either the azygous system or the superior vena cava inferior to its junction with the azygous vein leads to collateral blood flow through the coronary and portal veins into the inferior vena cava. This results in varices involving the entire length of the thoracic esophagus.

On contrast studies, esophageal varices are best demonstrated with the patient in the horizontal position because in the upright position gravity decreases distention of esophageal veins and can render varices invisible.

Box 1-3 Esophageal Varices: Direction Matters

Uphill varices are related to portal hypertension with resultant ascending varices.
Downhill varices result from obstruction of the superior vena cava with varicoid collateral veins descending along the upper esophagus toward the right heart.

The optimal technique for detecting varices is to have the patient take a single swallow of high-density barium. Continuous drinking may overcompress the varices; a single swallow usually demonstrates the smooth, serpentine submucosal masses typical of varices (Fig. 1-11). Mucosal relief views of the collapsed esophagus are also useful for demonstrating this appearance.

On CT, varices can appear as thickening of the esophageal wall or as adjacent lobulated soft tissue masses. Bolused intravenous (IV) contrast material may be necessary to differentiate enhancing varices from nonenhancing neoplastic or inflammatory disease. Angiography is also useful for demonstrating esophageal varices and may be combined with interventional techniques for treating acute variceal bleeding.

Cysts

Esophageal cysts may be congenital (foregut duplication cysts) or acquired (retention cysts). Duplication cysts are usually asymptomatic and, though usually discovered in childhood, are first noted in adults in 30% of cases (Figs. 1-12 and 1-13). They appear as a round or

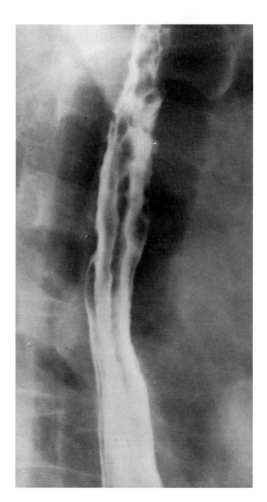

Fig. 1-10   Downhill varices. A 61-year-old patient with upper mediastinal mass, occluded superior vena cava and venous congestion (superior vena cava syndrome).

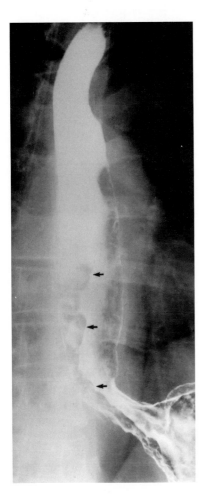

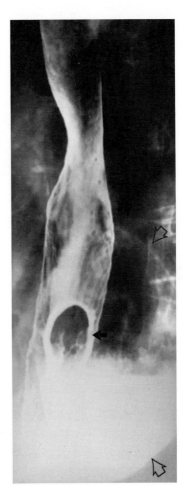

Fig. 1-11   Uphill varices. Typical serpiginous filling defects in distal esophagus *(arrows)* in patient with portal hypertension.

Fig. 1-12   Duplication cyst. Note communicating mouth of cyst *(arrow)* and the outer contours of the cyst *(open arrows)* demonstrating its size.

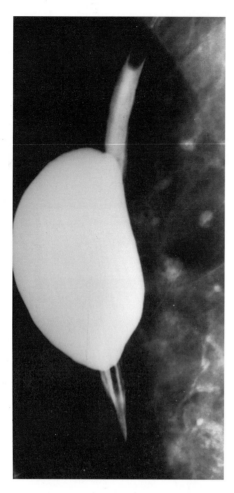

Fig. 1-13 Esophageal duplication cyst communicating with lumen and filling with barium on single-contrast examination.

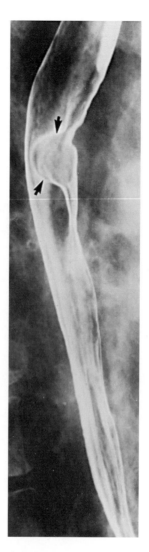

Fig. 1-14 Smooth submucosal mass *(arrows)* in the upper thoracic esophagus represents a leiomyoma.

ovoid, soft tissue density mediastinal mass on chest films, and as a submucosal or extrinsic mass on esophagrams. Retention cysts, rare lesions that arise from dilated mucous glands in the distal esophagus, have a similar radiographic appearance.

Neoplastic

Mesenchymal tumors

Stromal cell tumor, or leiomyoma, is the most common benign neoplasm of the esophagus. This smooth muscle tumor produces a focal rounded impression (Fig. 1-14). Although usually solitary, multiple leiomyomas of the esophagus occur in up to 3% of cases. Leiomyomas occasionally contain mottled calcifications.

Other benign submucosal tumors of the esophagus are uncommon. Like leiomyomas or stromal cell tumors, they arise from mesenchymal tissues and appear radiographically as smooth, rounded masses. These tumors include hemangiomas, lipomas, and neurofibromas.

Kaposi's sarcoma

Kaposi's sarcoma is a vascular tumor that was originally described as a rare cutaneous lesion affecting elderly men of Mediterranean descent. However, it is now recognized as a common lesion involving the skin, GI tract, and respiratory tract of patients with AIDS.

Fibrovascular polyp

Fibrovascular polyp, an unusual benign tumor, originates in the wall of the proximal esophagus and elongates to form a smooth intraluminal mass. This mass may extend inferiorly to occupy the entire esophageal lumen or may be regurgitated into the pharynx and cause asphyxiation.

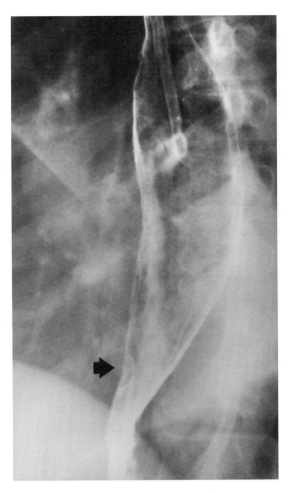

Fig. 1-15   Granular cell tumor of the distal esophagus.

Granular cell tumors

Granular cell tumors are rare submucosal tumors thought to have a neural origin, possibly Schwann cells. They occur in the GI tract as solitary small submucosal lesions usually involving the esophagus, although they have been reported in both the stomach and colon. Radiologically they are identical in appearance to any small submucosal mass (Fig. 1-15).

Lymphoma and metastases

Primary malignant neoplasms (sarcomas) and secondary malignancies (lymphoma, leukemia, and hematogenous metastases) are rare causes of discrete submucosal masses in the esophagus.

EXTRINSIC PROCESSES

Box 1-4 lists extrinsic abnormalities affecting the esophagus.

Box 1-4   Problems in the Neighborhood: Extrinsic Abnormalities Affecting the Esophagus
Cricopharyngeal spasm Vertebral osteophytes Thyroid enlargement Mediastinal masses Abnormal vessels, e.g., aberrant right subclavian artery, pulmonary sling Cardiac enlargement Ectatic thoracic aorta

Cervical Esophagus

Postcricoid defect is a normal indentation on the anterior aspect of the hypopharynx at approximately the level of the C4 vertebra. This was originally thought to represent a venous plexus but is now considered to result from redundant mucosa. This incidental finding may simulate a superficial neoplasm.

Incomplete relaxation of the cricopharyngeus muscle can cause transient extrinsic impression on the posterior aspect of the cervical esophagus at the level of the C5 or C6 vertebra. This localized esophageal dysmotility can cause significant dysphagia.

Anterior osteophytes of the cervical spine and, rarely, anterior herniation of an intervertebral disk may cause focal impressions on the posterior wall of the cervical esophagus. Focal or diffuse enlargement of the thyroid gland can deviate and compress the esophagus. Retropharyngeal tumor, hematoma, or abscess may displace the hypopharynx and cervical esophagus anteriorly. Cervical adenopathy and parathyroid enlargement may also lead to extrinsic compression of the cervical esophagus (Fig. 1-16).

Thoracic Esophagus

The most commonly noted normal extrinsic impressions on the thoracic esophagus are the aortic arch and left main bronchus (Fig. 1-17). Abnormal vessels, such as a right aortic arch, aneurysm or ectasia of the thoracic aorta, and aberrant right subclavian artery, may also compress or displace the esophagus (Figs. 1-18 and 1-19). On rare occasions, an aberrant left pulmonary artery arising from the right pulmonary artery and crossing the mediastinum to the left lung can produce an anterior focal impression on the esophagus about the level of the carina. This is known as the pulmonary sling.

Mediastinal adenopathy causes impressions along the anterior aspect of the midesophagus, and spinous

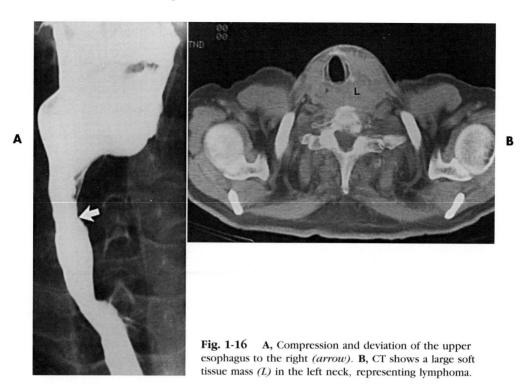

Fig. 1-16   A, Compression and deviation of the upper esophagus to the right *(arrow)*. **B,** CT shows a large soft tissue mass *(L)* in the left neck, representing lymphoma.

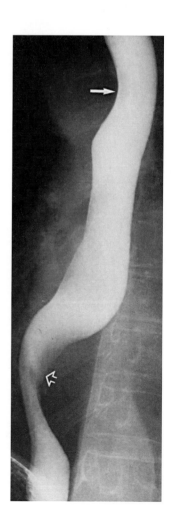

Fig. 1-17   Esophageal compression by the aortic arch *(arrow)* and tortuous descending thoracic aorta *(open arrow)*.

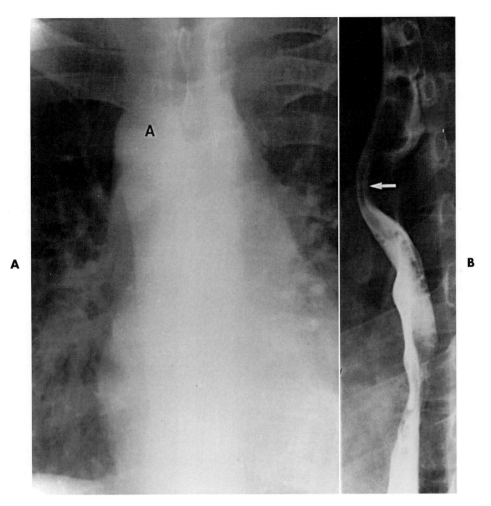

Fig. 1-18   **A,** Chest film shows a right aortic arch *(A)*. **B,** Lateral view from esophagram shows smooth posterior compression of the upper thoracic esophagus *(arrow)* by aberrant left subclavian artery.

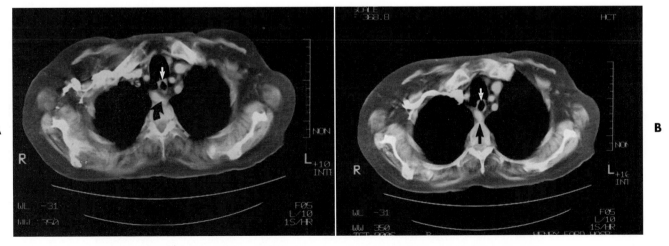

Fig. 1-19   **A,** Aberrant right subclavian artery. Note right subclavian artery *(curved black arrow)* swinging posterior to the esophagus *(white arrow)*. **B,** More inferior CT section, showing impression of the right subclavian artery *(black arrow)* on posterior wall of the esophagus *(white arrow)*.

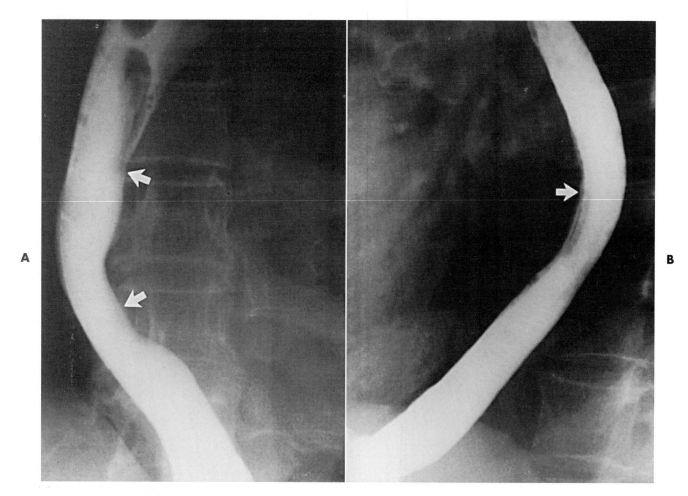

Fig. 1-20   **A,** Frontal and, **B,** lateral films show extrinsic compression of the distal esophagus *(arrows)* by an enlarged left atrium.

osteophytes result in one or more focal impressions on the posterior esophageal wall. Cardiac impressions on the esophagus can be focal (left atrial enlargement) or more diffuse (generalized cardiomegaly and pericardial effusion) (Fig. 1-20). An adjacent lung tumor or mediastinal mass may compress and deviate the esophagus; pulmonary volume loss as a result of fibrosis typically causes ipsilateral retraction of the esophagus. Noncommunicating duplication cysts can be seen as a mediastinal mass impressing the esophageal lumen (Fig. 1-21).

ULCERATIONS AND FISTULAS

Nonneoplastic

Infections

Infectious causes of esophageal ulceration include viruses, fungi, and bacteria. Viral esophagitis most often affects immunocompromised patients, particularly those with AIDS. Both herpes simplex virus and cytomegalovirus (CMV) cause solitary or multiple discrete shallow ulcers on a normal esophageal mucosal background (Fig.

1-22). The ulcers of CMV may be quite large. Human immunodeficiency virus itself has been reported to produce giant esophageal ulcers identical to those caused by CMV.

Tuberculous esophagitis usually occurs in patients with pulmonary or mediastinal tuberculosis and may result from contiguous extension of disease or from swallowing infected sputum. Esophageal ulcerations, sinus tracts, and nodularity are typically noted (Fig. 1-23). This is being reported with increasing frequency in patients with AIDS and may result in esophagorespiratory fistulas. Esophageal ulceration caused by atypical mycobacteria has also been described in AIDS.

In *Candida* esophagitis, confluence of fungal plaques may allow barium to penetrate between the plaques, resulting in pseudoulceration. True ulceration may also occur in severe esophageal candidiasis and can be focal or diffuse.

Inflammation (noninfectious)

Reflux esophagitis (Box 1-5) can cause erosions or ulcerations in the distal esophagus as a result of irritation

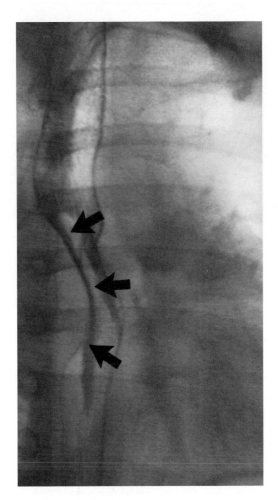

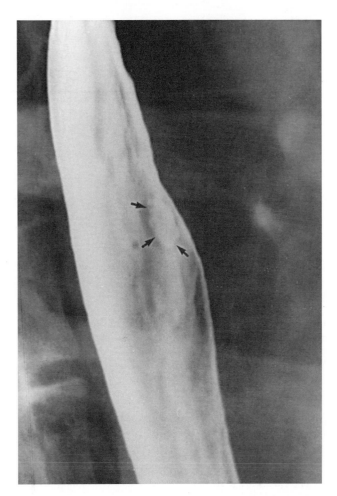

Fig. 1-21 Extrinsic compression of the midesophagus by a mediastinal mass. At surgery the mass proved to be a noncommunicating duplication cyst.

Fig. 1-22 Focal ulceration in the midesophagus *(arrows)* represents CMV esophagitis in a patient with AIDS.

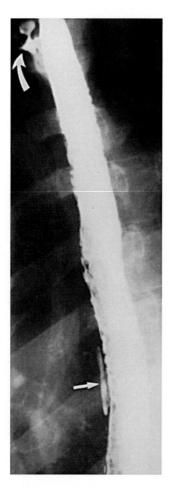

Fig. 1-23 Sinus tract *(curved arrow)* and longitudinal ulceration *(arrow)* in a patient with AIDS and mycobacterial esophagitis. (From Goodman P, Pinero SS, Rance RM, et al: Mycobacterial esophagitis in AIDS, *Gastrointest Radiol* 14:103, 1989.)

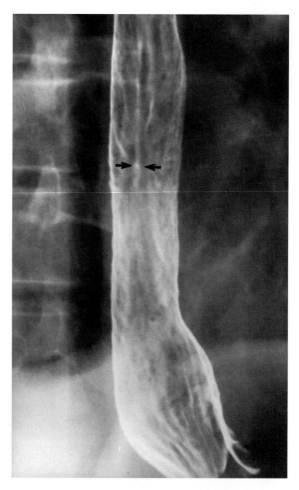

Fig. 1-24 Severe reflux esophagitis with diffuse nodularity, granularity, and linear longitudinal ulceration *(arrows)*.

Box 1-5 Radiological Signs of Reflux Esophagitis

Thickened distal folds, e.g., esophagogastric polyp
Benign strictures
Ulcers, usually linear and located distally
Hiatal hernias with spontaneous gastroesophageal
 reflux commonly seen but not absolutely necessary
 for diagnosis

---

of the esophageal mucosa by gastric acid (Figs. 1-24 and 1-25). Conditions predisposing to development of severe reflux esophagitis include bile reflux esophagitis, Zollinger-Ellison syndrome, and prolonged nasogastric intubation. Bile reflux esophagitis is a particularly severe form of reflux esophagitis seen most often in patients with previous partial or complete gastric resection in whom alkaline bile from the proximal small bowel refluxes into the esophagus. This may lead to esophageal ulceration and stricturing. This complication can be avoided by surgically diverting the flow of bile away from the gastric remnant or esophagus (revision of gastroduodenostomy or creation of Roux-en-Y enteroenterostomy). Zollinger-Ellison syndrome, when complicated by gastroesophageal reflux, may also lead to severe reflux esophagitis because of the acidic gastric fluid in this condition.

Prolonged nasogastric intubation, by not allowing complete closure of the lower esophageal sphincter around the indwelling tube, permits continuous reflux to occur. The tube also alters esophageal peristalsis, preventing rapid clearance of the refluxed material from the esophagus. This may eventually result in diffuse esophageal narrowing.

Barrett's esophagus is a condition in which esophageal squamous epithelium undergoes metaplasia to a

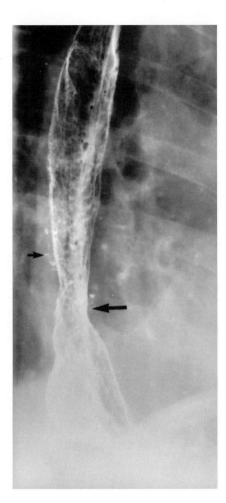

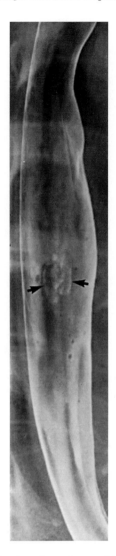

Fig. 1-25 Severe chronic reflux esophagitis. Note stricture *(large arrow)* and multiple pseudodiverticula *(small arrow).* Commonly associated with chronic reflux disease.

Fig. 1-26 Discrete ulcerations *(arrows)* in the midesophagus caused by the ingestion of antibiotic capsules.

gastric-type columnar epithelium. This occurs in about 10% of patients with reflux esophagitis and is thought to be directly related to reflux disease. Although Barrett's esophagus is usually seen in the distal esophagus (where reflux most often occurs), it may also involve the midesophagus or upper third of the esophagus with areas of intervening normal esophageal mucosa. Radiographic manifestations of Barrett's esophagus include mucosal nodularity, a reticular mucosal pattern (on double-contrast films), focal ulceration, and focal narrowing or stricture formation.

Certain oral medications may cause focal irritation and ulceration of the esophagus by prolonged contact with the esophageal mucosa (Fig. 1-26). This is most often seen with tetracycline and its derivatives and has also been reported with quinidine, potassium chloride, some nonsteroidal antiinflammatory agents, and several other medications. A capsule or tablet, especially when taken at bedtime with a small amount of water, may lodge in the esophagus at the level of the aortic arch or distal esophagus. The focal esophagitis will usually heal following discontinuation of the offending medication.

Corrosive esophagitis resulting from the ingestion of lye or other caustic substances often leads to severe edema and ulceration of the esophagus in the acute stage, followed by stricture formation after healing occurs. Contrast studies are not usually performed in the acute stage of a severe corrosive esophagitis.

In acute alcoholic esophagitis, superficial ulcerations are seen in the midesophagus and distal esophagus shortly after alcoholic binges.

Although the esophagus is relatively radioresistant, radiation therapy to the mediastinum may cause esophagitis and esophageal ulcerations. This occurs in the

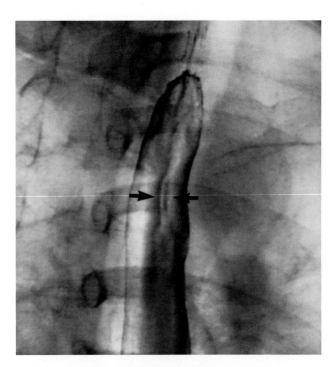

Fig. 1-27 Esophageal Crohn's ulcer. A 26-year-old patient with known small bowel Crohn's disease presents with odynophagia. Processed digital images from esophagram show to advantage a solitary linear Crohn's ulcer of proximal esophagus.

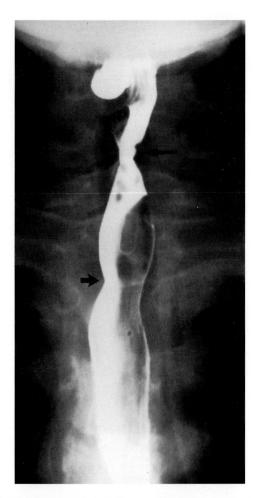

Fig. 1-28 Epidermolysis bullosa. At least two proximal esophageal strictures *(arrows)*.

acute stage and may lead to stricture formation following healing. The location of inflammatory changes conforms to the radiation port used.

Changes associated with radiation esophagitis are typically seen after doses of 4500 to 6000 rads over a 6- to 8-week period and are even more common following combination radiation therapy and chemotherapy. Following radiation therapy, esophagorespiratory fistulas may develop in patients with mediastinal adenopathy compressing the esophagus, presumably as a result of tumor necrosis induced by radiation. Similarly, patients who undergo external beam or intracavitary radiation therapy for primary esophageal carcinoma may develop necrosis of the tumor with subsequent ulceration or formation of an esophagorespiratory fistula.

Esophageal involvement occurs in approximately 3% of patients with Crohn's disease of the ileum or colon and may be seen as aphthous or longitudinal ulcers (Fig. 1-27). Crohn's disease of the esophagus rarely occurs in the absence of ileal or colonic disease.

Behçet's disease is an unusual condition of unknown etiology that is characterized by oral and genital ulcerations, ocular inflammation, and vascular thrombosis. Focal ulcerations have been reported in the esophagus, colon, and ileum.

Benign mucous membrane pemphigoid and epidermolysis bullosa are rare skin diseases that may be associated with ulcerations, webs, and strictures in the pharynx and esophagus (Fig. 1-28). As noted, the initial finding in these conditions is multiple mucosal nodules.

Eosinophilic esophagitis is a rare cause of esophageal ulcerations. This disease, like eosinophilic gastroenteritis, is associated with eosinophilic infiltration, peripheral eosinophilia, and a history of allergies. In addition to ulcerations, esophageal nodularity and stricture formation may occur in this disease.

Aortoesophageal fistula

Aortoesophageal fistula is an unusual complication of thoracic aortic aneurysms or aortic grafts. Erosion into the esophagus causes hematemesis, usually followed within hours to days by massive bleeding.

Trauma

Trauma may lead to ulceration, laceration, or perforation of the esophagus. This includes iatrogenic causes, such as instrumentation, endoscopic perforation of an esophageal diverticulum, and sclerotherapy of esoph-

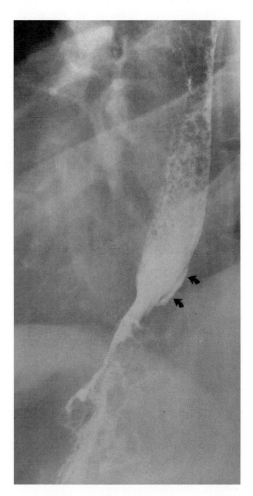

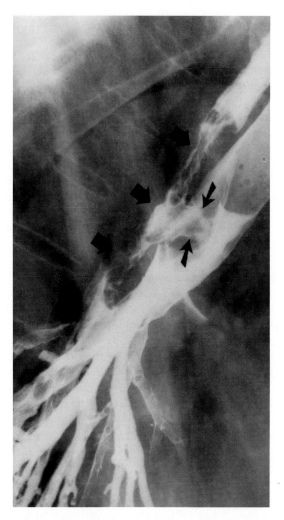

Fig. 1-29 Intraluminal sinus tract formation *(arrows)* after sclerotherapy treatment for varices.

Fig. 1-30 Tracheal-esophageal fistula in a 59-year-old male with a long destructive malignant lesion of the midesophagus *(large arrows)* and a wide fistulous communication *(curved arrows)* with the trachea.

ageal varices with resultant ulceration (Fig. 1-29). Taco chips or corn chips may lacerate the esophagus, and impacted foreign bodies may cause focal irritation and ulceration. Vomiting can lead to mucosal disruption (Mallory-Weiss tear) or transmural perforation (Boerhaave's syndrome) of the distal esophagus.

Neoplastic

Carcinoma, metastases, and lymphoma

Focal necrosis and ulceration are not unusual in primary squamous cell carcinoma of the esophagus. However, extensive ulceration (in which the tumor is almost completely ulcerated) is uncommonly seen radiographically. Primary esophageal adenocarcinoma arising in Barrett's epithelium may also undergo focal ulceration. Other malignant lesions that may appear ulcerated include metastases and lymphoma.

Additionally, fistulous communication between squamous cell carcinoma of the esophagus and the bronchial or tracheal airway can occasionally be seen with midesophageal lesions (Fig. 1-30).

DYSMOTILITY

Normal esophageal motility or peristalsis refers to the coordinated propulsion of a bolus from the pharynx to the stomach. This process is regulated by complex neuromuscular interactions and appears radiographically as a continuous, smooth, wavelike contraction. Whereas a primary wave is initiated by the act of swallowing, a secondary wave is produced in response to distention of the esophagus caused by refluxed stomach content.

Cervical Esophagus

Neuromuscular abnormalities

Diseases of striated muscle, such as dermatomyositis and muscular dystrophy, can affect motility of the cervical esophagus because this portion of the esophagus is composed of striated muscle rather than smooth muscle. Various neuromuscular abnormalities including brainstem infarction, multiple sclerosis, and pseudobulbar palsy can cause dysmotility of the cervical esophagus because swallowing function is controlled by the central nervous system, cranial nerves, and peripheral autonomic nerves. Myasthenia gravis, a disorder involving the neuromuscular junction, can also affect cervical esophageal motility.

Incomplete cricopharyngeal relaxation

The cricopharyngeus muscle, as the lower portion of the inferior constrictor muscle, forms the posterior wall of the pharyngoesophageal junction. During swallowing, the cricopharyngeus muscle normally relaxes to allow the food bolus to pass from the pharynx into the esophagus. If this muscle remains contracted during swallowing, it causes a smooth, rounded impression at the level of the C5-C6 disk space that may persist for a variable length of time (Fig. 1-31). This is an important cause of dysphagia and may lead to the formation of a Zenker's diverticulum by creating increased intraluminal pressure in the hypopharynx. Incomplete cricopharyngeal relaxation may develop as a protective mechanism in patients with gastroesophageal reflux to prevent aspiration of gastric contents. Prominence of the cricopharyngeus muscle can also be seen following laryngectomy.

Thoracic Esophagus

Scleroderma is a systemic disorder of connective tissue in which smooth muscle is replaced by fibrous tissue. In the esophagus, the proximal third that is composed of striated muscle is unaffected whereas the distal two thirds, composed of smooth muscle, displays abnormal motility. Typically the esophagus appears dilated and the gastroesophageal junction is widely patent. Gastroesophageal reflux is common and may be marked. Because of the long-standing reflux and the delayed clearance of refluxed material by the flaccid esophagus, reflux esophagitis usually develops. This may be severe, with resultant stricture formation or development of Barrett's esophagus. Mixed connective tissue diseases that often include scleroderma may also demonstrate these findings.

Achalasia (Box 1-6) is a disease of the myenteric plexus of the esophagus in which peristalsis is diffusely decreased or absent and the lower esophageal sphincter

fails to relax. The esophagus is often dilated and may appear on frontal chest films as an air- or fluid-filled tubular structure in the medial right hemithorax (with an air-fluid level present on upright films). Contrast studies show dilution of barium by retained fluid in the esophagus. Peristaltic contractions appear disordered in the early stage of the disease and diminished or absent in

---

Box 1-6   The Two Faces of Achalasia

Idiopathic achalasia—a neuromuscular abnormality of the lower esophageal sphincter of unknown etiology
Secondary achalasia—a neuromuscular abnormality of the lower esophageal sphincter caused by subtle malignant infiltration of the region of the gastroesophageal junction; can be easily confused with the idiopathic type

---

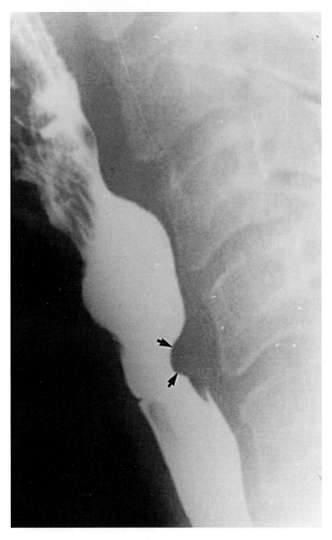

Fig. 1-31   Lateral view of the cervical esophagus shows prominence of the cricopharyngeus muscle *(arrows)*.

later stages. The distal esophagus demonstrates smooth, tapered narrowing caused by the contracted lower esophageal sphincter (Fig. 1-32). In the upright position, gravity may partially overcome the decreased peristalsis and the tightened sphincter to allow intermittent passage of small amounts of contrast material into the stomach. However, in the horizontal position, little, if any, contrast material passes into the stomach.

Primary or idiopathic achalasia usually has its onset in early adulthood and results in dysphagia, regurgitation, and other complications of esophageal stasis including bad breath, aspiration pneumonia, and esophageal candidiasis. In cases of long-standing achalasia, there is an increased incidence of squamous cell carcinoma of the esophagus, probably secondary to chronic mucosal irritation by retained food (Fig. 1-33). Diagnosis of superimposed carcinoma in achalasia is rarely made before the tumor has become large and invasive. Early radiological detection is limited by the patient's underlying chronic dysphagia, the markedly dilated esophageal lumen, and the presence of food and debris within the esophagus.

Secondary achalasia simulates primary achalasia but results from malignancy and usually has an abrupt onset later in life (Fig. 1-34). The decreased peristalsis and smooth tapering of the distal esophagus in secondary achalasia typically result from tumor infiltrating the myenteric plexus of the distal esophagus. This can occur in invasive gastric carcinoma, lymphoma, and metastatic disease involving the gastroesophageal junction. Other suggested pathogenetic mechanisms in secondary achalasia include paraneoplastic syndrome and central nervous system lesions affecting the vagal nerve nuclei.

Chagas' disease, an infectious disease seen in Brazil and other tropical areas, also mimics idiopathic achalasia. Chagas' disease is caused by *Trypanosoma cruzi,* a protozoan transmitted to humans by the reduviid bug, and affects the esophagus, duodenum, colon, and heart.

Diffuse esophageal spasm and related disorders (e.g., presbyesophagus and corkscrew esophagus) cause a spectrum of esophageal dysmotility. Disordered peristalsis is often reflected by the presence of tertiary waves (Fig. 1-35). These nonpropulsive, sometimes bizarre-appearing contractions may be associated with significant dysphagia.

Abnormal esophageal motility is one of the earliest findings in reflux esophagitis and in other inflammatory causes of esophagitis, such as radiation and caustic ingestion.

Systemic diseases that may cause esophageal dysmotility include myxedema, thyrotoxicosis, amyloidosis, and diabetes mellitus.

Drugs, particularly atropine and other anticholinergics, also can cause esophageal dysmotility.

NARROWED ESOPHAGUS

Narrowing of the esophagus may result from intrinsic or extrinsic causes. Narrowing can be further characterized as focal or diffuse, mild or severe, and smooth or irregular.

Neoplasms

Esophageal neoplasms, especially squamous cell carcinoma, are common causes of focal esophageal narrowing. The most typical appearance of esophageal squamous cell carcinoma on contrast studies is an abrupt irregular narrowing by an annular mass (Fig. 1-36). CT is used to evaluate the primary lesion and to determine depth of invasion and presence of regional adenopathy and distant metastases (Figs. 1-37, 1-38, and 1-39). Contiguous extension of tumor may involve the tracheobronchial tree, aorta, pleura, or pericardium and is

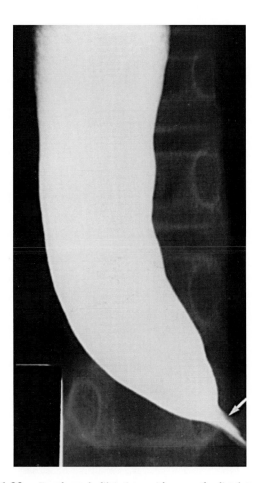

Fig. 1-32 Esophageal dilatation with smooth distal tapering *(arrow)* represents achalasia.

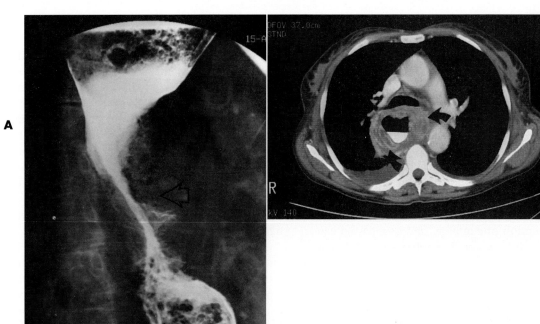

Fig. 1-33 Achalasia with complicating carcinoma.
A, Patient with long-standing achalasia and esophagram showing dilated atonic esophagus with midesophageal irregular stricture. **B,** CT of same patient demonstrates thickened infiltrated esophageal wall *(curved arrows)* at the level of the carina. Note air-fluid level in the esophagus.

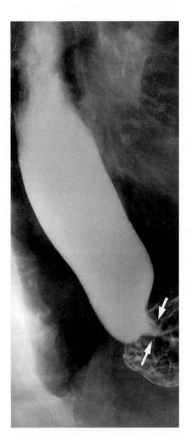

Fig. 1-34 Secondary achalasia. A 70-year-old male with recent history of dysphagia and weight loss. Esophagram shows tapered narrowing of distal esophagus *(arrows)*. However, the expected "beak" primary achalasia lacks a pointed tip and has some mild irregularity that, along with the history, makes it suspicious. Biopsy showed infiltrating carcinoma.

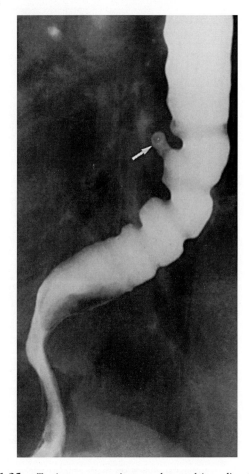

Fig. 1-35 Tertiary contractions and a pulsion diverticulum *(arrow)* in the distal esophagus.

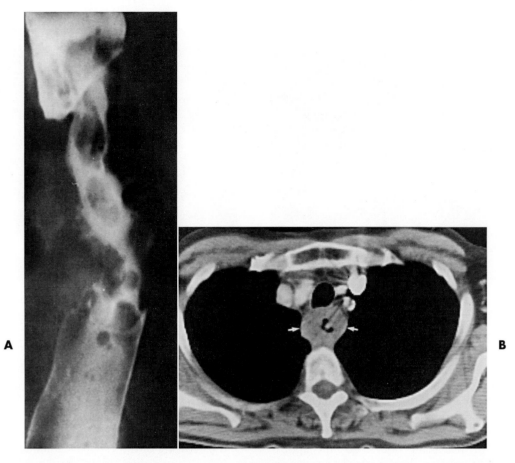

Fig. 1-36 **A,** Irregular narrowing in the upper thoracic esophagus represents squamous cell carcinoma. **B,** CT demonstrates marked circumferential wall thickening *(arrows)* as a result of tumor infiltration.

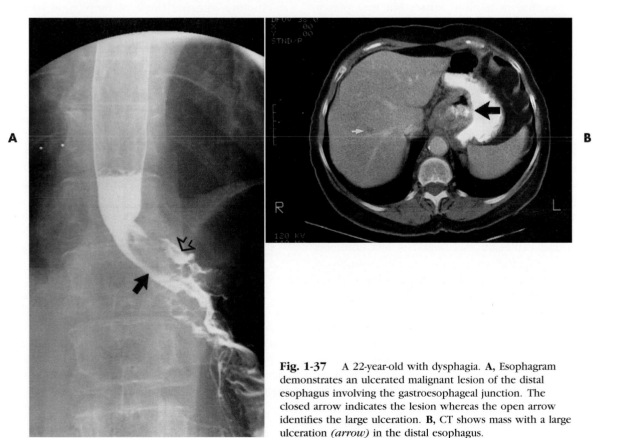

Fig. 1-37 A 22-year-old with dysphagia. **A,** Esophagram demonstrates an ulcerated malignant lesion of the distal esophagus involving the gastroesophageal junction. The closed arrow indicates the lesion whereas the open arrow identifies the large ulceration. **B,** CT shows mass with a large ulceration *(arrow)* in the distal esophagus.

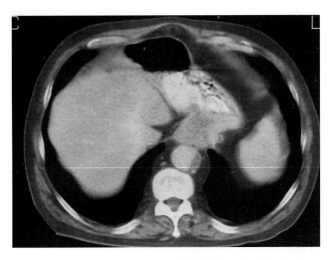

Fig. 1-38 A 74-year-old with malignant lesion in gastroesophageal junction. Note obvious low-attenuation mass with no ulceration.

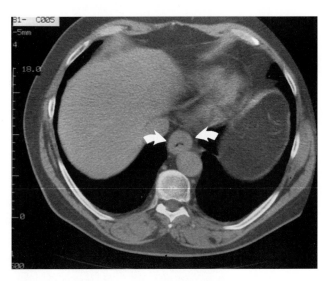

Fig. 1-39 Carcinoma of the distal esophagus. Note subtle CT appearance of lesion. Findings consist of wall thickening *(arrows)* and luminal narrowing.

demonstrated by infiltration of paraesophageal fat planes. However, this may be overestimated in the absence of fat planes secondary to cachexia or fibrosis. Lymphatic extension of tumors, though usually present when adjacent lymph nodes appear enlarged, may be underestimated (if malignant nodes do not appear enlarged) or, less commonly, overestimated (if nodes are enlarged because of benign disease).

MRI has been limited in evaluation of esophageal carcinoma because of motion artifact but may play a more important role with the development of cardiorespiratory gating techniques.

Esophageal adenocarcinoma arising in Barrett's epithelium can cause irregular luminal narrowing similar to that seen in squamous cell carcinoma (Fig. 1-40).

Metastatic disease to the esophagus occurs through contiguous or hematogenous spread of tumor. Direct invasion can involve the cervical esophagus (laryngeal carcinoma and thyroid carcinoma), midesophagus (lung carcinoma and mediastinal adenopathy), or distal esophagus (superior extension of gastric carcinoma). Radiographic findings include esophageal obstruction, displacement, narrowing, ulceration, and fistula formation. Hematogenous metastasis to the esophagus (breast carcinoma and malignant melanoma) is less common than contiguous spread but may also produce a variety of radiographic findings including focal narrowing and submucosal masses.

Lymphoma affects the esophagus in fewer than 1% of cases and is more often a result of extrinsic compression by mediastinal adenopathy than of intrinsic esophageal involvement. Esophageal lymphoma has many different radiographic appearances and may simulate achalasia, varices, contiguous extension of gastric carcinoma, and

hematogenous metastases (Fig. 1-41). It may also cause luminal narrowing or a polypoid mass, either of which may be associated with ulceration.

Leiomyomas or other benign esophageal neoplasms, when of sufficient size, can cause smooth compression and narrowing of the esophageal lumen.

Infection

Another intrinsic cause of esophageal narrowing is inflammatory stricture formation (Fig. 1-42). Infectious causes of stricturing include tuberculosis, candidiasis, and, rarely, syphilis.

Inflammation (Noninfectious)

Noninfectious inflammatory strictures may result from gastroesophageal reflux (and disorders associated with reflux), Barrett's esophagus, corrosive ingestion, and radiation (Figs. 1-43 to 1-47). Less common causes include Crohn's disease, benign mucous membrane pemphigoid, epidermolysis bullosa (Fig. 1-48), eosinophilic esophagitis, graft-versus-host disease, and prior sclerotherapy for varices.

Motility Abnormalities, Hematoma, and Extrinsic Compression

Motility abnormalities may focally narrow the esophagus by causing tertiary contractions (diffuse esophageal spasm) or incomplete relaxation of the distal esophageal sphincter (achalasia). Traumatic intramural hematoma of the distal esophagus can also cause focal narrowing.

Text continued on p. 30

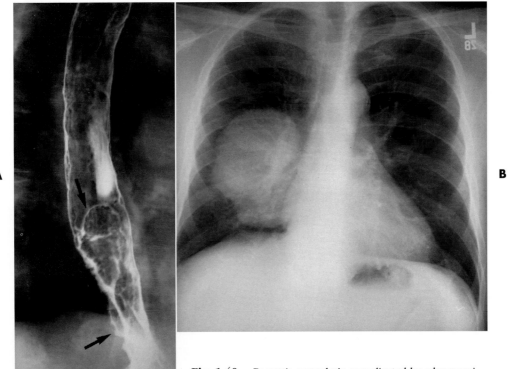

Fig. 1-40 Barrett's metaplasia complicated by adenocarcinoma. **A,** A 60-year-old patient with known scleroderma presents with dysphagia, weight loss, and fatigue. Esophagram demonstrates ulcerated mass lesion *(arrows)* of distal esophagus. Biopsy confirmed malignant lesion and evidence of Barrett's metaplasia. **B,** Admission chest film shows large pulmonary metastatic lesion.

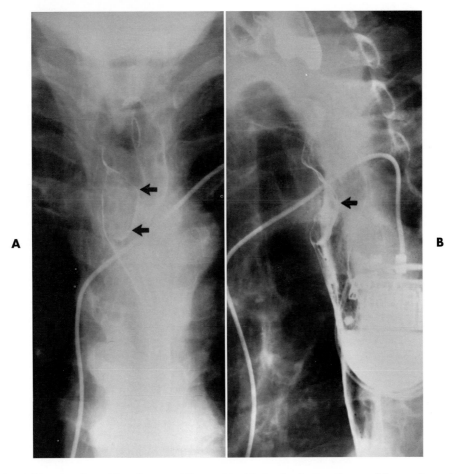

Fig. 1-41 Esophageal lymphoma. A 70-year-old with dysphagia. Lymphoma of the esophagus by biopsy and surgical resection. Lymphomatous lesion has unusually well-defined margins. On en face view **(A)** it looks like mucosal lesion *(arrows)*, whereas on profiled view **(B)** it could be a mucosal or submucosal lesion *(arrow)*.

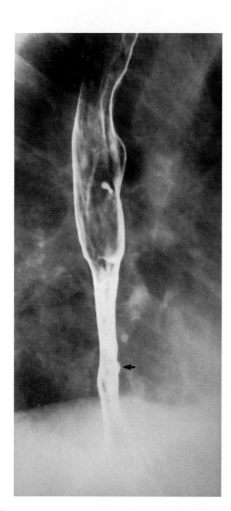

Fig. 1-42   Long esophageal stricture. A 47-year-old with a long history of chronic reflux esophagitis. Barium esophagram shows a long benign stricture with ulceration *(arrow)*.

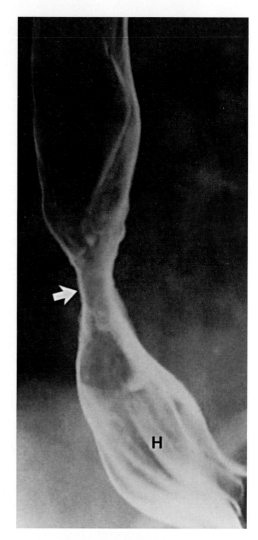

Fig. 1-43   Narrowing of the distal esophagus *(arrow)* proximal to an axial hiatal hernia *(H)* represents a reflux stricture.

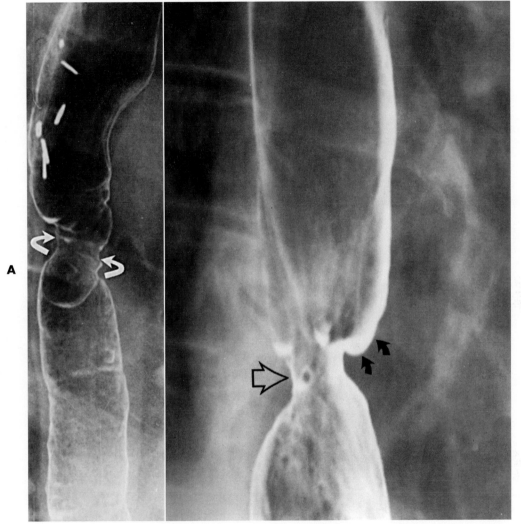

Fig. 1-44   Inflammatory strictures. **A,** Short narrowing in the midthoracic esophagus *(curved arrows)* represents a Barrett's stricture in a patient with long-standing scleroderma. The surgical clips are from a previous sympathectomy. **B,** Patient with chronic benign esophageal stricture *(open arrow)* with "overhanging edge" *(black arrows)*. This radiological sign, where a cul-de-sac of the prestrictured esophagus is projected below the level of the stricture, is indicative of benignity and chronicity. It is the reverse of the "shoulder" sign seen in malignant lesions.

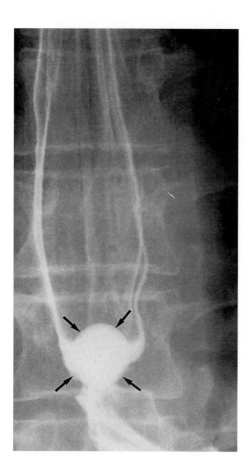

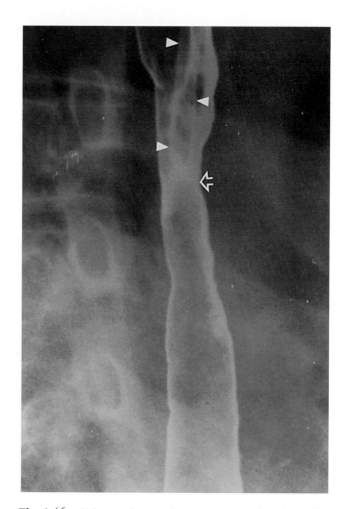

Fig. 1-45 A 13-mm barium tablet *(arrows)* lodges above a distal esophageal stricture with the patient in upright position.

Fig. 1-46 Tube esophagram demonstrates a midesophageal lye stricture *(open arrow)*. The tube *(arrowheads)* lies proximal to the stricture.

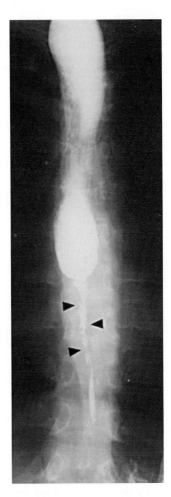

Fig. 1-47 Long, irregular narrowing of the distal esophagus *(arrowheads)* resulting from lye ingestion.

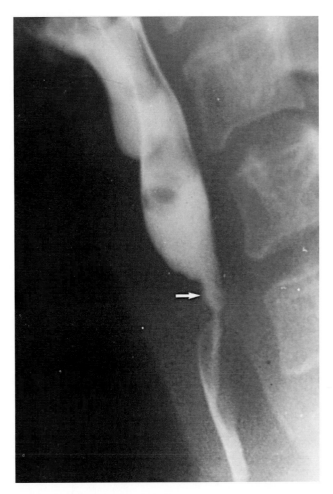

Fig. 1-48 Lateral view of the cervical esophagus shows a focal stricture *(arrow)* in a patient with epidermolysis bullosa.

Extrinsic compression by adjacent benign or malignant processes typically causes smooth, eccentric narrowing.

DILATED ESOPHAGUS

Esophageal Distention, Mechanical Obstruction

Dilatation of the esophagus most often occurs proximal to a mechanical obstruction, either a neoplasm or an inflammatory stricture. Extrinsic compression or intraluminal obstruction (food impaction) can also result in esophageal dilatation proximally.

Esophageal Distention, No Obstruction

In the absence of mechanical obstruction, the esophagus may appear diffusely dilated secondary to motility disorders (achalasia and scleroderma), drugs (anticholinergics), and systemic diseases (myxedema, thyrotoxicosis, amyloidosis, and diabetes mellitus). Saccular dilatations of the esophagus are an uncommon manifestation of scleroderma and other connective tissue diseases. This appears similar to the saccular dilatation more typically seen in the small bowel and colon in these disorders.

Esophageal Distention, Focal

Focal dilatation of the esophagus can result from expansion around a bulky, intraluminal neoplasm, such as a mesenchymal sarcoma or spindle-cell carcinoma. It can also occur following various operations including Heller's myotomy (distal esophagus) and resection of esophageal duplication cyst (midesophagus). Retraction of the esophagus secondary to pulmonary scarring typically results in focal esophageal dilatation.

DIVERTICULA

Zenker's Diverticula

Zenker's diverticulum is a herniation of mucosa and submucosa through a defect in the posterior aspect of the pharyngoesophageal junction. This defect occurs in an area of potential weakness (Killian's dehiscence) in the midline between horizontal and oblique fibers of the inferior constrictor muscle (Fig. 1-49). Zenker's diverticulum most likely results from increased intraluminal pressure in the hypopharynx and may be associated with incomplete relaxation of the cricopharyngeus muscle. When small, Zenker's diverticulum extends directly posteriorly and is best visualized in the lateral projection

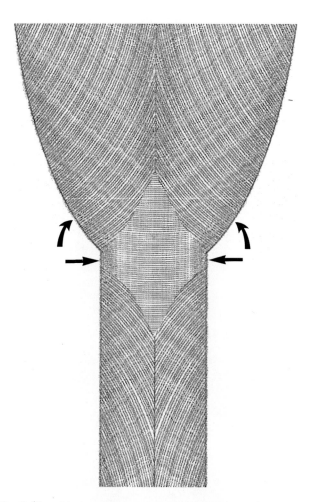

Fig. 1-49   Diagram of the posterior wall of the hypopharynx and cervical esophagus illustrates the horizontal fibers *(arrows)* and oblique fibers *(curved arrows)* of the inferior constrictor muscle.

on contrast examination (Fig. 1-50). With continued increased pressure, the diverticulum may enlarge and extend laterally. Complications associated with Zenker's diverticulum include dysphagia, bad breath, and aspiration pneumonia, and iatrogenic perforation of the diverticulum at endoscopy is a recognized danger. Less commonly, diverticula can arise from the lateral aspects of the pharyngoesophageal junction.

Midesophageal Diverticula

Midesophageal diverticula often occur at the anterior aspect of the esophagus at the level of the carina (Fig. 1-51). These may represent traction diverticula resulting from retraction of the esophageal wall by healed granulomatous disease of the mediastinum. However, recent studies suggest that most midesophageal diverticula are caused by increased intraluminal pressure and therefore represent pulsion diverticula. On contrast examination, traction diverticula, which contain a muscular wall,

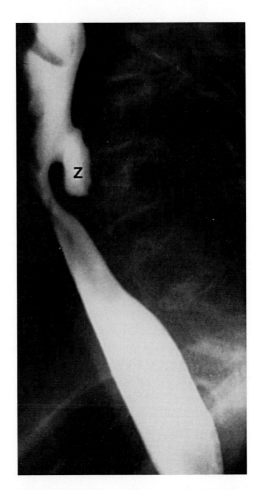

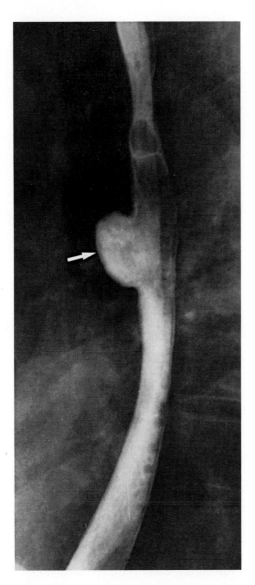

Fig. 1-50 Lateral view of the cervical esophagus shows a Zenker's diverticulum *(Z)*.

Fig. 1-51 Anterior midesophageal diverticulum *(arrow)*.

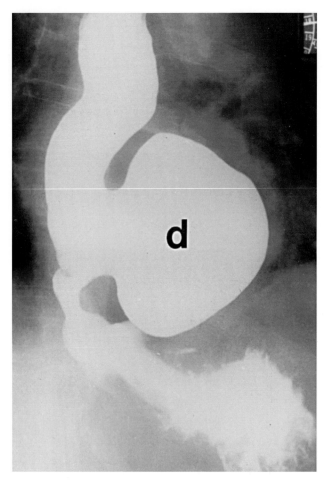

Fig. 1-52 Large epiphrenic diverticulum *(d)*.

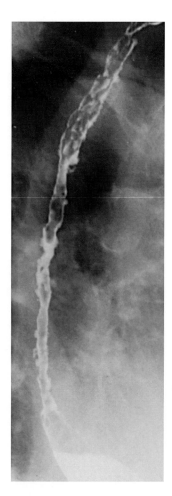

Fig. 1-53 Long stricture of the thoracic esophagus with numerous intramural pseudodiverticula.

typically have an angular contour and can contract, whereas pulsion diverticula, which lack a muscular wall, have a rounded configuration and do not contract.

Epiphrenic Diverticula

Epiphrenic diverticula are located in the distal esophagus near the gastroesophageal junction (Fig. 1-52). These pulsion diverticula result from abnormal intraluminal pressure and may be associated with tertiary contractions of the esophagus. Accidental entry of the endoscope into an epiphrenic diverticulum may lead to perforation.

Intramural Pseudodiverticula

Esophageal intramural pseudodiverticulosis is an unusual condition in which dilated mucous glands in the esophageal wall may simulate true diverticula on contrast studies (Fig. 1-53). The pseudodiverticula are usually flask shaped and of uniform depth. They may be solitary or multiple, and distribution may be segmental or diffuse. This condition is most often associated with esophageal strictures, although the diverticula may be located proximal or distal to the stricture site. Intramural pseudodiverticulosis usually occurs as a rare sequela of esophagitis. There may be an association between this process and esophageal malignancies.

Intraluminal (Artifactual) Diverticula

Intraluminal esophageal diverticulum represents a transient artifact that results from barium mixing with retained fluid or debris in the esophagus. This appears similar to an intraluminal duodenal diverticulum ("windsock") on contrast examination but is not associated with an intraluminal membrane.

FOLDS

Normal

Longitudinal folds extend along the entire length of the esophagus and are best demonstrated on collapsed views. Transverse folds also occur normally, although

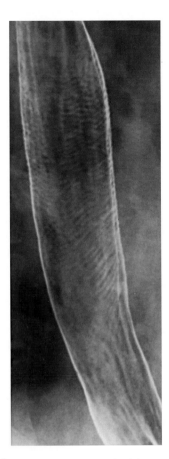

Fig. 1-54   Thin transverse folds (feline esophagus).

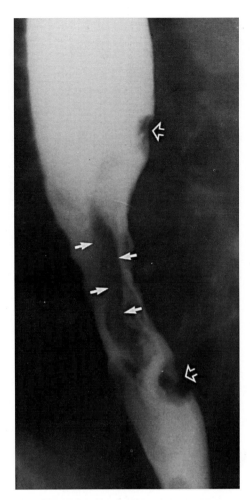

Fig. 1-55   Thickened longitudinal fold *(arrows)* and mural masses *(open arrows)* in the distal esophagus represent varicoid carcinoma.

they are seen less frequently than longitudinal folds. These thin, transient folds represent contraction of the muscularis mucosa of the esophageal wall (Fig. 1-54). This is sometimes referred to as a feline esophagus because the transverse folds resemble those seen normally in the esophagus of a cat.

Thickened

Thickening of longitudinal and transverse folds as a result of edema and inflammation has been described as an early finding in reflux esophagitis and may occur in other forms of esophagitis as well. Esophageal varices may appear as thickened folds but are differentiated by their tortuosity and changeability with position and esophageal distention.

Varicoid carcinoma is a form of esophageal carcinoma in which submucosal spread of tumor causes esophageal folds to appear thickened (Fig. 1-55). Esophageal lymphoma is a rare neoplasm that may also produce thickening of esophageal folds because of submucosal spread of tumor. Unlike varices, the deformity seen in varicoid carcinoma and esophageal lymphoma is fixed.

WEBS, HERNIAS, AND RINGS

Webs

Webs are incomplete membranes that appear as thin, transverse filling defects on contrast studies (Fig. 1-56). These most often occur at the anterior aspect of the proximal cervical esophagus and are less often circumferential. Webs can occur spontaneously or secondary to scarring from benign mucous membrane pemphigoid and epidermolysis bullosa. They can also develop in graft-versus-host disease, a complication of bone marrow transplantation in which host tissues are attacked by donor lymphocytes. In Plummer-Vinson syndrome, cervical esophageal webs are associated with iron-deficiency anemia and dysphagia (Fig. 1-57). Distal esophageal webs may result from reflux esophagitis.

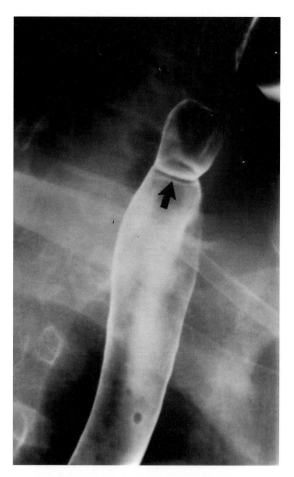

Fig. 1-56   Esophageal web. This 40-year-old patient complained of "pills sticking." Esophagram shows circumferential web in proximal esophagus.

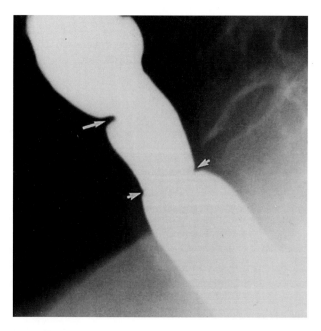

Fig. 1-57   Lateral view of the cervical esophagus demonstrates an anterior web *(arrow)* and a circumferential web *(short arrows)* in a patient with dysphagia and microcytic anemia.

Hernias

A hiatal hernia represents an extension of the stomach into the chest through the esophageal hiatus. In the more common axial or sliding hiatal hernia, the gastroesophageal junction lies more than 2 cm above the diaphragm. This type of hernia is frequently associated with gastroesophageal reflux.

Although hiatal hernias usually involve only the proximal portion of the stomach, the entire stomach may herniate into the chest, resulting in an intrathoracic stomach (Fig. 1-58). The stomach assumes an inverted position in the chest with the greater curvature located superiorly and the lesser curvature inferiorly. Subsequently, the proximal portion of the stomach may return through the esophageal hiatus to its normal position below the diaphragm, leaving the distal portion within the chest. Complications of intrathoracic stomach include obstruction, volvulus, and perforation.

Paraesophageal hernias account for less than 5% of all hiatal hernias and are not associated with gastroesophageal reflux. In this type of hernia, the gastroesophageal junction is located below the diaphragm, but the gastric fundus partially extends upward through the esophageal hiatus or a diagrammatic defect to the left of the distal esophagus (Figs. 1-59 and 1-60).

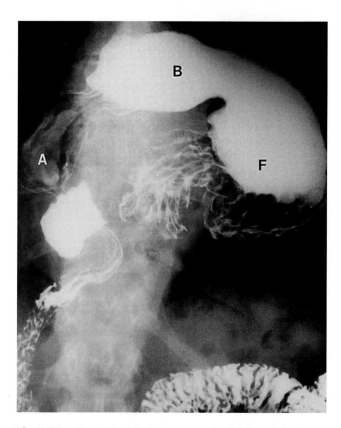

Fig. 1-58   Large hiatal hernia contains the fundus *(F)*, body *(B)*, and antrum *(A)* of the stomach.

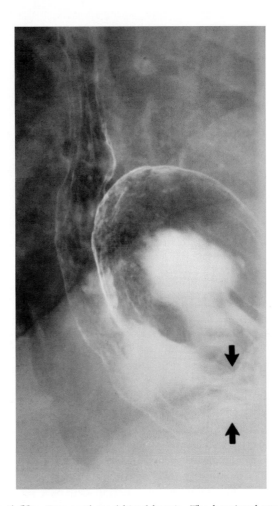

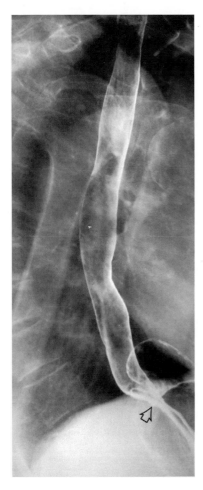

Fig. 1-59 Paraesophageal hiatal hernia. The herniated portion of the stomach protruding upward through the diaphragmatic hiatus next to the gastroesophageal junction *(arrows)*.

Fig. 1-60 Paraesophageal hernia. The herniated segment of the stomach protrudes upward in a diaphragmatic defect near the hiatus.

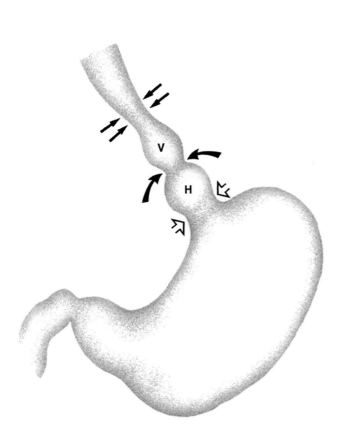

Fig. 1-61   Diagram of the distal esophagus and stomach illustrates esophageal vestibule *(V)*, axial hiatal hernia *(H)*, A-ring *(arrows)*, B-ring *(curved arrows)*, and diaphragmatic impressions *(open arrows)*.

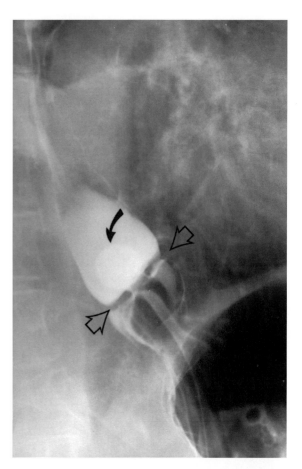

Fig. 1-62   Small hiatal hernia with obstructing B-ring (Schatzki ring) *(open arrows)* and luminal narrowing. Note the 12.5-mm barium tablet held up above the obstruction *(curved arrow)*.

A mixed or combined hiatal hernia demonstrates features of both the axial and paraesophageal types, with the gastroesophageal junction located above the diaphragm and the gastric fundus lying alongside the distal esophagus.

Rings

Rings represent areas of narrowing in the region of the esophageal vestibule, which is the distal end of the esophagus that normally appears slightly distended (Fig. 1-61). The muscular ring (A-ring) is a variable smooth, broad narrowing at the superior aspect of the vestibule. This rarely causes dysphagia and most likely results from transient muscle contractions.

The more commonly noted mucosal ring (B-ring) is a persistent thin, transverse constriction at the inferior aspect of the esophageal vestibule in the region of the gastroesophageal junction. The mucosal ring is smooth and symmetrical and rarely causes dysphagia unless

measuring less than 13 mm in diameter. A narrowed mucosal ring that causes dysphagia is known as a Schatzki ring. Mucosal rings are commonly associated with hiatal hernias and are most easily visualized when the esophagogastric junction is distended during contrast examination in the horizontal position (Fig. 1-62). The maximal diameter of the ring can best be determined by having the patient swallow a 13-mm barium tablet while standing. The tablet will lodge above a Schatzki ring but will pass through a nonstenotic mucosal ring into the stomach.

Although the mucosal ring occurs at the gastroesophageal junction, it does not necessarily correspond to the histological squamocolumnar junction (Z line) (Fig. 1-63). This is true in Barrett's esophagus, where metaplasia of the distal esophageal epithelium may cause the Z line to be located proximal to the esophagogastric junction. The Z line is sometimes visualized on double-contrast films as a thin, serrated line in the distal esophagus.

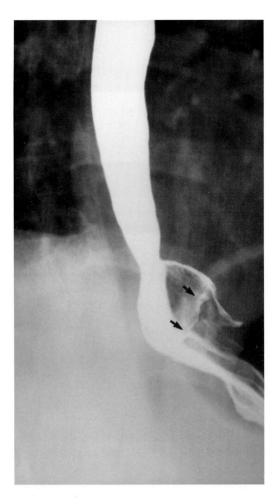

Fig. 1-63 Z line. Occasionally a fortuitous finding on a double-contrast esophagram. The Z line *(arrows)* represents the squamocolumnar junction.

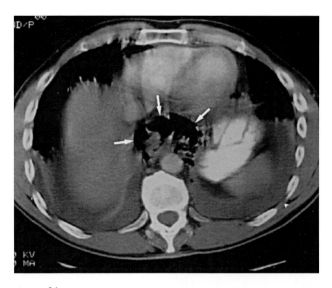

Fig. 1-64 CT shows a large amorphous air collection *(arrows)* in the posterior mediastinum in a patient with esophageal rupture.

TRAUMA AND FOREIGN BODIES

Mallory-Weiss Tear

Mallory-Weiss tear represents a mucosal disruption in the distal esophagus, usually resulting from prolonged or severe vomiting. This causes hematemesis and is sometimes identified on double-contrast films as a thin linear collection of barium in the distal esophagus. Mallory-Weiss tear usually heals spontaneously within several days.

Intramural Hematoma

Esophageal intramural hematoma represents hemorrhage in the submucosal layer of the esophageal wall. This usually occurs by extension of a mucosal tear and appears on contrast examination as a smooth submucosal mass.

Perforation

Boerhaave's syndrome

Boerhaave's syndrome is also usually caused by persistent or severe vomiting but represents transmural perforation of the distal esophagus. This causes mediastinitis and requires immediate surgical repair of the esophageal perforation. Delay in surgical treatment of Boerhaave's syndrome is associated with a high mortality rate. Chest films show mediastinal emphysema, and water-soluble contrast examination of the esophagus demonstrates extravasation of contrast material into the mediastinum (Fig. 1-64).

Instrumentation

Traumatic perforation of the esophagus may also result from penetrating injuries (e.g., knife or bullet wounds) and instrumentation, either surgical (inadvertent laceration during intrathoracic surgery) or nonsurgical (routine endoscopy, dilatation procedures, and stent placements) (Figs. 1-65 and 1-66).

Foreign bodies

Ingested foreign bodies, such as chicken bones or fish bones, may lodge in the cervical or thoracic portions of the esophagus and cause focal irritation or perforation (Fig. 1-67). Taco chips and corn chips have been reported to cause mucosal laceration of the esophagus. Ingestion of sharp metallic objects, such as pins or nails, may also cause laceration or perforation of the esophagus.

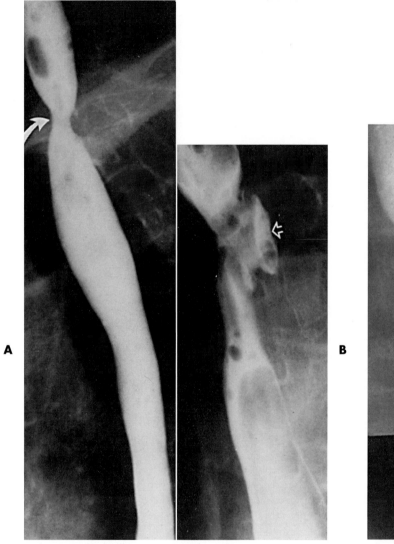

A

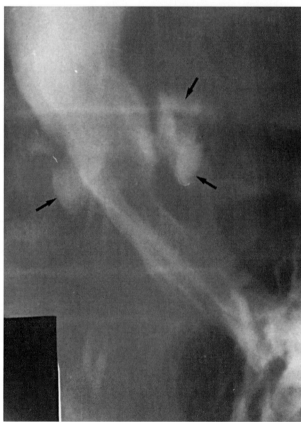

B

Fig. 1-65   **A,** Short stricture *(curved arrow)* following radiation and chemotherapy for squamous cell carcinoma of the lower cervical esophagus. **B,** Focal collection of contrast material *(open arrow)* at the site of previous stricture represents perforation secondary to endoscopic dilatation procedure.

Fig. 1-66   Water-soluble contrast examination shows two focal collections of contrast material *(arrows)* adjacent to the distal esophagus. These represent perforations following endoscopic dilatation for achalasia.

Food Impaction

Food impaction (Box 1-7) usually occurs when a poorly chewed piece of meat lodges in the esophagus. Although the underlying esophagus may on rare occasions be normal, strictures or other causes of esoph-

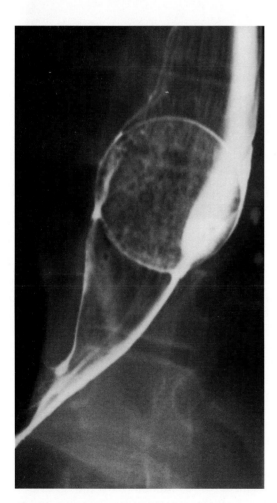

| Box 1-7 | Food Impaction: A Sign/Symptom, Not A Disease |

Food impaction occurs in the majority of cases in the distal esophagus at the gastroesophageal junction. Consider the cause of food impaction! Almost all cases of food impaction have some underlying esophageal abnormality such as inflammatory strictures or obstructing B-rings. It is rare for esophageal cancer to present with food impaction.

ageal narrowing can usually be implicated in the predisposition to the development of a food impaction. Contrast studies in cases of food impaction usually demonstrate a completely or partially obstructing intraluminal mass (Figs. 1-68 and 1-69). Glucagon, anticholinergic medications, and ingestion of effervescent granules have been used with varying success to dislodge impacted food boluses from the esophagus. Ingestion of enzymes or other meat tenderizers is no longer recommended because of complications including esophageal perforation.

POSTOPERATIVE ESOPHAGUS

Nonsurgical Procedures

A variety of surgical and nonsurgical procedures have been developed for treatment of esophageal diseases.

Bougienage and balloon dilatation

Bougienage consists of passage of a graded series of dilators into the esophagus to distend a stricture or other narrowed area. Balloon or pneumatic dilators contain a segment that can be placed at the site of narrowing and

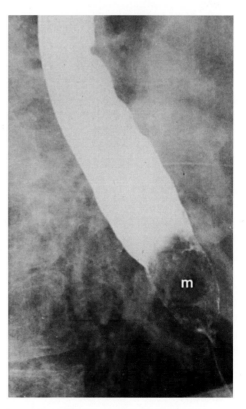

Fig. 1-67   Esophageal foreign body. This 19-year-old mentally retarded patient swallowed a play ball that partially occludes the distal esophagus.

Fig. 1-68   Large piece of meat *(m)* in the distal esophagus causes almost complete obstruction.

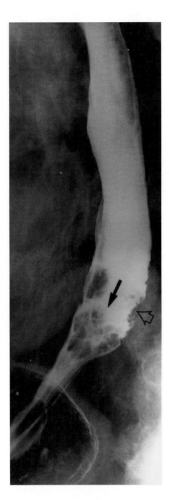

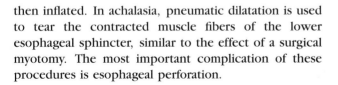

Fig. 1-69   Patient with carcinoma of distal esophagus. An esophagram has the appearance of food impaction *(arrow),* which is actually a tumor. Note destroyed mucosa *(open arrow).*

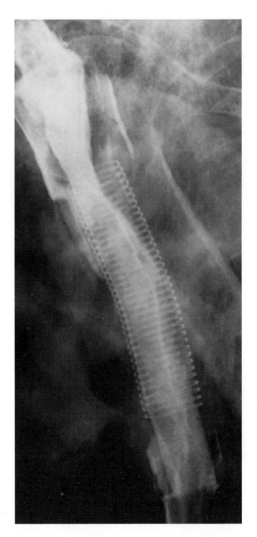

Fig. 1-70   Esophageal stent in a patient with advanced esophageal carcinoma.

then inflated. In achalasia, pneumatic dilatation is used to tear the contracted muscle fibers of the lower esophageal sphincter, similar to the effect of a surgical myotomy. The most important complication of these procedures is esophageal perforation.

Stent placement

Endoscopically guided stent placement is often used to maintain patency of the esophagus in patients with esophageal carcinoma (Fig. 1-70). Obstruction and migration of the tube and esophageal perforation are recognized complications of this palliative procedure.

Laser therapy

Laser therapy is another endoscopic palliative procedure, in which a laser beam (Nd:YAG laser) is used to destroy tumor tissue and thereby widen an obstructed esophageal lumen. This can lead to esophageal perforation or esophagorespiratory fistula.

Sclerotherapy

Sclerotherapy is sometimes used in the treatment of esophageal varices. Sclerosing agents are injected directly into the varices, causing fibrosis and obliteration of the varices. Complications of sclerotherapy include inflammation, ulceration, stricturing, fistula formation, and perforation.

Gastric balloon

Placement of a balloon into the gastric fundus (Sengstaken-Blakemore tube) is used to control variceal bleeding through a tamponading effect. However, incorrect placement of the tube with inflation of the balloon in the distal esophagus may cause esophageal perforation.

Surgical Procedures

Myotomy

Surgical esophageal myotomy has been used to treat both idiopathic achalasia (Heller's myotomy) and incomplete cricopharyngeal relaxation (cricopharyngeal myotomy). Extensive myotomy of the thoracic esophagus is sometimes performed in severe diffuse esophageal spasm (DES) that is unresponsive to other treatments and in idiopathic muscular hypertrophy of the esophagus, a rare condition characterized by diffuse marked thickening of the esophageal musculature. In these procedures, the abnormally contracted or thickened muscle is surgically incised.

Interposition

Various types of surgical interpositions can be performed in conjunction with esophageal carcinoma or extensive stricture formation. Stomach, colon, or jejunum can be used for this purpose. Contrast studies and CT are useful for demonstrating postoperative complications, both early (anastomotic leak, perforation, obstruction as a result of edema) and late (anastomotic stricture and recurrent tumor).

Fundoplication

Fundoplication and related surgical procedures can be used to reduce hiatal hernias and prevent associated gastroesophageal reflux. In fundoplication (Nissen, Mark IV [Belsey], and Hill types), a portion of the gastric fundus is wrapped around the distal esophagus (Fig. 1-71). This fundal wrap prevents reflux by compressing the distal esophagus and may appear as a pseudotumor on routine contrast studies and CT. Complications include obstruction if the wrap is too tight and persistent reflux if it is too loose. The Angelchik device, a ringlike structure filled with silicon, can be used in place of a fundal wrap but is associated with additional complications, including migration of the device into the abdominal or thoracic cavity and erosion into the gastric lumen.

Sugiura procedure

The Sugiura procedure is a complex surgical procedure used for treating esophageal varices. This extensive operation includes esophageal transection with devascularization of the distal esophagus and proximal stomach. Postoperative contrast studies typically reveal indentation at the distal esophageal suture line.

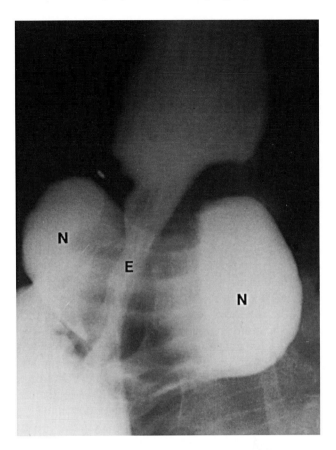

Fig. 1-71   Distal esophagus *(E)* is compressed by Nissen's fundoplication *(N)*.

Box 1-8   Dysphagia: The Radiologist's Dilemma

Always consider dysphagia to be a serious problem. Assume and look for a mechanical or dynamic basis for the symptom.

An appropriate clinical swallowing history and constitutional history is essential.

For purposes of evaluation, the swallowing function begins at the lips and terminates at the stomach.

THE RADIOLOGICAL EVALUATION OF DYSPHAGIA

Dysphagia (Box 1-8) is a serious symptom and should be evaluated thoroughly. There are few instances in radiology in which history-taking skills are as necessary as in the workup of these patients. The radiologist must be prepared to take time and elicit the history of the dysphagic symptom. This is necessary for two reasons. The first reason is to confirm the dysphagia. It is not uncommon for patients to complain of a sensation in the throat during or even after swallowing, but have no difficulty in swallowing solids or liquids. In other instances, coughing episodes, postnasal drip, or heartburn is presented to the radiologist as a clinical history of dysphagia. These are potentially important symptoms; however, it is important that the radiologist establish by history the presence or absence of true dysphagia (the inability or difficulty in passing the food bolus from mouth to stomach) or odynophagia (painful swallowing).

The second reason for eliciting the history of the dysphagic symptom is to determine a suitable radiological examination. Although the radiological evaluation of dysphagia requires basic evaluation of the morphology and function of the oral pharynx, esophagus, gastroesophageal junction, and proximal stomach, quite often it will be necessary to tailor the examination to fit the diagnostic problem. Additionally, the radiologist does not want to do anything that might harm the patient or increase patient discomfort. A patient presenting with weight loss or dysphagia to solids may not require the full biphasic examination with carbon dioxide granules and high dense barium, which could potentially be aspirated. Moreover, patients with moderate to severe odynophagia will experience considerable aggravation of their pain when CO_2 granules are used. Furthermore, a thorough history might suggest the problem to be of oral pharyngeal origin, in which a videotape recording, if available, should be used. After taking the history and performing the clinical evaluation, the radiologist can plan the form that the radiological study will take in order to optimize diagnostic opportunity and diminish complications.

If there is any question as to what might be encountered, we recommend a "test swallow" of approximately 5 ml of thin barium. Patients with possible high-grade mechanical obstruction, esophageal-airway fistula, or history suggestive of significant aspirations might be candidates for a test swallow. This test swallow will not seriously degrade the routine study that might follow.

A concise but complete swallowing history allows the radiologist to tailor the examination and in most instances also allows the experienced radiologist to predict the nature of the abnormality prior to the study.

History

The following should be considered:

1. Is it truly dysphagia? Does food "get stuck"? Does the patient have to work at getting the food down, (e.g., require fluids to force it down)?
2. What type of dysphagia is it? Is it dysphagia to liquids, solids, or both? In general, liquid dysphagia may suggest motility abnormalities, whereas dysphagia to solids tends to point to mechanical difficulties.
3. What are the duration and constancy of symptoms? Persistent dysphagia is clearly more worrisome than symptoms that are intermittent. Are the symptoms progressive? Progressive solid dysphagia is a serious concern. This is particularly true when it is associated with constitutional changes such as weight loss, decreased energy, and decreased appetite.
4. Are there accompanying constitutional changes? Has the patient experienced weight change? Has appetite been affected? Has eating pattern been altered? Those patients who experience a slow progression of dysphagia that requires them to avoid certain foods (e.g., meat) or puree their food are indicating potentially serious problems. However, one should be cautious when inquiring about eating habits. Many patients with chronic benign esophageal strictures have come to terms with their swallowing limitations and have altered their eating habits accordingly. They may consider their eating patterns perfectly normal and unchanged. One occasionally has to put very specific questions to the patient. Consider the following real-life exchange between a radiology resident prior to an examination and a 62-year-old patient with a prior history of a chest tumor currently complaining of intermittent heartburn for approximately 1 year.

Resident: Do you ever notice food getting stuck while eating?
Patient: No.
Resident: Do you ever have any problems swallowing?
Patient: No.
Resident: Do you ever notice the feeling of food getting stuck in your neck or upper abdomen?
Patient: No.
Resident: Do you have any pain when you swallow?
Patient: No.

The subsequent UGI disclosed a moderate lower esophageal stricture that had a benign appearance. The radiology resident was encouraged to question the patient in more detail. After the radiological examination, the following interview proceeded as follows:

Resident: So, you never notice any problems with swallowing?
Patient: No.
Resident: Food never seems to get stuck when you swallow?
Patient: No.
Resident: Any problems with swallowing, say, steak?
Patient: Actually, steak seems to get stuck.
Resident: What about other meats?
Patient: Usually. I seem to have problems whenever I swallow meat or bread because it usually gets stuck, so I avoid those foods. Sometimes when I take my vitamins in the morning, they seem to get stuck. Apart from that, I don't have any problems.

A conversation such as this would not be unique. There is no suggestion that the patient was deliberately intending to mislead or deceive the resident. Some patients are anxious or frightened about the procedures. The skills of history taking, which are learned, and hopefully mastered, in medical school, should be retained and frequently used by radiologists.

Radiological Evaluation

The radiological evaluation consists of five parts. Clinical history may emphasize one part over another; however, all parts of the examination should be included to some extent in every radiological dysphagia workup.

I. Oral pharyngeal airway
In this part of the examination the following observations are to be made:
1. Morphology.
   • Size of the oral pharyngeal airway. Is the airway dilated?
   • Shape and size of the epiglottis.
2. Bolus organization in transit in the mouth and on the tongue.
   • Is the bolus well organized on the tongue?
   • Is there spillage into the buccal cavity?
   • Is there spillage of contrast into the oral pharynx prior to the initiation of swallow?
3. Normal triggering of the autonomic swallowing reflex.
   • Is there a prompt and rapid triggering of the swallowing reflex when the bolus touches the posterior pharyngeal wall?
   • Delays of the triggering of the swallowing reflex should be noted.
4. Contraction, elevation of the soft palate, and exclusion of the nasopharynx.
   • Does the soft palate effectively occlude the nasopharynx during swallowing?
   • Is there any nasopharyngeal reflux?
5. Pharyngeal contraction.
   • Is the pharyngeal contraction symmetrical? Is there weakness in the contraction? Is the weakness unilateral or bilateral? Contrast tends to flow to the weak side in situations in which the pharyngeal contraction is asymmetrically weak.
6. Excursion of the laryngeal-hyoid complex and the posterior-inferior tipping of the epiglottis. These are the mechanisms of airway protection, the former being especially important.
   • Is swallowing accompanied by the normal upward and outward movement of the laryngeal hyoid complex?
   • Does the epiglottis tilt posteriorly and inferiorly with the bolus?

7. Relaxation of the cricopharyngeal muscle. The cricopharyngeal constitutes the upper esophageal sphincter.
   • During maximum bolus distention, does this area completely open?
It should be noted that some patients show a mild cricopharyngeal impression during maximum bolus transit. However, if the luminal compromise is less than 25% during maximum distention, it is always asymptomatic and of no clinical consequence.

Posterior impressions caused by cervical spine osteophyte formation are also a common finding but almost never result in dysphagia and should be ignored. The only exception might be the large bridging osteophytes of diffuse idiopathic skeletal hyperostosis (DISH) or large posttraumatic osteophytes.
8. Postswallow residual.
   • Is there residual barium in the hypopharynx following the swallow?
   • If so, estimate the amount (small, moderate, or large).
9. Aspiration. This is defined as contrast that is inhaled into the airway and descends below the laryngeal vestibule and the cords. Contrast that does not pass the vestibule is referred to as penetration.
   • If aspiration is present, record type and amount present. Is there a spontaneous cough reflex with aspiration?
Three types of aspiration can be identified:
• Preswallow aspiration. When patients spill barium over the posterior tongue into the oral pharynx or into the valleculae prior to the initiation of swallowing and immediately aspirate the bolus, it is referred to as preswallow aspiration. This is also the most serious type of aspiration, and most examinations will be terminated at this point.
• Swallowing aspiration. This is the most common form of aspiration. Failure to completely protect the airway may result in some aspiration during swallowing. This type of aspiration can be transient (e.g., in poststroke patients) and may be treated by the speech pathologist with varying therapeutic maneuvers.
• Postswallow aspiration. This occurs when the pharyngeal contraction is incomplete or incompetent if the cricopharyngeal muscle fails to fully relax. The resultant residual can be aspirated as the multifunctional oral pharynx (eating, breathing, and phonation) switches to breathing mode and contrast is subsequently aspirated.

II. Esophagus: tube morphology
This is accomplished by the biphasic examination, in which one evaluates such things as structure, filling

defects, barium collections suggesting ulcers or diverticula, and extrinsic impressions.

III. Esophageal dynamics

The presence and gross evaluation of the primary wave is observed. The presence of secondary or tertiary waves is also noted.

Whereas primary waves are striping waves triggered by the swallowing reflex, secondary waves are triggered by luminal distention and relate to reflux contrast from the stomach or poorly cleared contrast from the esophagus. Tertiary waves are nonpropulsive contractions of the esophagus, frequently seen in the elderly with otherwise normal esophageal dynamics. Hence, the condition is referred to as presbyesophagus. This is not pathology. The presence of tertiary waves as the *only* form of esophageal contraction is abnormal.

Esophageal dynamics are best evaluated with gravity eliminated as a factor and with the patient in the recumbent position (right anterior oblique being the optimal position). The primary wave must be evaluated with a single swallow. Multiple swallows will obliterate the primary wave ahead of it. This is a normal protective mechanism, but it could be misinterpreted as dynamic abnormality.

IV. Gastroesophageal junction

This is the most common site of esophageal disease and requires careful attention. One should never make judgments about the gastroesophageal junction based upon air contrast upright views. Invariably the gastroesophageal junction is pulled downward by gravity and by the weight of the stomach and its contents (especially if that content is barium). The need for single-contrast evaluation of the esophagus in the recumbent position is best demonstrated at the gastroesophageal junction. Occasionally, small hiatal hernias, B-rings, ulcers, thickened folds, and even small neoplastic lesions may be subtle or not seen on the upright air contrast views but effectively demonstrated on the single-contrast recumbent views (Fig. 1-72).

Additionally, it is important to note the absence or presence of gastroesophageal reflux and to quantify it to some extent. It is natural to occasionally reflux acidic stomach content into the esophagus. The protective mechanisms are (1) the secondary wave striping the acid back into the stomach, and (2) the cricopharyngeus, which protects the oral pharynx from refluxed gastric content. Failure of the secondary wave to clear the esophagus rapidly and completely increases the risk of reflux esophagitis. Failure of the cricopharyngeus to bar the way of refluxed acid into the oral pharynx can result in confusing and occasionally deadly consequences. Patients may complain of sore throat or hoarseness in the morning or awake with alarming coughing fits during the night as reflux and aspiration occur. Sometimes the aspiration is in tiny amounts, silent and continuous, which can result in either pneumonia or bronchospasm. These patients may be treated with antibiotics and/or antiasthmatic medication, when in fact the underlying problem is gastroesophageal reflux. Quantifying gastroesophageal reflux is somewhat subjective. In the lower third of the esophagus it may be called "small." Reflux to the midesophagus can be termed "moderate," whereas reflux up the entire esophageal column to the level of the cricopharyngeus would be considered "large." However, to emphasize again, it is not the presence of reflux that is important, but the effectiveness of the protective mechanisms, namely the clearing function of the secondary wave and the protective function of the cricopharyngeus muscle.

V. Cardiofundal region of the stomach

The cardia and fundus of the stomach should be included as part of the dysphagic workup. Neoplastic lesions in these areas not directly affecting the gastroesophageal junction have been seen in patients presenting with dysphagia, for which no other cause of dysphagia is evident.

Conclusion

Two additional issues require attention in the radiological workup of dysphagia. The first issue to consider is the type of contrast agent. Barium is always the contrast agent of choice for any patient who presents with a dysphagia history and in whom there is no suspicion of an esophageal tear or leak.

Water-soluble contrast has little or no role in this radiological examination. Since many of these patients can aspirate, it is preferable that barium be the aspirated agent rather than the water-soluble iodine-based contrast agents. The latter can cause chemical pneumonitis and even pulmonary edema.

In patients with relatively healthy lungs, barium aspiration is relatively harmless. It should be pointed out that it was only four to five decades ago that radiological bronchography was performed using barium as the contrast agent. In patients with chronic lung disease, barium may be seen for a protracted period of time in the lungs, but it is still unquestionably preferable to water-soluble contrast and its complications.

The second issue to consider is the modified barium swallow. This is sometimes referred to as a dynamic swallowing study and is performed in the radiology department in conjunction with a speech pathologist. Because swallowing is a function that commences at the lips and tongue and ceases in the stomach, it is necessary for the radiologist to be completely involved in these types of examinations. This is important not only to provide professional fluoroscopic imaging and manage-

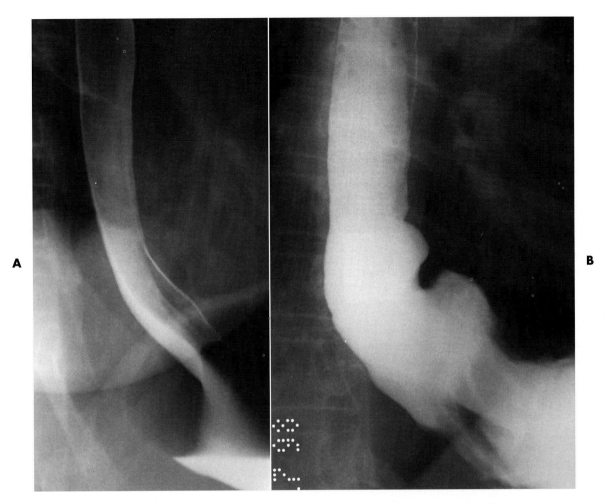

Fig. 1-72   The gastroesophageal junction. **A,** Demonstration of gastroesophageal junction during upright double contrast views in patient with complaint of heartburn. The junction looks normal. **B,** The same patient recumbent during single-contrast phase of the biphasic examination. Note hiatal hernia not seen on the upright view.

ment of radiation safety issues, but also to ensure that whenever possible a lesion of the esophagus, gastroesophageal junction, or proximal stomach is not missed because only the oral pharynx is evaluated.

The speech pathologist's role in the examination is to evaluate the patient's capacity for oral feeding and to plan strategies relative to that issue. These examinations should not be performed to evaluate for dysphagia unrelated to central nervous system incidents, degenerative muscle diseases, or neurological diseases. If they are, it is the radiologist's responsibility to do what is necessary for a proper radiological evaluation. This is particularly true if the oral pharyngeal phase of the evaluation is normal.

SUGGESTED READINGS

Balthazar EJ, Naidich DP, Megibow AJ, et al: CT evaluation of esophageal varices, *AJR* 148:131-135, 1987.

Bleshman MH, Banner MP, Johnson RC, et al: The inflammatory esophagogastric polyp and fold, *Radiology* 128:589-593, 1978.

Bova JG, Dutton NE, Goldstein HM, et al: Medication-induced esophagitis: diagnosis by double-contrast esophagography, *AJR* 148:731-732, 1987.

Buchholz D: Neurologic causes of dysphagia, *Dysphagia* 1:152-156, 1987.

Buecker A, Wein BB, Neuerburg, JM, et al: Esophageal perforation: comparison of use of aqueous and barium-containing contrast agents, *Radiology* 202:683-686, 1997.

Calenoff L, Rogers LF: Radiologic manifestations of iatrogenic changes of the esophagus, *Gastrointest Radiol* 2:229-237, 1977.

Carter MM, Kulkarni MV: Giant fibrovascular polyp of the esophagus, *Gastrointest Radiol* 9:301-303, 1984.

Chasen MH, Rugh KS, Shelton DK: Mediastinal impressions on the dilated esophagus, *Radiol Clin North Am* 22:591-605, 1984.

Curtis DJ: Radiographic anatomy of the pharynx, *Dysphagia* 1:51-62, 1986.

Donner MW, Bosma JF, Robertson DL: Anatomy and physiology of the pharynx, *Gastrointest Radiol* 10:196-212, 1985.

Donner MW, Saba GP, Martinez CR: Diffuse diseases of the esophagus: a practical approach, *Semin Roentgenol* 16:198-213, 1981.

Ekberg O, Nylander G: Dysfunction of the cricopharyngeal muscle: a cineradiographic study of patients with dysphagia, *Radiology* 143:481-486, 1982.

Fisher MS: Metastasis to the esophagus, *Gastrointest Radiol* 1:249-251, 1976.

Freeny PC, Marks WM: Adenocarcinoma of the gastroesophageal junction: barium and CT examination, *AJR* 138:1077-1084, 1982.

Gedgaudas-McClees RK, Torres WE, Colvin RS, et al: Thoracic findings in gastrointestinal pathology, *Radiol Clin North Am* 22:563-589, 1984.

Gelfand DW, Ott DJ: Anatomy and technique in evaluating the esophagus, *Semin Roentgenol* 16:168-182, 1981.

Ghahremani GG, Rushovich AM: Glycogenic acanthosis of the esophagus: radiographic and pathologic features, *Gastrointest Radiol* 9:93-98, 1984.

Gilchrist AM, Levine MS, Carr RF, et al: Barrett's esophagus: diagnosis by double-contrast esophagography, *AJR* 150:97-102, 1988.

Goldstein HM, Zornoza J, Hopens T: Intrinsic diseases of the adult esophagus: benign and malignant tumors, *Semin Roentgenol* 16:183-197, 1981.

Grishaw EK, Ott DJ, Frederick MG, et al: Functional abnormalities of the esophagus: a prospective analysis of the radiographic findings relative to age and symptoms, *AJR* 167:719-723, 1996.

Halber MD, Daffner RH, Thompson WM: CT of the esophagus. I. Normal appearance, *AJR* 133:1047-1050, 1979.

Halvorsen RA, Thompson WM: Computed tomography of the gastroesophageal junction, *Crit Rev Diagn Imaging* 21:183-228, 1984.

Halvorsen RA Jr, Thompson WM: CT of esophageal neoplasms, *Radiol Clin North Am* 27:667-685, 1989.

Heiken JP, Balfe DM, Roper CL: CT evaluation after esophagogastrectomy, *AJR* 143:555-560, 1984.

Jones B, Kramer SS, Donner MW: Dynamic imaging of the pharynx, *Gastrointest Radiol* 10:213-224, 1985.

Kawamoto K, Yamada Y, Utsunomiya T, et al: Gastrointestinal submucosal tumors: evaluation with endoscopic US, *Radiology* 205:733-740, 1997

Laufer I: Radiology of esophagitis, *Radiol Clin North Am* 20:687-699, 1982.

Lepke RA, Libshitz HI: Radiation-induced injury of the esophagus, *Radiology* 148:375-378, 1983.

Levine MS, Caroline DF, Thompson JJ, et al: Adenocarcinoma of the esophagus: relationship to Barrett mucosa, *Radiology* 150:305-309, 1984.

Levine MS, Chu P, Furth EE, et al: Carcinoma of the esophagogastric junction: sensitivity of radiographic diagnosis, *AJR* 168:1423-1426, 1997.

Levine MS, Loevner LA, Saul SH, et al: Herpes esophagitis: sensitivity of double-contrast esophagography, *AJR* 151:57-62, 1988.

Levine MS, Moolten DN, Herlinger H, et al: Esophageal intramural pseudodiverticulosis: a reevaluation, *AJR* 147:1165-1170, 1986.

Levine MS, Rubesin SE, Herlinger H, et al: Double-contrast upper gastrointestinal examination: technique and interpretation, *Radiology* 168:593-602, 1988.

Love L, Berkow AE: Trauma to the esophagus, *Gastrointest Radiol* 2:305-321, 1978.

Marx MV, Balfe DM: Computed tomography of the esophagus, *Semin Ultrasound CT MR* 8:316-348, 1987.

Mauro MA, Parker LA, Hartley WS, et al: Epidermolysis bullosa: radiographic findings in 16 cases, *AJR* 149:925-927, 1987.

Olmsted WW, Lichtenstein JE, Hyams VJ: Polypoid epithelial malignancies of the esophagus, *AJR* 140:921-925, 1983.

Olmsted WW, Madewell JE: The esophageal and small-bowel manifestations of progressive systemic sclerosis, *Gastrointest Radiol* 1:33-36, 1976.

Ott DJ, Gelfand DW, Wu WC, et al: Esophagogastric region and its rings, *AJR* 142:281-287, 1984.

Owen JW, Balfe DM, Koehler RE, et al: Radiologic evaluation of complications after esophagogastrectomy, *AJR* 140:1163-1169, 1983.

Phillips LG, Cunningham J: Esophageal perforation, *Radiol Clin North Am* 22:607-613, 1984.

Rubesin SE, Glick SN: The tailored double-contrast pharyngogram, *Crit Rev Diagn Imaging* 28:133-179, 1988.

Rubesin S, Herlinger H, Sigal H: Granular cell tumors of the esophagus, *Gastrointest Radiol* 10:11-15, 1985.

Schneider R: Tuberculous esophagitis, *Gastrointest Radiol* 1:143-145, 1976.

Seaman WB: Pathophysiology of the esophagus, *Semin Roentgenol* 16:214-227, 1981.

Zboralske FF, Dodds WJ: Roentgenographic diagnosis of primary disorders of esophageal motility, *Radiol Clin North Am* 7:147-162, 1969.

Stomach and Duodenum

EXAMINATION TECHNIQUES

The biphasic-contrast examination of the stomach is considered to be the radiological examination of choice at present. This technique consists of examining the stomach, utilizing both double-contrast and single-contrast technique (Box 2-1).

In most cases, the stomach examination is combined with the esophagus study. Following the ingestion of effervescent granules and high-density barium and the double-contrast evaluation of the esophagus in the upright position, the patient is quickly lowered into a supine recumbent position. To avoid excessive spillage of the contrast into the small bowel, this should be done promptly after the last esophageal film has been obtained. With the patient in the supine position, a quick fluoroscopic evaluation of the stomach will indicate to the fluoroscopist whether gastric distention is adequate, and if a sufficient amount of barium is retained within the stomach to continue with the examination or whether remedial measures may be necessary at this time.

If the stomach is adequately distended and contains sufficient barium, the patient is then rotated one to two times to achieve gastric coating. By rotating patients to the left, it is felt that less barium is spilled into the small bowel. The gastric mucosa is covered by a surface layer of mucus that must be washed away by the barium to achieve optimum mucosal coating and detail. Inadequate washing of the barium over the mucosal surface or residual food and secretions will degrade mucosal coating and cause the examination to be limited. Following rotation of the patient, the stomach is again fluoroscopically evaluated for the quality of the mucosal coating.

The menu of spot radiographs obtained varies among different institutions. Generally, a supine film of the stomach is obtained when adequate coating has been achieved. The patient is turned sharply to the right into a steep right posterior oblique or right lateral position, where air-contrast views of the cardia and fundus are obtained. Under fluoroscopic control, the patient is then turned back into the supine position and slightly to the left to thin out the barium pool in the antrum. As the barium flows from the antrum into the proximal stomach, a thin layer of barium is left in the antrum, achieving

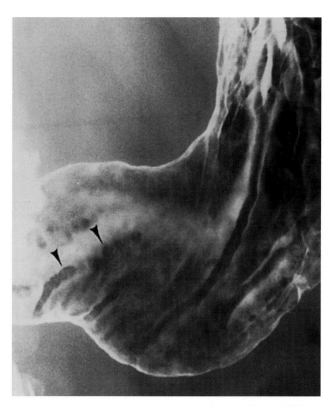

Fig. 2-1   Utilizing flow technique, tiny superficial erosions are seen along one of the folds of the distal stomach. Edema around the erosions results in a beaded appearance of the fold *(arrows)*.

the "flow technique" (Box 2-2), which is an excellent method for demonstrating subtle mucosal findings, such as tiny nodules and linear or punctate erosions (Fig. 2-1). A spot film is obtained at this point. The patient is again turned to the left, and air-contrast views of the antrum and duodenum are obtained. This series of maneuvers basically represents the double-contrast portion of the stomach examination. Additional films and maneuvers may be necessary to completely demonstrate all areas within the stomach and the duodenal bulb and sweep.

At this point the patient is turned to a recumbent right anterior oblique (RAO) position and ingests low-density barium. A limited evaluation of oropharyngeal function may be obtained during this phase. Esophageal dynamics are also studied, and barium distended views of the gastroesophageal junction are obtained. The latter constitutes an important part of the stomach evaluation. With sufficient barium within the stomach and antrum and duodenal bulb, RAO or prone compression views of the antrum and duodenal bulb are obtained. This maneuver is as important in the upper gastrointestinal (UGI) series today as it was 50 years ago. Occasionally, ulcers that are either unfilled during the earlier part of the examination or not well demonstrated can be easily seen with compression views of the antrum and duodenal bulb.

Occasionally, the duodenal bulb and, possibly, the distal antrum will be in a posterior position. In some cases, the bulb will lie almost directly behind the distal antrum. This makes compression of the area somewhat difficult. It also makes air-contrast views of the bulb and antropyloric region difficult as well. In such an instance, the fluoroscopist may utilize angulation of the tube, if this facility is available. However, most fluoroscopic suites have tableside type of fluoroscopy. In such a situation, the fluoroscopist can turn the patient on the left side and firmly position a bolster, which may represent an inflated compression paddle or a balloon against the left costochondral margin. The patient, under fluoroscopy, is then moved down into a left anterior oblique (LAO) position, compressing the abdomen as the patient rolls to the left and toward the table. This is often sufficient compression to push away the antrum of the stomach and allow the duodenal bulb and pyloric channel to be demonstrated (Fig. 2-2).

The use of glucagon in UGI studies has been advocated and practiced for over a decade. Small doses of glucagon have been shown to be effective in improving the demonstration of the antrum and duodenal bulb. However, many centers have now ceased this practice, and no intravenous (IV) injection is given before the examination. No objective evidence shows that this

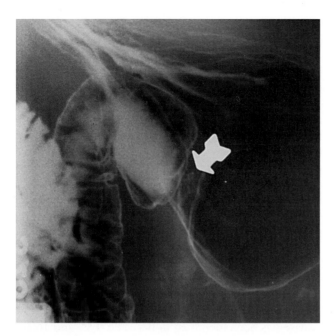

Fig. 2-2 LAO view with compression demonstrates the profiled pyloric channel and duodenal bulb. A small pyloric channel ulcer, not seen on other views, is demonstrated *(arrow).*

results in any decreased sensitivity in the detection of disease in these areas. Without the use of an antiperistaltic agent, such as glucagon, gastric contractions may be observed and evaluated.

The last part of the examination consists of rotating the patient again to evaluate for the possibility of spontaneous gastroesophageal reflux. We tend not to use any extraordinary methods for inducing reflux. Valsalva maneuvers, abdominal compression, and bolstering have all been described. Virtually any patient can be made to reflux with sufficient effort. The significance of this reflux is doubtful. However, the rotation of a patient that results in a spontaneous and significant amount of reflux is probably important. This often simulates what happens when the patient rolls over in bed at night and experiences gastric reflux and associated symptoms. It should be remembered that the lack of demonstrated reflux may not necessarily rule out gastroesophageal reflux as the cause of the patient's symptoms.

In many instances, instead of the standard biphasic examination, a single-contrast study using low-density barium will be performed. Although this should represent a minority of cases, there are acceptable indications for a single-contrast examination. In elderly or debilitated patients who are unable to stand or who cannot roll or provide the compliance necessary for a double-contrast evaluation of the stomach, a single-contrast examination is an alternative. In patients with suspected gastric outlet obstruction, single-contrast examination will suffice. In patients who have had surgery or procedures involving use of instrumentation and in whom

there is any question of perforation or leakage, a water-soluble single-contrast examination is indicated.

When faced with the decision as to whether a single-contrast or biphasic examination should be undertaken, the radiologist should be guided by the same axiom that applies to the radiological evaluation of the colon—a limited single-contrast evaluation is better than a limited double-contrast evaluation of the organ.

Helical computed tomography (CT) is extremely useful in evaluating for known or suspected malignant lesions of the stomach. The extent of perigastric involvement and spread to adjacent organs can usually be demonstrated with this type of imaging. Magnetic resonance imaging has been extremely limited to date in evaluation of the stomach and plays little or no role in the diagnostic imaging workup of patients with gastric disease. Endoscopic ultrasound with a rotating transducer placed on the tip of a specially prepared endoscope has been useful in the evaluation of malignant diseases of the stomach. It is shown to be superior to CT in evaluating the extent of gastric wall involvement and limited perigastric spread and adenopathy, which may not be evident on CT. For evaluation of liver metastatic involvement, however, helical CT of the liver with pre-IV and post-IV contrast remains the examination of choice.

The following sections approach the differential diagnosis of gastric disease, based on the dominant radiological problems seen on barium examinations. It closely reflects the way cases are actually encountered in a daily clinical practice. However, it should be kept in mind that the same condition may be discussed under several categories, reflecting the different manifestations or stages of the same disease process.

STOMACH

Gastric Outlet Obstruction Resulting in Gastric Distention

Peptic ulcer disease
The most common cause of gastric outlet obstruction in adults is peptic ulcer disease involving the antrum, the pyloric channel of the stomach, and the first portion of the duodenum. This complication, however, is seen in only 5% of patients with peptic ulcer disease. Duodenal bulb and pyloric channel ulcers are responsible for over 80% of the cases in which it does occur. Luminal narrowing usually results from the combined changes of chronic and acute inflammation and ulceration. These patients commonly have a long history of peptic ulcer disease and recurrent peptic ulcers. It is unusual for gastric outlet obstruction to be the presenting complaint in a patient without a history of peptic ulcer disease. In such an instance, other possibilities, particularly malignancy, should be considered.

The most common presenting symptoms are vomiting, abdominal pain, and upper abdominal distention. Less prominent findings may include weight loss and anorexia.

The distention of the stomach in patients with chronic peptic ulcer disease is a gradual process in which symptoms can be present for several months or years before diagnosis. As a result, the size of the stomach, when seen on plain films of the abdomen, can be surprisingly large. Over a period of time, the capability of the stomach to distend is remarkable (Fig. 2-3). It may appear on plain films as a huge, confusing, mottled, or soft tissue mass in the upper abdomen. At other times, the amount of distention can be less and a discernible dilated stomach can be identified. The mottled appearance of the dilated stomach is the result of the accumulation of secretions and the residue of numerous meals (Fig. 2-4). There may be diminished gas distally, although complete obstruction is unusual and air is generally seen in the small bowel and colon. In fact, they may have a normal appearance, except for depression of the transverse colon. Upright films will demonstrate an air-fluid level within the stomach. The presence of an air-fluid level within the duodenum is helpful in distinguishing between delayed outflow of gastric content secondary to gastric or duodenal obstruction.

The plain films are often diagnostic, and barium studies can be undertaken, not necessarily to confirm outlet obstruction, but rather to attempt to identify the site (duodenal or gastric) and the nature of the obstructing process (Fig. 2-5). Gastric dilatation and delayed flow into the small bowel will be the major findings. Ulcers may or may not be seen. Residual food will, generally, make the examination limited. The contrast of choice in the absence of free intraperitoneal air is barium. The large amount of residual fluid within the stomach of most of these patients, along with the propensity for frequent vomiting, makes the use of water-soluble contrast relatively contraindicated.

Other inflammatory causes
Crohn's disease
In various studies, gastric involvement with Crohn's disease has been identified in between 0.5% and 10% of patients. The most common pattern of severe gastric involvement with Crohn's disease is a narrowed, somewhat rigid stomach (Fig. 2-6). On rare occasions, involvement of the distal antrum, in particular the pyloric channel, can result in gastric obstruction.

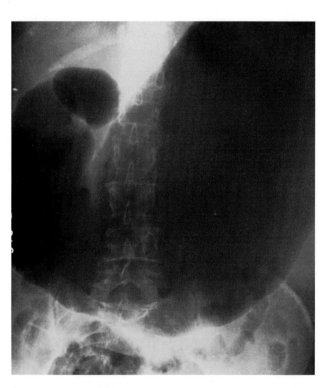

Fig. 2-3 Plain film of the abdomen demonstrates massive air distention of the stomach and duodenal bulb.

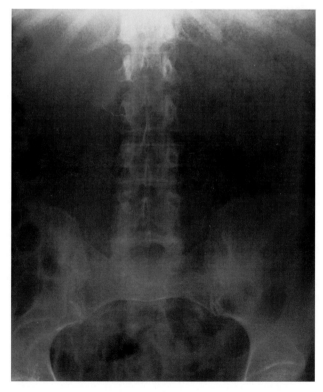

Fig. 2-4 A large, mottled mass occupying the entire upper abdomen and displacing air-filled loops of bowel laterally and inferiorly represents a grossly distended stomach filled with food debris and secretions.

Pancreatitis

Patients with severe pancreatitis may present with degrees of gastric outlet obstruction. This is generally secondary to contiguous involvement of the adjacent structures with the inflammatory changes. In the stomach, wall thickening, edema, and spasm can lead to luminal compromise.

Corrosive materials

Patients ingesting corrosive materials, particularly acids, can present with severe inflammatory changes in the distal antrum, especially along the lesser curvature, and luminal stricturing can occur, either acutely or chronically. The radiological features of such a lesion may be indistinguishable from malignancy.

Other causes

Other unusual inflammatory causes of gastric outlet obstruction include radiation gastritis, tuberculosis, and syphilis. The changing pattern of disease prevalence and the recent increased incidence of both of these latter diseases in the population could conceivably result in an increased incidence of gastric involvement. However, because modern treatment regimens usually limit the severity of these diseases commonly seen in previous decades, the number of cases with severe involvement of the stomach and potential gastric outlet obstruction will probably not increase and will remain extremely rare.

Malignancy

Carcinoma, especially of the scirrhous variety, involving the antrum or pyloric region, commonly results in gastric outlet obstruction (Fig. 2-7). In addition, carcinoma of the head of the pancreas with adjacent spread involving the gastric antrum can compromise gastric outflow. These two tumors are probably the most common causes of gastric outlet obstruction resulting from neoplastic diseases. On rare occasions, lymphoma can result in outlet obstruction. However, lymphomas,

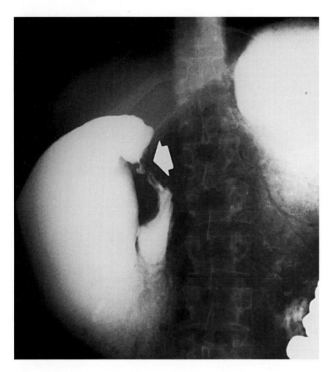

Fig. 2-5 UGI examination in a patient presenting with chronic abdominal pain and distention demonstrates a grossly distended stomach with ulceration in the pyloric channel *(arrow)* and the duodenal bulb.

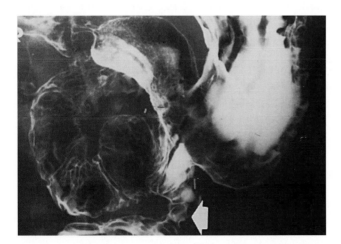

Fig. 2-6 UGI examination demonstrates a contracted stomach and a gastrojejunostomy. There is also fold thickening and narrowing of the efferent loop below the anastomosis *(arrow)*. All the observed inflammatory changes both in the stomach and adjacent small bowel are due to Crohn's disease.

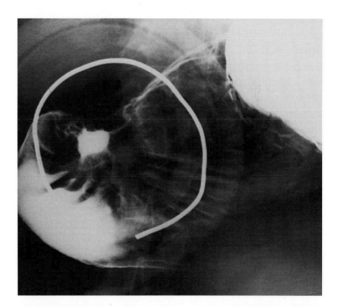

Fig. 2-7 Ulcerating mass with a central barium collection occupies the distal prepyloric region of the stomach resulting in gastric outlet obstruction. The lesion was found to be adenocarcinoma of the stomach.

especially the non-Hodgkin's lymphomas, tend to be somewhat pliable tumors, and infrequently cause obstruction, even when the tumor traverses the pyloric channel and involves the duodenal bulb. However, on rare occasions, a polypoid mass involving the distal stomach and pyloric channel can result in mechanical obstruction by the presence of its sheer bulk in the most anatomically narrowed region of the stomach.

Gastric bezoars

Generally, gastric bezoars (Box 2-3) do not obstruct. Indeed, they may be asymptomatic for long periods of time (Fig. 2-8). However, on occasion, the bezoar may act as an occluding agent in a ball-valve type of obstructive process within the stomach. Postgastrectomy patients are most susceptible to bezoar formation and gastric distention. Although a small number of patients may demonstrate degrees of outlet obstruction, distention of the stomach or gastric remnant is often a result of the increasing size of the bezoar. The most common bezoar encountered is the phytobezoar, composed of fiber, plant matter, leaves, and roots. These are usually smaller and more compact than hair bezoars (trichobezoars). They are also more abrasive and the incidence of associated peptic ulcer is higher with phytobezoars. They are the most common type of bezoar encountered following gastric surgery. Occasionally, a bezoar representing an overgrowth of fungi and yeast is also encountered in postoperative patients. The susceptibility of postoperative patients to bezoar formation probably relates to the accompanying vagotomy and diminished ability of the stomach to empty.

Trichobezoars or hairballs are the second most commonly occurring gastric bezoar. They represent a congealed collection of hair enmeshed with mucus and decaying food material. They are always black in appearance and have a characteristic odor. They can be asymptomatic and can attain great size with resultant gastric dilatation. They tend to be found in younger female patients. Incidences are higher in institutionalized patients and those with psychiatric disturbances.

A type of bezoar commonly encountered in medical literature is the persimmon bezoar. This is generally

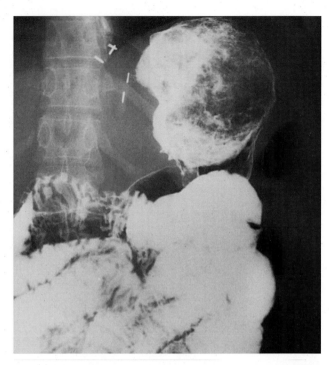

Fig. 2-8   Gastric bezoar is demonstrated in a postoperative stomach.

unrelated to gastric surgery and is named for the native American persimmon tree. The fruit of the persimmon tree, although possessing little fiber, has considerable pulp quantity. Unripe persimmon fruit has a well-known astringent property. The interaction of the astringent and the stomach acid results in a coagulum or gelatinous pulpy mass within the stomach and can occasionally result in acute gastric outlet obstruction. Other uncommon types of bezoars that have been reported include food bezoars, actually representing forms of phytobezoars. Some cases of bezoar formation in the stomach relating to the ingestion of vegetable fiber powder and psyllium have been reported. This is, no doubt, related to postoperative stomachs, abnormal gastric emptying, and inadequate amounts of ingested fluids along with the vegetable powders.

Foreign body bezoars, although previously uncommon and almost exclusively seen in children or emotionally disturbed individuals, are being brought to the public's notice as individuals attempting to smuggle illegal drugs into the country have discovered new and lucrative uses for condoms. However, in such individuals, the problem of gastric outlet obstruction fades into insignificance in the light of the relatively high incidence of condom leakage or rupture.

Antral diaphragms

Antral diaphragms are thin, well-defined, symmetrical mucosal webs seen in the distal portion of the antrum

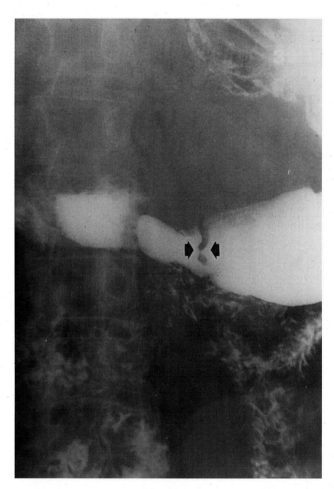

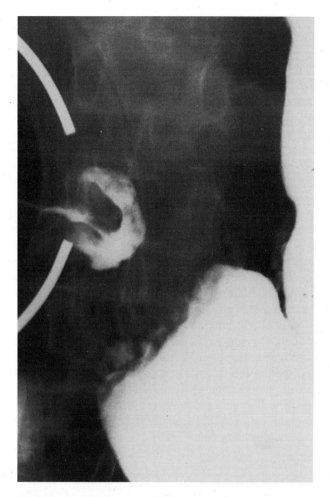

Fig. 2-9   UGI study demonstrates a thin, incomplete weblike structure in the antrum of the stomach representing an antral web *(arrows)*.

Fig. 2-10   UGI examination from a patient with gastric outlet obstruction demonstrates mass effect in the pyloric region with elongated pyloric channel and possible ulceration along the course of the channel.

compromising the antral lumen to varying degrees. Many feel that they are congenital because of the lack of histological evidence of scarring in some patients. However, the origins of the antral web or diaphragm still remain unclear. Not all antral diaphragms are congenital in nature. The history of chronic peptic inflammatory disease in many of these patients seriously suggests the possibility that some of these antral diaphragms may in reality be narrowed, well-defined bands of scarring. The circumferential healing of gastric ulcers is well known.

Most antral diaphragms are not associated with obstruction. However, where the lumen is sufficiently compromised, degrees of gastric obstruction may be encountered. Generally, luminal narrowing of 1.5 cm or less will be symptomatic. Careful fluoroscopic evaluation of the motility through this region, as well as the use of a 12.5-mm barium tablet, is helpful in establishing the degree of luminal compromise.

Fluoroscopically, these must be demonstrated as fixed, weblike areas of narrowing in the antral portion of the stomach (Fig. 2-9). The degree of circumferential involvement may or may not be complete.

Pyloric stenosis

In the adult, pyloric stenosis is a confusing entity. Whether it represents a true congenital pyloric stenosis or is an unusual sequela of peptic inflammatory disease is unclear. Most of the patients with the radiological findings of adult hypertrophic pyloric stenosis have concomitant peptic inflammatory disease. However, presentation with significant gastric outlet obstruction is unusual. The radiological findings have been described as mass effect in the pyloric region with an elongated pyloric channel measuring two to three times its normal length. A bulging mass in the base of the duodenum or antrum is commonly seen with this process (Fig. 2-10). This should not be confused with prolapsed gastric mucosa, which is a transient finding in patients with antral gastritis. Prolapsing gastric mucosa is rarely, if ever, associated with gastric outlet obstruction.

A small number of patients will demonstrate a small triangular outpouching of the antrum along the greater curvature, just proximal to the pyloric channel, called Twining's recess. This outpouching represents a protrusion of mucosa between the hypertrophied circular torus muscles of the distal antrum. Twining's recess has been frequently associated with adult hypertrophic pyloric stenosis.

Gastric volvulus

Gastric volvulus is an unusual condition in which the stomach undergoes a torsion abnormality as a result of twisting on itself. This twisting can occur around the luminal axis of the stomach (organoaxial) or around its mesentery on a plane perpendicular to its luminal axis (mesenteroaxial). These configurations almost always occur as a result of large hiatal hernias with migration of a large amount, if not all, of the stomach into an intrathoracic location (Fig. 2-11).

Surprisingly, unless the degree of torsion is significant enough to result in luminal obstruction, these patients exhibit few symptoms. When obstruction does occur, it becomes a surgical emergency as a result of compromise of the blood supply. Patients will present with severe upper abdominal pain, severe chest pain, constant vomiting, and obstructive interference in attempts to pass a nasogastric tube.

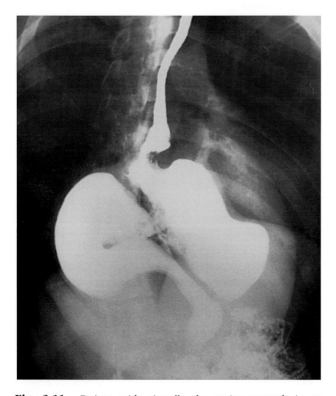

Fig. 2-11   Patient with virtually the entire stomach in an intrathoracic position. There is an organoaxial configuration, although the stomach is not obstructed at this time.

Plain films of the abdomen and chest will reveal typical findings of dilated air-filled proximal segments of the stomach either in the chest or upper abdomen. Barium studies will demonstrate the abnormal positioning of the stomach as a result of the torsion abnormality. Attempts should be made to identify the relative positions of the lesser and greater curvature.

Duodenal Obstruction Resulting in Gastric Distention

Gastric distention and impaired outflow resulting from obstructive disease in the proximal duodenum are probably more common than those resulting from primary gastric disease. The most common of the duodenal processes resulting in a gastric outlet obstruction is peptic ulcer disease. Severe pancreatitis and pseudocysts with secondary involvement of the duodenum can also result in obstruction. In addition, pancreatic malignancy commonly invades the duodenum. Primary duodenal malignancy is rare but does commonly present as obstruction with gastric distention. Other processes, such as lymphoma, duodenal adenoma, annular pancreas, superior mesenteric artery syndrome, as well as intraluminal diverticulum, can also result in obstruction. These entities are covered in more detail in the duodenal section of this chapter.

Gastric Atony without Obstruction

Neuromuscular abnormalities

In scleroderma (progressive systemic sclerosis), the entire bowel can be involved with the neuromuscular degenerative processes, resulting in diminished gut motility and subsequent stasis. As a result, it is possible for gastric distention to be observed in some of these patients. More commonly, distention of the esophagus, colon, and duodenum is encountered.

Chronic idiopathic intestinal pseudoobstruction

For similar reasons thought to relate to diffuse neuromuscular dysfunction throughout the gut, chronic idiopathic intestinal pseudoobstruction can also result in an abnormal gut motility, stasis, and distended portions of the gut. Although the small bowel and colon would predominate in this disorder, a small number of patients may manifest gastric distention as well.

Central nervous system and electrolyte abnormalities

Patients with more central neurological abnormalities, such as tabes dorsalis or bulbar poliomyelitis, may develop degrees of gastric distention.

Significant electrolyte and acid-base imbalances can commonly produce a transient distention of the colon and stomach with the impairment of contractility of the smooth muscle of the gut, probably secondary to hypokalemia.

Drug-induced atony

Gastric atony can also be drug induced and is often associated with atropine-like anticholinergic medications. Elderly and bedridden patients are particularly susceptible to drug-induced gastric atony. The use of glucagon may, on rare occasions, induce acute gastric atony. This has been reported in a few patients receiving glucagon for routine UGI examinations. Patients with diabetes mellitus and significant degrees of diabetic peripheral neuropathy may manifest prominent gastric atony as a result of diminished neuromuscular function.

Agonal atony

Acute massive gastric distention can be seen on abdominal radiographs of patients who are preterminal. The presence of this finding carries a bleak prognosis for survival beyond the next 48 hours. The exact cause of this finding is unclear. It may relate to severe and irreversible electrolyte imbalance or may be associated with major cardiovascular collapse. These patients are severely ill and almost always unconscious. Clinical findings will be limited to a distended tympanic upper abdomen. Nasogastric decompression will not alter the outcome. The radiological finding is but a reflection of the catastrophic systemic events that are occurring simultaneously.

Other considerations

Another diagnostic consideration when one is faced with the radiological finding of gastric atony is aerophagia, not an unusual occurrence in patients undergoing acute severe emotional stress. Patients who have recently ingested large amounts of carbonated drinks may demonstrate gas in a distended stomach on plain films of the abdomen. The gas, however, should also be well distributed throughout the remainder of the gut. Other considerations include porphyria and lead poisoning, both of which can result in degrees of gastric distention. In addition, degrees of gastric atony may be encountered in pregnant patients.

In patients with severe spinal deformity, chronic gastric distention has been described. The exact cause of this is not clear.

Contracted or Narrowed Stomach

A contracted narrow stomach (Box 2-4) has been historically referred to as the linitis plastica (leather bottle) stomach. This generally implies that all or a large part of the stomach is involved by the pathological process, which results in a rigid, narrowed, contracted lumen. When not all of the stomach is involved, it is the proximal portion of the stomach that is generally spared.

The problem of a contracted, narrowed stomach gives rise to the consideration of diffuse infiltrative changes in which the normal pliability and peristaltic activity of the stomach wall are impaired or absent. Any process that can excite desmoplastic or fibrotic reaction within the gastric tissues, whether it be neoplastic or inflammatory in nature, can result in such a radiological appearance.

Scirrhous carcinoma

The original description of the linitis plastica stomach was associated with an infiltrating scirrhous (desmoplastic) type of primary malignancy of the stomach. Although there are varied presentations of gastric carcinoma, the most common appears to be focal gastric wall thickening with or without ulceration. However, diffuse infiltrative wall thickening, which will result in a contracted, narrow stomach, is not uncommon and generally has been identified in patients with less-differentiated tumors and poorer prognoses (Fig. 2-12). There is also some evidence to suggest that this form may be more common in younger patients (Fig. 2-13).

The mortality rate and incidence of gastric cancer has declined steadily in the United States since 1940. Environmental factors that have been implicated in an increased incidence of gastric carcinoma in some parts of the world include an increase in salt consumption, increased ingestion of smoked meat and fish products and nitrosamines, and a questionable increase in the incidence in patients on long-term cimetidine therapy, as well as chronic *Helicobacter pylori* gastritis. Some possible precancerous situations include pernicious anemia, chronic atrophic gastritis (which may be a reflection of chronic *H. pylori* infection), gastric adenomas, and possibly long-term postgastrectomy patients.

The infiltrative form of gastric carcinoma results in diffuse thickening and rigidity of the stomach wall. The

---

Box 2-4 The Case of the Tapering Tube: The Contracted or Narrowed Stomach

Carcinoma, scirrhous type
Metastatic disease (especially breast and lung)
Chronic gastritis
Corrosive gastritis
Crohn's disease (ram's horn sign)
Zollinger-Ellison syndrome
Eosinophilic gastritis
Radiation
Sarcoidosis
Syphilis

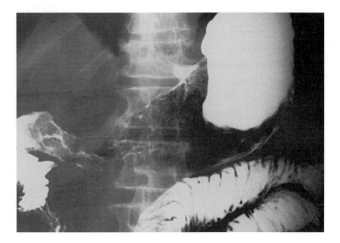

Fig. 2-12 Gastric carcinoma involving the distal half of the stomach with narrowing, irregularity, and rigidity as a result of the desmoplastic changes induced by the neoplasm.

involved stomach has a tubular appearance, and a normal fold pattern is not discernible. At fluoroscopy, no peristaltic activity can be detected in the involved area. The infiltrating process usually starts in the pyloric antral region and extends proximally. It is unusual for the tumor to cross the pyloric channel into the duodenum.

Barium studies reveal the expected narrow, tubular, rigid, aperistaltic appearance of the involved portion of the stomach. Ulcerations may be present. A fold pattern is either absent or clearly abnormal. CT is particularly helpful in evaluation of gastric carcinoma and will demonstrate extension beyond the gastric wall, involvement of the adjacent perigastric, peripancreatic, and retroperitoneal lymph nodes, in addition to aiding in the evaluation of liver metastatic lesions (Fig. 2-14).

Metastatic disease

Metastatic lesions to the stomach have a varied appearance. However, a common appearance is diffuse infiltrative scirrhous involvement of the stomach that is indistinguishable from primary scirrhous carcinoma. The two major primary sites are breast and lung.

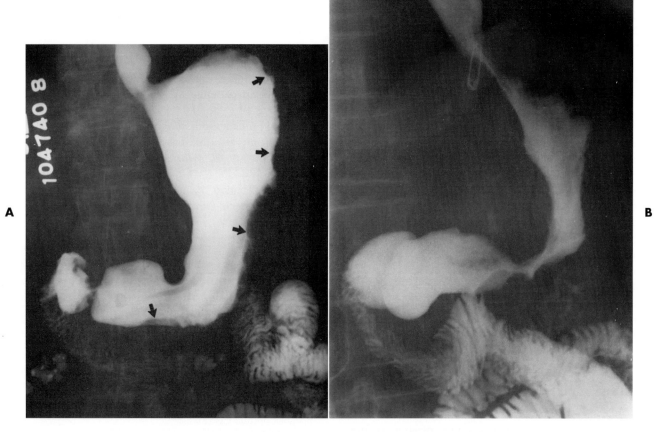

Fig. 2-13 Linitis plastica. **A,** Patient presents with abdominal pain and weight loss. UGI demonstrates irregularity and rigidity of stomach wall along greater curve *(arrows)*. Patient refused treatment. **B,** Follow-up examination 11 months later discloses progression of the disease and typical appearance of linitis plastica with narrowing and rigidity of almost the entire stomach.

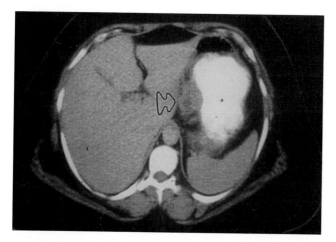

Fig. 2-14   CT image obtained at the level of the gastric cardia demonstrates mass lesion involving the posterior stomach wall, as well as an involvement of the medial wall and gastrohepatic ligament *(arrow)*.

Metastatic disease from the breast involving the stomach has been described in 10% to 15% of patients. In over half of these patients, the appearance of gastric involvement is of linitis plastica.

Involvement of the stomach by carcinoma of the pancreas as a result of contiguous spread, especially when it involves the distal stomach, can also give an appearance of a narrow, rigid antrum. These changes are usually regional and not widespread throughout the stomach, such as may be found in the primary or secondary hematogenous scirrhous lesions of the stomach.

Corrosive gastritis

Patients who ingest strong corrosive materials, such as alkaline caustic agents, tend to have more esophageal damage than stomach damage. On the other hand, the ingestion of strong acids appears to involve the stomach to a greater extent. This is particularly true in the distal antrum and along the lesser curvature. However, the antrum and body can be involved circumferentially, giving a narrowed, rigid appearance. This can be seen in both the acute and chronic stages with accompanying ulceration and mass effect. Following healing, permanent stricturing and rigidity of the distal stomach are common findings, indistinguishable from infiltrating gastric carcinoma.

Extrinsic compression of the stomach

A retrogastric or retroperitoneal process resulting in sufficient compression or invasion of the stomach to result in a narrowed or contracted stomach is unusual.

However, a large retroperitoneal tumor, such as leiomyosarcomas or liposarcomas, could result in such an appearance. In addition, significant splenomegaly associated with hepatomegaly could sufficiently com-

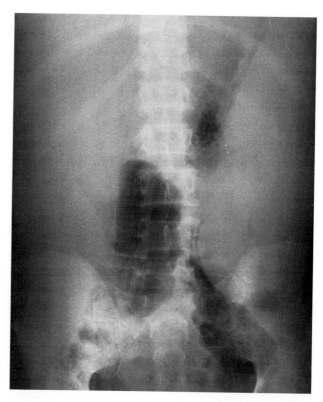

Fig. 2-15   Patient with massive hepatosplenomegaly demonstrates central compression of air-filled stomach on plain film of the abdomen.

press the stomach to give a very narrowed appearance (Fig. 2-15). A large, left upper quadrant mass, such as a subphrenic abscess, could result in a similar appearance, with the gastric spasm resulting from adjacent inflammation. A large pancreatic mass, such as a pseudocyst, can compress the stomach posteriorly and give the impression of a narrowed lumen (Fig. 2-16). Other pancreatic lesions that could result in such an appearance include nonfunctioning islet cell tumors of the pancreas, which can grow to great size, acute or chronic pancreatitis, and cystadenomas of the pancreas.

Lymphoma

Although the common appearance of lymphoma is generally wall thickening, mass effect, and ulceration, the occasional lymphomatous lesion of the stomach can be diffusely infiltrative and result in severe desmoplastic reaction, so that the radiological appearance is identical to scirrhous adenocarcinoma (Fig. 2-17). This is especially seen in the Hodgkin's-type lesion. CT evaluation for lymphoma has become the imaging mainstay for this lesion and is particularly useful for evaluation of wall thickening, perigastric nodal disease, and liver, spleen, and renal involvement (Fig. 2-18). Recently, there is some evidence that intraluminal endoscopic ultrasound may be more sensitive in detecting both intramural and perigastric disease.

Crohn's disease

Severe involvement of the stomach with Crohn's disease causing narrowing and rigidity of the stomach is unusual. The classical appearance of the narrow distal stomach and widened normal proximal stomach has given rise to the historical description of the "ram's horn" stomach of Crohn's disease. This stenotic involvement of severe disease in the distal stomach may or may not result in gastric outlet obstruction. The presence of Crohn's disease in the stomach is almost always associated with involvement of the small bowel or colon. Involvement of the stomach in patients with Crohn's disease should be differentiated from peptic ulcer disease, which has been shown to be increased in patients with Crohn's disease.

Zollinger-Ellison syndrome

Zollinger-Ellison syndrome results from the presence of a non–beta islet cell tumor of the pancreas that continuously secretes gastrin. The high levels of this hormone result in an increased stimulus of the gastric parietal cells to form and secrete hydrochloric acid, resulting in marked hyperacidity of the stomach and proximal small bowel. The severe inflammatory changes involving the stomach are usually manifest by multiple ulcerations, thickened folds, and hypersecretion. However, the presence of chronic inflammation throughout the stomach, particularly in the distal stomach, can result in a narrowed, contracted appearance. Additional radiological findings that may suggest the diagnosis include proximal small bowel ulcerations and history of recurrent intractable ulcer disease.

Up to 50% of the islet cell lesions are malignant with metastatic disease present within the liver. In addition, the primary neoplasms are generally small with 90% of them being less than 2 cm, and many of these are not detectable on routine CT scanning. In approximately 60% of cases, the lesions are multiple. The lesions may be detected on angiographic studies of the pancreaticoduodenal region as a result of their hypervascularity. For the same reason, they may be detected during the arterial phase of bolus injection of this area on CT

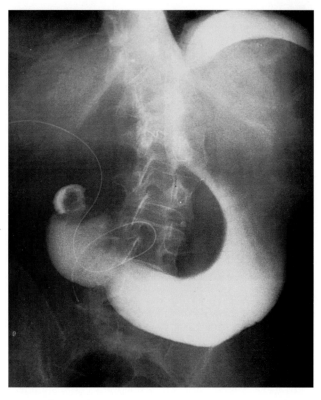

Fig. 2-16 UGI examination demonstrates large extrinsic impression on the fundus and proximal body of the stomach from huge pancreatic pseudocyst.

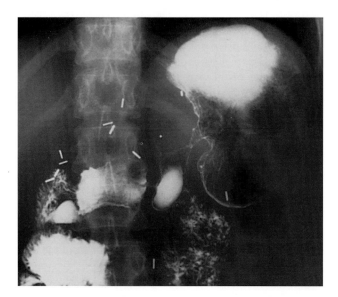

Fig. 2-17 UGI examination of patient with Hodgkin's disease of the stomach. Note the marked narrowing and irregularity of the distal stomach.

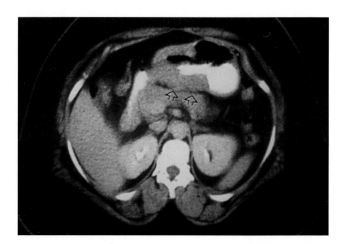

Fig. 2-18 CT image through the distal stomach demonstrates marked focal wall thickening *(arrows)* as a result of lymphomatous infiltration of the stomach.

scanning using thin (2- to 4-mm) contiguous sections through the pancreas. The procedure of choice has been to remove the entire target organ, which is represented by the parietal cell–containing portions of the stomach.

Eosinophilic gastritis

Eosinophilic infiltration of the muscular layers of the distal stomach can result in a narrowed, contracted antrum and body (Fig. 2-19). The appearance can be similar to that of malignancy. Patients usually have an associated peripheral eosinophilia and a history of food allergies. The infiltration can result in erosions, ulceration, and subsequent anemia. Affected patients may also demonstrate elevated immunoglobulin E levels. Involvement of the proximal small bowel may be present, although isolated gastric involvement is not unusual. The disorder usually responds well to daily doses of steroids.

Postradiation

A narrowed, contracted stomach may also be the sequela of radiation injury to the stomach. Radiation doses involving the stomach usually greater than 4000 rad result in an acute inflammatory response with resultant healing that may include extensive fibrosis.

Sarcoidosis

Although involvement of the gastrointestinal (GI) tract in sarcoidosis is unusual, the stomach is the most commonly affected site. Often the patients are asymptomatic. In chronic severe involvement, the possibility of contracture and narrowing of the stomach increases (Fig. 2-20).

Hepatic artery infusion chemotherapy

The increasing use of hepatic artery infusion of chemotherapeutic and cytotoxic agents has resulted in increased incidence of resultant inflammatory changes within the stomach. Despite attempts to control the flow of the chemotherapeutic agents and to reduce deleterious flow to the stomach, the vascular arterial anatomy in the region of the celiac axis can be quite variable, and on occasion some of the agent is delivered to the gastric wall with resultant marked inflammatory changes. The inflammatory changes tend to regress with the termination of the therapy.

Phlegmonous gastritis

This entity, although common in the early part of the century, is very uncommon today. It is a bacterial infection and invasion of the stomach that results in marked thickening of the stomach wall and mucosa. Most reported cases are associated with alpha-hemolytic streptococci, although other organisms, including staphylococci, pneumococci, and some of the more common

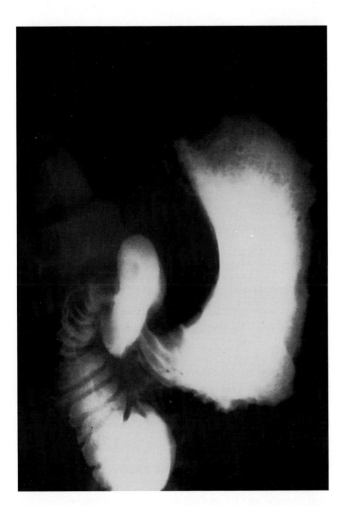

Fig. 2-19   UGI study of patient with eosinophilic gastroenteritis demonstrates a contracted and rigid stomach with some irregularity along the greater curvature. The findings could easily be interpreted as malignant infiltration.

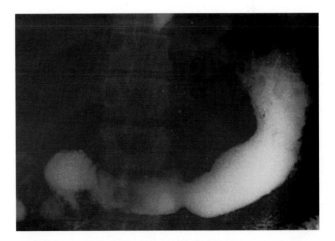

Fig. 2-20   UGI study of patient with diffuse involvement of the stomach with sarcoidosis, resulting in a tubular, narrowed stomach.

gram-negative organisms, have also been demonstrated. Often, when there is associated emphysematous gastritis, clostridial organisms or gram-negative bacteria have been implicated. The exact underlying cause of this condition is unclear, although many have been suggested, including ischemia, ulceration, gastric malignancy, and ingestion of corrosive material. The treatment consists of vigorous antibiotic therapy and prompt surgical intervention.

Tuberculosis

Involvement of the stomach with tuberculosis is rare but can occur, particularly in the pyloric antral region. Wall thickening, rigidity, and a contracted lumen may be demonstrated.

Syphilis

Involvement of the stomach with syphilis is rare, although this manifestation is seen from time to time. Involvement may be identical to that of peptic ulcer disease with erosive changes, ulceration, and thickened folds. Additionally, a contracted, narrowed, deformed stomach has been described in chronic involvement.

Thickened Gastric Folds

In the normal, adequately distended stomach, the folds in the fundal region usually measure approximately 1 cm or less in thickness. As they descend toward the body and antrum of the stomach, the folds become increasingly narrow and ribbonlike until the prepyloric antral folds are found to be 5 mm or less in diameter. The folds should be symmetrical without nodularity, focal thickening, or areas of discontinuity. The fold pattern in the region of the gastric cardia and along the greater curvature of the body can be complex and at times difficult to evaluate.

Focal thickening
Peptic gastritis

Peptic gastritis can present as widespread diffuse thickening of the gastric folds, although the much more common presentation is fold thickening in the antrum and possibly the distal body (Fig. 2-21). The folds can be nodular. There may or may not be ulceration or evidence of erosions. However, folds that are beaded in appearance generally will have small erosions along their course (Fig. 2-22). The beading process is secondary to the focal edematous changes around the erosions. These erosions may commonly be seen on double-contrast study. Meticulous attention to detail and use of flow technique will often demonstrate them.

When the involvement is throughout the stomach, some consideration should be given to Zollinger-Ellison syndrome, particularly if there is duodenal and proximal small bowel involvement (Fig. 2-23).

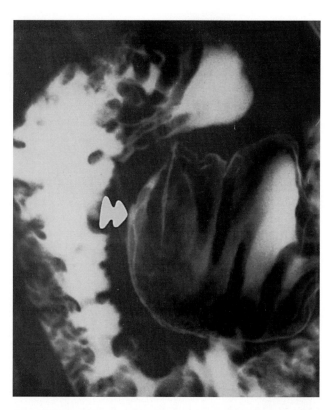

Fig. 2-21 Spot film from gastric antrum demonstrates transverse thickened gastric folds representing peptic gastritis. A tiny shallow ulcer is seen along the greater curvature *(arrow)*.

Aspirin and NSAID-induced gastritis

The increasing use of aspirin and the availability of over-the-counter nonsteroidal antiinflammatory drugs (NSAIDs) will increase the frequency of aspirin- and NSAID-induced gastritis (Fig. 2-24). These changes tend to be localized in the antral and body region, although diffuse involvement is possible. Although most of the damage caused by these drugs relates to local mucosal irritation and erosions, the process appears to be more complicated. Alterations, as a result of aspirin-induced changes in the gastric mucosal barrier, have been described along with loss of blood across the barrier unrelated to ulcer or erosion formation. There also appear to be higher incidences of peptic ulcer disease. Patients with chronic rheumatic disease taking significant doses of aspirin have a 50% increased incidence of gastric erosions and a 20% increase in gastric ulcers (Fig. 2-25). The use of enteric-coated forms of aspirin is helpful in dealing with the local and erosive effects. However, it probably has little impact on the systemic effect of the drug on the stomach wall. Aside from the emergence of *H. pylori* as the major factor in the development of gastritis and peptic ulcer disease, NSAIDs and aspirin are probably the next most important factor.

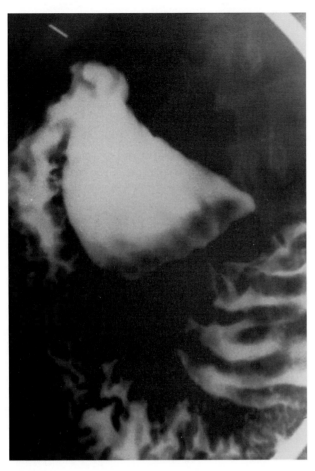

Fig. 2-22 Spot film from the gastric antrum and duodenum demonstrates thickened, beaded appearance of the folds in the gastric antrum, almost always associated with tiny erosions along the folds.

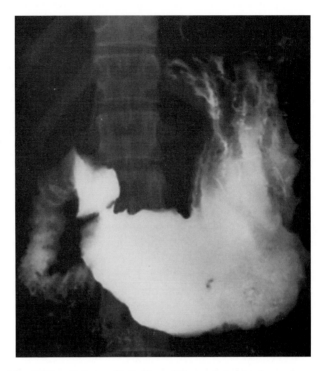

Fig. 2-23 Patient with Zollinger-Ellison syndrome shows abnormalities of the stomach on UGI study with diffuse fold thickening, hypersecretion, and multiple small ulcers.

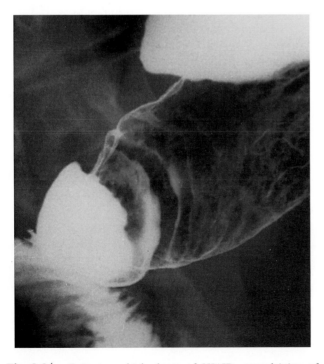

Fig. 2-24 Patient on high doses of NSAID, complaining of abdominal pain. UGI study demonstrates transverse thickened folds in the antrum of the stomach.

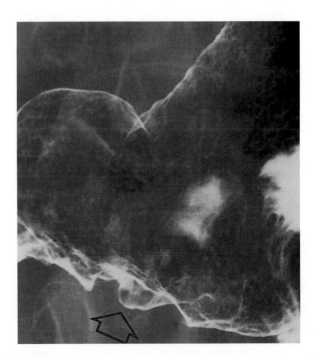

Fig. 2-25 UGI study of patient with abdominal pain and bleeding being treated with high doses of aspirin for arthritic disease. An area of mass, with irregularity and ulceration, is seen along the greater curvature of the stomach *(arrow)*. The ulcer does not project beyond the confines and is extremely suspicious. Biopsy was entirely benign. Patient improved rapidly with withdrawal of the medication.

Corrosive gastritis

Ingestion of acid-corrosive materials can give rise to focal inflammatory changes within the distal stomach. The appearance can be varied, but focal fold thickening is one manifestation. This is often associated with ulceration.

Hypertrophic gastritis

Hypertrophic gastritis is thought to represent a widening of the folds secondary to mucosal hyperplastic changes of the epithelial cells (Fig. 2-26). The etiology and prevalence of this entity is controversial, and the changes are thought to relate to chronic inflammation. It may be focal or diffuse and tends to be chronic in nature. In a patient with thickened gastric folds, possibly associated with hyperacidity and without a significant history of alcohol ingestion, hypertrophic gastritis is a differential consideration. Other types of gastritis can present with focal thickening of the fold pattern and include such things as herpetic gastritis and gastric candidiasis.

Helicobacter gastritis

In the early 1980s, researchers in Australia isolated *H. pylori* from the stomach and suggested the possibility of a relationship between the bacteria, gastritis, and peptic ulcer disease. Since then the literature has abounded with additional research regarding the role of *H. pylori* in an array of gastrointestinal diseases. It is clear that the isolation of the bacteria and the exploration of its potential role in the pathogenesis of disease have been among the most important developments in gastroenterology in the past two decades. Today there is general consensus that *H. pylori* is linked etiologically to the development of certain types of gastritis and most peptic ulcer disease. The inoculation of volunteers' stomachs with the organism and the subsequent development of mucosal inflammation, as well as the resolution of disease following the eradication of the organism, have provided fundamental scientific evidence of the etiological relationship. However, some interesting questions remain. The prevalence of the organism is widespread and can be found in the stomachs of many asymptomatic patients. In most instances there may be evidence of some mucosal inflammation, but only a small number will develop symptomatic peptic ulcer disease. Although prior to the 1980s the stomach was thought to be a sterile environment, the presence of this organism in the human stomach has been known since the early days of microbiology and bacteriology in the late nineteenth century. Moreover, in patients with the organism in the stomach, there is no evidence of bacterial proliferation or invasiveness common to most bacterial infections. Is *H. pylori* the one and only issue in peptic disease, or is it a major factor in a multifactorial pathological process?

How does the organism cause mucosal damage? Research in this area has suggested three possible mechanisms (Box 2-5):

1. Local tissue injury. The bacteria produce several toxins that may cause local mucosal damage. Among these is urea, which is the basis for the current breath test for the presence of the organism.

2. Elevated gastrin levels with resultant increased acid secretion. *H. pylori* may contribute to elevated gastrin levels by interfering with the cellular process that limits the amount of gastrin being produced. Although the research in this area has been interesting, it is presently inconclusive and contradictory, as there is also evidence that *H. pylori* decreases gastric acid.

3. Focal mucosal immune response. *H. pylori* appears to recruit white blood cells (WBCs) to the mucosa, possibly resulting in the inflammatory response.

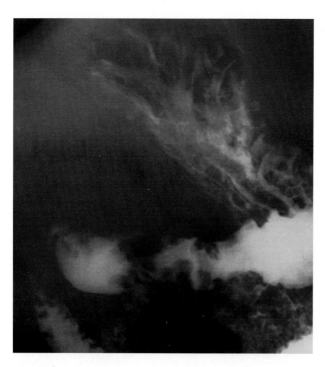

Fig. 2-26 UGI study of patient with history of chronic abdominal pain demonstrating diffuse fold thickening throughout the stomach. Biopsy showed epithelial hyperplastic changes of hypertrophic gastritis.

Box 2-5 H. Pylori: Theories on Mechanisms of Mucosal Tissue Damage

May cause focal tissue injury due to bacteria-produced toxins.

May cause elevated gastric levels and resultant increase acid secretion.

May cause local mucosal inflammation by increasing presence of white blood cells focally.

It should also be noted that *H. pylori* has been implicated in more than peptic inflammatory disease. It is now considered an important risk factor in the development of gastric carcinoma. The organism is frequently seen with gastric carcinoma and is most prevalent in those geographical locations and ethnic groups that have known high incidences of gastric carcinoma. Some have suggested that harboring the bacteria in the upper gut from an early age is an important factor in determining risk for malignancy. Indeed, the World Health Organization has designated *H. pylori* as a Class 1 carcinogen.

H. pylori has also been determined to be the cause of the rare low-grade gastric mucosa-associated lymphoid tissue (MALT) lymphoma. It has been reported that the eradication of the bacteria alone without any other treatments can lead to regression of the gastric MALT lymphoma in the majority of patients.

H. pylori can be diagnosed by a variety of means, of which the gold standard is considered to be endoscopic biopsy of the stomach. This can be achieved either by staging the specimen with Giemsa, silver, or Genta stains to demonstrate the organism or by "rapid urease tests," which indicate the presence of the bacteria through color change when exposed to the biopsy specimen. The diagnosis can also the made through serological testing or the urea breath test. The latter is about 95% sensitive and can be read in 10 to 30 minutes. What is the role of radiology in the diagnosis of *H. pylori* gastritis or ulcer disease? On the surface the UGI, even the high-quality double-contrast technique, appears to offer little and is of no value with respect to the presence or absence of the bacteria. However, in the ever-accelerating era of cost containment and capitated health care, the UGI examination may actually make a significant contribution to the diagnosis and treatment of *H. pylori* disease of the stomach and duodenum. As mentioned above, the UGI cannot detect the presence of the bacteria, but if quality double-contrast work is undertaken, it is very good in detecting gastritis, both erosive and nonerosive. Enlarged gastric folds or nodular folds are a common finding on the double-contrast UGI examination. Although these findings cannot establish the absence or presence of *H. pylori,* the bacteria have been found in approximately 50% of patients with enlarged folds. This provides the radiological examination a place in a diagnostic algorithm that can provide effective diagnosis and treatment of *H. pylori* infection of the stomach in a less costly and less invasive manner than an endoscopic survey on potential multitudes of patients. Thickened or nodular folds in the gastric antrum appear to be the best indicators of the possible presence of *H. pylori.* In such patients, without symptoms or signs that might suggest malignancy, a test for *H. pylori* can be undertaken. If positive, eradication therapy can be commenced and a repeat UGI may be undertaken to assess for change. If folds have returned to normal, no further workup or treatment is indicated. If folds remain enlarged or are increasing in size, the patient undergoes endoscopy. In such an algorithm much refinement is possible. Nevertheless, the potential exists for considerable savings. The very low risk of carcinoma and its decline with the eradication of the bacteria have not resulted in the need for widespread endoscopic screening. Unless double-contrast UGI examinations are of consistently high quality, however, the resurgence of the radiological examination as an important factor in the workup of *H. pylori* will not occur. It may happen only sporadically in areas where GI radiology is practiced with consistent excellence. The radiological community would be well advised to note the exceptional opportunity and act accordingly.

The most widely utilized treatment for the eradication of *H. pylori* consists of a bismuth-based triple therapy. This usually consists of a 2-week course of colloidal bismuth, metronidazole, and tetracycline or amoxicillin and cessation of NSAIDs if possible.

Carcinoma

Irregular focal thickening is an unusual presentation of carcinoma of the stomach (Fig. 2-27). The most common presentation tends to be a mass with ulceration. However, thickened irregular folds, usually limited to one portion of the stomach and indistinguishable from gastric lymphoma, are not a rare finding in gastric carcinoma (Fig. 2-28).

Lymphoma

The most common presentation of lymphoma is a thickened, distorted, nodular gastric fold pattern (Fig. 2-29). This may or may not be associated with a mass effect or ulceration. There may be a degree of residual

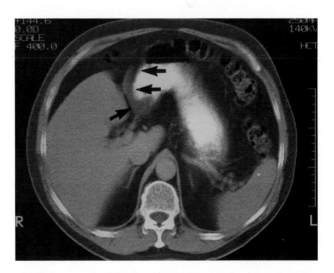

Fig. 2-27   Patient with weight loss and decreased appetite. CT of upper abdomen demonstrates focal wall thickening along the greater curvature of the distal stomach *(arrows)*. Biopsy showed adenocarcinoma of the stomach.

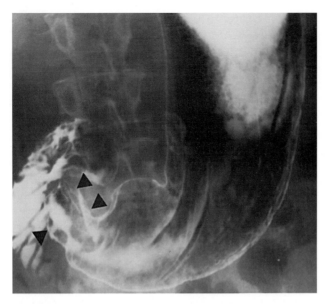

Fig. 2-28 UGI study of patient with abdominal pain and weight loss demonstrates some slight narrowing of the distal stomach with thickened nodular folds through the area *(arrowheads)*. Biopsy confirmed the diagnosis of gastric carcinoma.

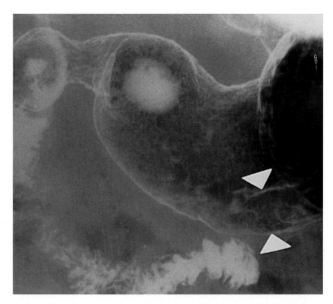

Fig. 2-30 UGI examination of patient with history of breast cancer. There are chronic changes seen in the distal stomach. However, there is an area of focal fold thickening and nodularity *(arrowheads)* that proved to be a focal metastatic lesion.

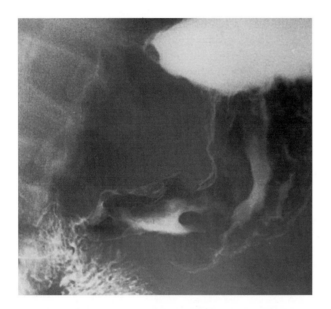

Fig. 2-29 Patient with diffuse lymphomatous involvement of the stomach demonstrates marked thickening and nodularity and distortion of the folds throughout the distal two thirds of the stomach.

distensibility and pliability that may help distinguish lymphoma from carcinoma. However, the definitive diagnosis will require biopsy. Extension across the pyloric channel into the duodenal bulb tends to be more common with lymphoma than carcinoma, although one should bear in mind that lymphoma represents 5% or less of gastric malignancies. Thus, in actuality, most lesions

that cross that pylorus are adenocarcinomas. Associated findings that may be seen with lymphoma include extrinsic masses associated with aggregates of lymphomatous nodes or an enlarged spleen.

Pseudolymphoma

Lymphoreticular hyperplasia of the stomach (pseudolymphoma or lymphoreticular gastritis) can present with findings of focal fold thickening. These benign lesions almost always have the radiological appearance of malignancy with most common findings being mass and ulceration. However, cases of infiltrative lesions with associated focal fold thickening have been reported. Anemia is a common finding, and the average age is slightly younger than that seen in gastric carcinoma.

Metastatic disease

Metastatic disease presenting with focal fold thickening is unusual but does occur (Fig. 2-30). This may be seen in the early metastatic involvement of the stomach with breast or lung lesions. Leukemic involvement of the stomach may result in a focal or diffuse thickening of gastric folds. Direct contiguous spread of carcinoma of the pancreas to the stomach can also produce a radiological pattern of focal gastric fold thickening along the greater curvature.

Crohn's disease

Crohn's involvement of the stomach may manifest in fold thickening in the antral region. Superficial erosions may also be detected.

Pancreatitis

A relatively common cause of fold thickening within the distal stomach relates to inflammatory disease in the

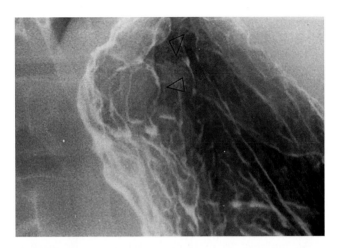

Fig. 2-31 Patient with gastric varices demonstrates area of focal fold thickening and nodularity. Note the smooth mucosal surface over the affected area *(arrowheads)*.

adjacent pancreas. Folds along the greater curvature of the body and in the antrum may be enlarged and nodular, as a result of contiguous inflammatory changes. More severe disease may result in more widespread gastric changes.

Ménétrier's disease

Ménétrier's disease is a relatively rare condition of unknown etiology. It is characterized by prominence and tortuosity of the gastric mucosal fold pattern. At one time, this was thought to be an antral sparing process, although recently degrees of antral involvement have been demonstrated. The preponderance of changes, however, appears to be in the proximal stomach. The process is associated with increased protein loss from the stomach and diminished gastric acid production. The disease is generally detected between 30 to 60 years of age and tends to be more common in men. Presenting complaints include epigastric pain, anorexia, and weight loss. The radiological pattern demonstrates a large tortuous fold pattern predominantly proximally and, in most cases, with sparing of the antrum. There will also be some evidence of hypersecretion within the stomach.

Gastric varices

Gastric varices can readily cause apparent thickening of the gastric folds, particularly in the proximal fundal region of the stomach (Fig. 2-31). These are commonly seen in association with significant portal hypertension and in patients with splenic vein thrombosis. The radiological findings usually are those of a smooth, thickened, proximal fold pattern most prominent in the fundus, but they can be seen more distally. Esophageal varices can be demonstrated by increasing the venous distention of the varices through various techniques associated with patient positioning and respiration.

These techniques tend to be less useful in gastric varices, and this is particularly the case in those patients with splenic vein thrombosis.

Eosinophilic gastritis

The stomach is commonly involved in this relatively rare disorder. The predilection appears to be for the gastric antrum, although the entire stomach may be involved. The disease results in eosinophilic infiltrates of the mucosal and muscular layers of the stomach. Radiological manifestations are generally those of thickened rugal fold pattern predominantly distally. Clinical features are nonspecific, and the patients may present with early satiety, nausea, or vomiting. Involvement of the small bowel is helpful in making the diagnosis, and thickened folds will be demonstrated in the proximal small bowel wall. However, isolated gastric involvement is relatively common. In patients with thickened gastric folds, small bowel involvement, peripheral eosinophilia, abdominal pain, history of food allergies, and no evidence of parasitic GI infestation, the diagnosis of eosinophilic gastritis should be considered.

Partial gastrectomy

In patients with long-term gastric resection, particularly Billroth II procedure, the presence of thickened folds within the gastric remnant is common. The exact etiology of this is unclear. It is believed by some to represent the sequela of chronic bile reflux. The long-term significance is also not absolutely clear. Whether this predisposes these individuals to a "stump carcinoma" of the gastric remnant is uncertain.

Diffuse thickening

Box 2-6 summarizes the causes of diffuse gastric fold thickening.

Gastritis

Virtually all forms of gastritis, including hypertrophic gastritis and phlegmonous gastritis, can diffusely involve the entire stomach. Alcoholic gastritis, although occasionally manifesting as a regional gastritis, most commonly is diffuse in its presentation.

Pancreatitis

Occasionally, with severe involvement of the length of the pancreas, the secondary inflammatory changes involving the adjacent stomach may involve the entire length of the stomach.

Eosinophilic gastritis

Although involvement of the stomach with eosinophilic gastritis is often limited to the antrum, all parts of the stomach may be involved.

Ménétrier's disease

Although Ménétrier's disease is more commonly seen involving the proximal stomach, it can also involve the entire stomach, giving a diffusely thickened rugal fold pattern throughout.

Amyloidosis

GI involvement by amyloid is not uncommon, although involvement of the stomach appears to be rare. Diffuse infiltrative changes may be present throughout the stomach with resultant thickening of the rugal fold pattern. This probably represents the most well-known presentation of gastric amyloid. Other presentations include focal changes, such as mass and ulceration. Involvement of the stomach with amyloid can be either a result of primary systemic amyloidosis, secondary amyloidosis, or even isolated amyloid deposition.

The secondary type of amyloidosis is associated with some chronic underlying disease that predisposes to amyloid formation and deposition in tissues. The most common antecedent diseases include rheumatoid arthritis, tuberculosis, bronchiectasis, and chronic lung disease. The site of amyloid involvement is usually the reticuloendothelial system. Primary systemic amyloid is a condition in which no underlying disease is thought to be present. The GI system involvement with amyloid is more commonly seen with the primary systemic type. Isolated amyloid deposition, sometimes referred to as amyloid tumor, involves a single site or organ. This is probably a variant of the primary type. A fourth type of amyloidosis that should be considered and in which gastric involvement is probably extremely unusual would be amyloid formation associated with multiple myeloma.

Diminished Gastric Folds

Normal aging

The problem of diminished gastric folds continues to be a radiological dilemma. Correlation between diminished fold pattern, as seen on the UGI study and endoscopy, and histological biopsy is often poor.

In many patients a diminished fold pattern will be apparent, which will primarily involve the fundus and, to a lesser degree, the body and antrum. It is often seen in older patients, and in a majority of cases, it represents normal aging processes. Various population studies have suggested that mild to moderate atrophy and associated fold diminution are seen in patients over 50 years of age. It has been suggested that 50% of patients over age 50 will show some degree of these changes within the stomach. Histologically, this is found to be a mild superficial and atrophic type of gastritis, with the atrophic component increasing with age. There is often accompanying intestinal metaplasia, which also appears to be age-dependent. The relationship of these findings with *H. pylori* gastritis remains to be elucidated.

These findings of diminution of fold pattern may be accompanied by prominence in the areae gastricae pattern, but these findings are controversial and not well understood. The radiologist should not presume serious disease or increased risk of malignancy on the basis of these findings. In most cases, where the stomach is otherwise normal, a simple descriptive phrase, such as "the stomach has a mild atrophic appearance with some diminution of the fold pattern," will suffice. Diagnosis of atrophic gastritis should be avoided unless the stomach is totally devoid of folds.

Partial gastrectomy

After partial gastrectomy, the development of gastritis is inevitable. Widened folds may be evident in most postgastrectomy patients. On the other hand, a diminished or absent fold pattern may also be seen in a smaller number of postgastrectomy patients. In some of these patients, no folds will be discernible. These changes are more marked in the Billroth II type of anastomosis. The etiology of these types of gastritis is unclear. The same bile or alkaline reflux gastritis suggested for prominent gastric folds has also been offered as an etiology for the atrophic appearance of the gastric remnant as well. The long-term sequela of this type of gastritis is also uncertain. The increased incidence of postgastrectomy "stump carcinoma" has been documented in the literature, but the association is not without some controversy. It is not clear what, if any, role chronic gastritis of the gastric remnant plays in the development of carcinoma in the gastric remnant 10 to 25 years following surgery. Nor is it clear if manifestations of atrophic changes in the gastric stump or prominent gastric folds in the residual stomach indicate an increased risk in these patients (Fig. 2-32).

Gastric ulcers

Gastric ulcers, particularly of chronic variety, tend to be associated with diminished fold pattern throughout the stomach and particularly in the antrum. Histologically, it is often atrophic superficial gastritis with intestinal metaplasia commonly accompanying the atrophic changes.

Pernicious anemia

Addisonian pernicious anemia is a serious hematological condition that is characterized by a megaloblastic type of anemia and near absolute achlorhydria. The Schilling test demonstrates the impaired absorption of vitamin B_{12} from the gut and is a result of the diminished ability to secrete intrinsic factor. The stomach will demonstrate severe fundal atrophy, giving rise to the "bald fundus." The remainder of the stomach will demonstrate diminished or complete absence of a fold pattern (Fig. 2-33). The stomach will remain distensible and pliable at fluoroscopy. Peristaltic activity is diminished but not absent. Histological examination will demonstrate severe mucosal atrophy, gastritis, and intestinal metaplasia. It is not unusual to see inflammatory changes within the antrum, in which case thickened folds, possibly erosions, may be encountered in a patient who otherwise presents with an absence of fold pattern throughout the remainder of the stomach.

Gastric cancer

Cancers found in the gastric antrum and body are often associated with extensive changes of fundal atrophic gastritis and prominent intestinal metaplastic changes. This association is of questionable significance in that the intestinal metaplastic changes have been shown to be present in the aging population and the degree and severity appear to correlate directly with age. However, the increased risk of gastric carcinoma in

patients with the atrophic changes of the stomach, secondary to pernicious anemia, are well known. It has been estimated that such patients have three times the risk of developing gastric cancer than the normal population. A patient with severe atrophic changes throughout the stomach and an absolute absence of gastric fold pattern presents something of a dilemma to the radiologist. Although both the supporting and disputing evidence are controversial, such patients should probably be considered at higher risk for the development of gastric carcinoma and referred for endoscopic evaluation and sample biopsy of various portions of the stomach.

Extrinsic Masses

A number of possible perigastric processes can result in an extrinsic compression defect on the stomach. The most common of these is simply an enlarged liver, particularly the left lobe. Splenomegaly can also result in a significant impression. Other processes, particularly those arising from the pancreas, such as tumors, pseudocysts, and other forms of pancreatic cystic disease, also result in gastric impression. Large retroperitoneal, retrogastric lymph node masses, as well as hematomas or abscesses, can give a picture of a posterior wall

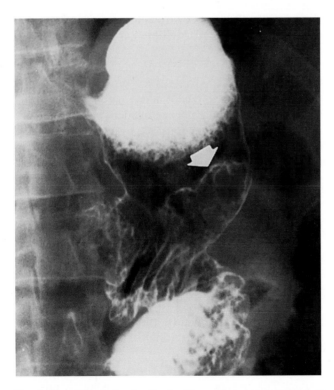

Fig. 2-32 UGI study of patient with previous gastric Billroth II resection. The gastric stump is devoid of folds. An area of focal nodularity and elevated mucosa is seen just above the anastomosis *(arrow)* that proved to be carcinoma of the gastric stump.

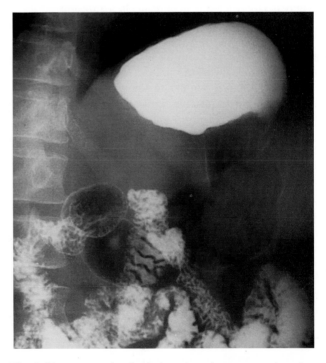

Fig. 2-33 UGI study of elderly patient demonstrates complete absence of gastric folds, giving the stomach a marked atrophic appearance.

impression on the stomach. Occasionally, a marked aortic aneurysm impresses the stomach, and neoplastic lesions arising from the region of the splenic flexure of the colon can result in gastric impression. Huge renal or adrenal masses can also displace the stomach.

Small Solitary Masses (<2 cm)

Gastric polyps

Solitary gastric polyps are not common. Varied studies have put the incidence between 0.6% and 3%. Benign spindle cell tumors are the most common type of neoplastic polyps seen in this category, with leiomyomas the most frequent lesions seen. However, lipomas, hemangiomas, and neurofibromas do occur. These lesions tend to be small and solitary. They can, on occasion, grow to large size and commonly undergo surface ulceration. However, autopsy studies have suggested that the incidence of multiple leiomyomas of the stomach may be higher than previously believed. A leiomyoma originates in the smooth muscle of the stomach wall and apparently can remain for a prolonged period of time as a small intramural submucosal process. If enlargement does occur, it may grow toward the gastric lumen or toward the serosal side of the bowel wall and develop as an exophytic lesion. Most leiomyomas tend to occur in the proximal part of the stomach.

In general, it has been a clinical assumption that leiomyomas less than 2 cm tend to be asymptomatic, whereas larger lesions may result in symptoms.

Lipomas of the stomach are rare and generally small and asymptomatic. When they do become symptomatic, it is almost always a result of GI bleeding. These usually occur in the distal stomach.

Glomus tumors, similar to leiomyomas in histology, although more commonly found in other sites, such as skin, can also occur in the stomach. The usual reported site is in the distal stomach and the most common manifestation is GI bleeding.

Ectopic pancreas

These lesions are most commonly encountered within the stomach, with the next most common site being the duodenum. However, polypoid lesions representing ectopic pancreatic rests have been described from the esophagus to the ileum.

The incidence is variable, ranging from 1% to 14% in autopsy series. It appears to be more common than other benign polypoid conditions of the stomach, including leiomyoma.

Radiographically, these polypoid lesions are usually less than 2 cm in size and generally located in the distal prepyloric antral region of the stomach. The surface of the lesion may be smooth or slightly lobulated. There may be a central depression or umbilication representing

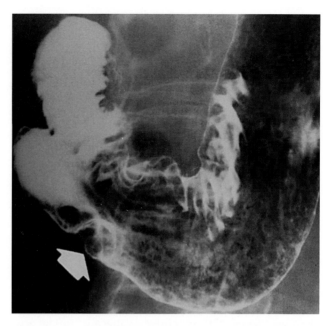

Fig. 2-34 Marginal polypoid lesion is seen along the greater curvature of the antrum *(arrow)*. Endoscopic evaluation and biopsy showed this to be ectopic pancreatic tissue.

a rudimentary duct opening in approximately 50% of the cases (Fig. 2-34).

Most of these lesions are discovered incidentally in patients with nonspecific or vague GI complaints. Occasionally, the surface of the ectopic pancreatic rests may ulcerate and bleed. Multiple gastric pancreatic rests are uncommon.

Adenomas

Unlike the colon, where adenomatous polyp formation is common, the presence of adenomas in the stomach is unusual. Adenomatous polyps in the stomach also appear to be more predisposed to malignant degeneration. Like colonic adenomas, the potential for malignant degeneration increases with size. Although generally uncommon, adenomatous polyps are more common in stomachs that contain gastric carcinoma. The incidence has been reported to be near 60%.

Most of these lesions are sessile, although pedunculated polyps may be seen (Fig. 2-35). The most common site appears to be in the distal stomach. Tubular adenomas, which are the most common adenomas in the colon, tend to be the least common of the gastric adenomas. More frequently, the more dangerous varieties, such as villous or tubulovillous adenomas, are encountered.

Solitary polyps are more common than multiple lesions. The presence of multiple lesions should raise the question of one of the polyposis syndromes.

The radiological appearance is usually that of a mucosal lesion. It may be smooth or villous in its

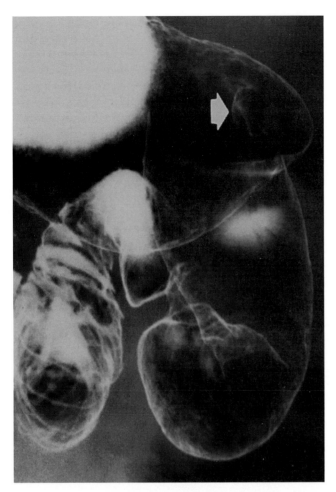

Fig. 2-35   A smooth, polypoid lesion *(arrow)* is seen on the anterior wall of the stomach at the junction of the body and antrum. Endoscopy showed it to be a gastric adenoma.

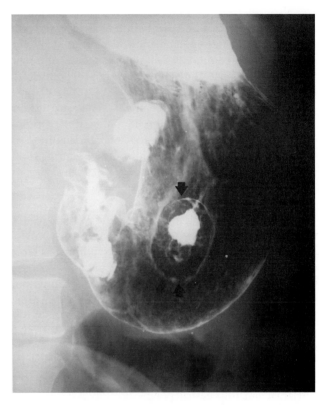

Fig. 2-36   Gastric metastatic lesion. A rounded, well-defined gastric mass *(arrows)* with a central barium collection proved to be a metastatic lesion from the breast.

appearance. Ulceration can occur. Most solitary adenomas are incidental findings, and the vast majority of the lesions are less than 2 cm.

Metastatic lesions

Metastatic lesions to the stomach resulting in solitary, small filling defects are not common but do occur. Metastatic melanoma is probably the most frequently encountered lesion and can on occasion present as a single, small filling defect with typical surface ulceration and "bull's-eye" appearance. Solitary, small lesions secondary to metastatic spread of breast or lung lesions may be seen rarely (Fig. 2-36).

Inflammatory fibroid polyps

These nonadenomatous polyps are characterized by an arrangement of fibrous and connective tissues infiltrated with sheets of eosinophils. These lesions are also known as eosinophilic granulomas. The lesions apparently are unrelated to eosinophilic gastroenteritis. There

is no history of food allergies nor is there peripheral eosinophilia. The lesion is usually solitary and less than 2 cm in size. It has no distinctive appearance radiologically and is seen as a smooth, sessile polypoid filling defect in the distal stomach (Fig. 2-37). Patients are usually asymptomatic, and these lesions are rarely associated with any significant symptoms. The possibility of erosions on the surface of the lesion and subsequent bleeding does exist.

Carcinoids

These lesions usually do not involve the stomach and are seen in this organ in fewer than 3% of cases. They may be seen as small mucosal polypoid lesions in the antrum, often solitary. A more common appearance is that of a larger fungating lesion involving the antral portion of the stomach, which may be radiologically indistinguishable from an ulcerating carcinoma. Approximately 25% of gastric carcinoids will have associated metastatic disease.

Multiple Small Masses

Hyperplastic polyps

The hyperplastic polyp is the most common cause of small polypoid filling defects within the stomach. They are also referred to as regenerative and sometimes inflammatory polyps and are believed to represent the sequelae of chronic inflammation. They are small and sessile and are commonly multiple in nature, although they can be solitary. They tend to be seen predominantly in the antral region (Fig. 2-38).

The hyperplastic polyp is not a neoplastic lesion. Malignant degeneration is virtually unheard of. Despite this, there is a well-documented increase in the incidence of coexisting hyperplastic polyps found in stomachs harboring gastric carcinoma.

Adenomas

The finding of multiple gastric adenomas not related to one of the polyposis syndromes is rare. Gastric polyps are reported in most of polyposis syndromes. More commonly they are seen in familial polyposis coli and Gardner's syndrome. Although these adenomatous polyps have a high malignant potential within the colon, malignant degeneration of adenomatous gastric polyps in patients with either Gardner's or familial polyposis syndrome is exceedingly rare.

Hamartomas

Hamartomatous gastric polyps develop in the stomach almost exclusively in patients with Peutz-Jeghers or Cronkhite-Canada syndromes. They are multiple, generally small, and seen in conjunction with the more common presentation of small bowel polyps and mucocutaneous pigmentation changes. There is relatively little malignant potential related to hamartoma formation. Although a slight increase in small bowel cancer has been reported in patients with Peutz-Jeghers syndrome, there is no known increase in gastric cancer.

Multiple hamartoma syndrome (Cowden's disease) is a rare condition manifested by hamartomatous polyps within the stomach and elsewhere within the GI tract, along with associated thyroid and breast lesions. The GI polyps are almost always hamartomatous, although simple hyperplastic polyps have been reported.

Hemangiomas

Rarely, multiple hemangiomas are seen within the stomach, occasionally associated with typical calcification. The blue rubber bleb nevus syndrome (Bean syndrome) is rare. This is inherited as a sporadic, autosomal-dominant trait in some families. It is mani-

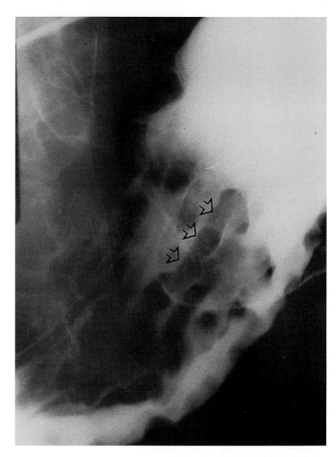

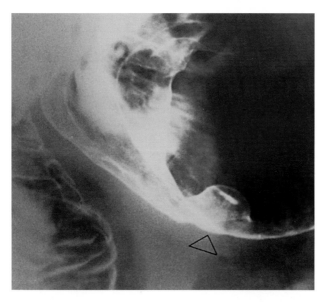

Fig. 2-37 A patient with a solitary eosinophilic granuloma of the stomach *(arrowhead)* located along the greater curvature of the antrum. The lesion is smooth and mucosal in appearance. A small, linear ulceration is seen on the surface.

Fig. 2-38 UGI study demonstrates numerous, rounded filling defects throughout the body and antrum of the stomach *(arrows)* that on endoscopic evaluation proved to be multiple hyperplastic polyps.

fested by mucosal hemangiomas, mostly reported in the stomach and associated with GI bleeding. These are always seen as multiple, small filling defects.

Peptic erosions

Multiple, small filling defects may be identified in patients with multiple gastric erosions. This finding relates to the edematous raised mucosa around the site of the punctate ulceration (Fig. 2-39). On single-contrast examination, these may appear as multiple, small filling defects predominantly in the distal stomach. Good quality double-contrast examination will almost always demonstrate the punctate ulceration present in the center of the filling defect. Quite often these erosions line up on the folds of the body and antrum of the stomach.

Candidiasis

With the increasing pool of immunocompromised patients in the health care system today, there is an increasing incidence of gastric candidiasis. This may present, as in the esophagus, with multiple, rounded filling defects throughout the stomach, which if untreated, can go on to the ulcerative hemorrhagic stage commonly seen in the esophagus.

Large Solitary Masses

Adenomas

Solitary gastric adenomas greater than 2 cm are extremely uncommon but do occur and carry a high risk of malignancy. Larger adenomatous polyps within the

stomach have more likelihood of being pedunculated (e.g., on a stalk).

Stromal cell tumors (leiomyomas)

Although multiple leiomyomas (now called stromal cell tumors) of the stomach have been reported, the solitary lesion is more common. These lesions can be quite large and the patients are often asymptomatic (Fig. 2-40). Occasionally, stromal cell tumors can continue to grow within the gastric wall and reach sizable proportions. The stromal cell tumor greater than 5 cm in diameter is quite likely to be a malignant stromal cell tumor (leiomyosarcoma). These tumors often outgrow their blood supply and undergo central necrosis, often leading to large barium-filled cavities within the tumor mass (Fig. 2-41). The ulcerations are usually centrally located in the tumor mass. Although stromal cell tumors appear to have a predilection for the proximal stomach, they have been described throughout the stomach. These tumors carry a relatively good prognosis, and distal metastasis is rare. Direct extension to the adjacent spleen, liver, and pancreas does occur. Lymph node spread is unusual. Symptoms are produced usually when the lesions are quite large, and patients most commonly present with bleeding. Occasionally, obstruction or even perforation may be presenting features.

Because of the tendency for these lesions to grow in an exophytic manner, CT is helpful in identifying the limits of the tumor mass. Barium studies may demonstrate wall abnormalities and may possibly be evidence of extrinsic mass relating to the exophytic component of the lesion (Fig. 2-42).

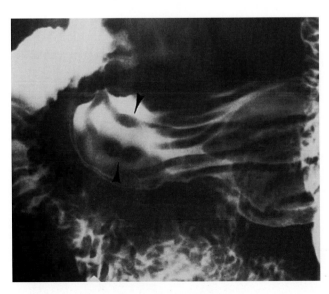

Fig. 2-39   Focal swelling and beaded appearance *(arrowheads)* are demonstrated in the distal stomach of this patient as a result of tiny superficial erosions and the associated edema surrounding each erosion.

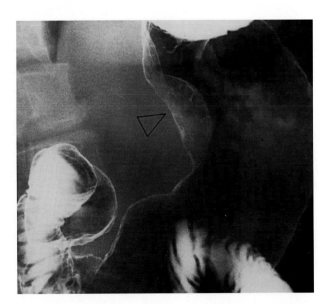

Fig. 2-40   Large, smooth submucosal mass *(arrowhead)* is seen arising from the lesser curvature of the body of the stomach. This represents a large gastric stromal cell tumor (leiomyoma).

Metastatic lesions

Again, the usual presentation of metastatic lesions is multiple polypoid or infiltrative lesions within the stomach. Occasionally, a larger, isolated metastatic lesion will be encountered. This is most likely to occur in metastatic melanoma (Fig. 2-43).

Duplication cysts

Gastric duplications are rare and may present in various sizes and configurations. A solitary filling defect

within the stomach, usually along the greater curvature, is one presentation. Alternatively, the cyst may communicate with the lumen and present as a large diverticulum-like barium collection along the margin of the stomach.

Polypoid carcinomas

Approximately a quarter of gastric carcinomas present as polypoid mass lesions growing into the gastric lumen. These polypoid lesions may or may not be ulcerated on their surface (Fig. 2-44). In addition, there may be an adjacent spread along the wall. It is thought that about a third of all malignant gastric carcinomas will manifest all of the characteristics of polypoid, ulcerative, and infiltrating types.

Discrete isolated polypoid lesions tend to carry the best prognosis. The most common sites tend to be in the distal portion of the stomach, although in patients with gastric atrophy, proximal regions are more involved.

Jejunal gastric intussusception

This complication is occasionally encountered after the Billroth II partial gastrectomy. Intussusceptive changes occur within the adjacent jejunum, and retrograde progression of the intussusception results in a large filling defect within the gastric remnant. This has a typical radiographic appearance on barium studies of a large intragastric mass with evidence of a fold pattern within it that may or may not have the typical "coil spring" appearance. There is usually a significant degree of obstruction to the distal flow of barium.

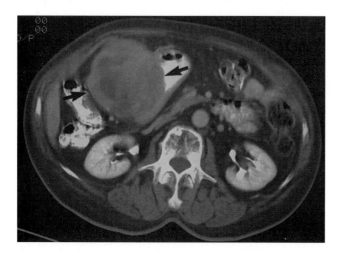

Fig. 2-41 Malignant stromal cell tumor of the distal stomach. CT shows a large lesion arising from distal stomach *(arrows)* composed of mixed density with tissue necrosis within tumor.

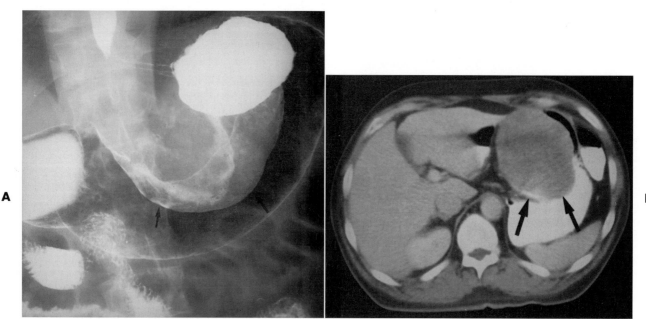

A

B

Fig. 2-42 Malignant stromal cell tumor. **A,** UGI examination demonstrates huge gastric mass arising from lesser curve *(arrows)*. Note smooth mucosal surface over mass. **B,** CT scan shows large soft tissue mass (arrows) with significant exophytic component.

Gastric bezoars

Small, asymptomatic bezoars can be seen as a filling defect within the stomach. These are usually less than 2 cm and mobile.

Multiple Large Masses

Metastatic disease

As already suggested, metastatic disease to the stomach can be eclectic in appearance. Multiple, large nodular lesions can be seen in metastatic melanoma. On occasion, metastatic lesions arising from breast and lung lesions may present in such a fashion. Quite often these types of metastatic lesions are sharply circumscribed and have the typical "bull's-eye" or "target lesion" appearance when associated with central ulceration. The lesions, particularly melanoma, may remain silent for some time and increase in size. Bleeding will usually be the first manifestation of gastric involvement.

Stromal cell tumors (leiomyomas)

Stromal cell tumors can, on rare occasion, occur in the stomach as multiple, large submucosal masses. These lesions can grow to large sizes, and the patient can be entirely asymptomatic. The usual presentation is bleeding associated with ulceration on the surface of one of the stromal cell tumors.

Neurogenic tumors

Neurofibromas occur as isolated tumors of the stomach. However, they can be multiple, and in a patient with generalized neurofibromatosis, there may be involvement of the stomach with multiple neurofibromata. Apart from the possibility of ulceration and bleeding, these are generally asymptomatic.

Kaposi's sarcoma

Kaposi's sarcoma is a vascular endothelial tumor that was described approximately 100 years ago. There has been significant resurgence in the incidence with the advent of the acquired immunodeficiency syndrome (AIDS) epidemic. Involvement of the GI tract is common and probably the most frequent site of involvement after the skin. It is estimated that 40% to 50% of patients with Kaposi's sarcoma lesions of the skin have GI involvement. Nearly any level of the GI tract may be involved, from the pharynx to the rectum, although most are in the upper tract. The GI lesions are almost always seen in homosexual males. Gastric involvement can be either diffuse or in the form of large discrete nodules (Fig. 2-45). The nodules may or may not have central ulceration. CT is helpful in defining the extent of wall involvement and the presence or absence of perigastric disease. The lesions themselves are generally asymptomatic, although they can bleed.

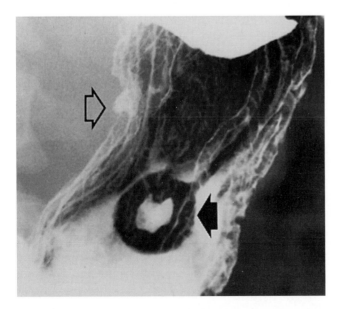

Fig. 2-43 UGI study of patient with known lung cancer in which at least two bull's-eye metastatic lesions to the stomach are demonstrated. The classic appearance of a mass with an ulcerated, barium-filled center is seen en face *(closed arrow)*, whereas the same type of lesion is seen profiled *(open arrow)*.

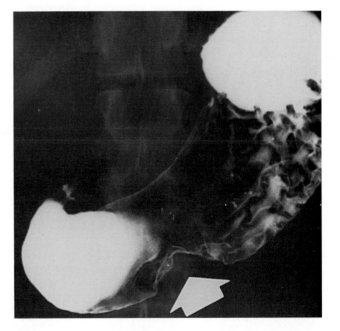

Fig. 2-44 A polypoid carcinoma is seen arising from the greater curvature of the stomach at the junction of the antrum and body *(arrow)*.

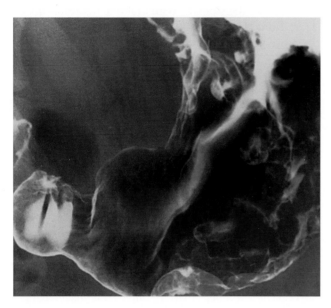

Fig. 2-45   Patient with Kaposi's sarcoma of the stomach demonstrates numerous rounded, ulcerated masses of the stomach.

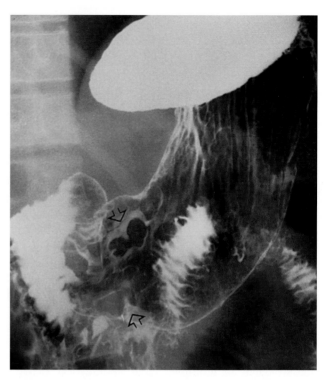

Fig. 2-46   Lymphoma of the stomach presenting as multiple polypoid lesions in the antrum *(arrows)*.

Lymphoma

Primary lymphoma of the stomach is much less common than adenocarcinoma and accounts for about 5% of malignant lesions of the stomach. As with gastric adenocarcinoma, the patients may present with nonspecific complaints of abdominal pain, nausea, vomiting, and weight loss. The radiological manifestations of lymphoma can be quite variable. Ulcerating, infiltrating types of lesions are common, as well as multiple polypoid filling defects within the stomach (Fig. 2-46). Unfortunately, lymphoma can imitate numerous conditions, and radiological differentiation can be difficult. When faced with multiple large nodules in the stomach, factors that favor the possibility of lymphoma include relative preservation of the pliability of the stomach, associated fold thickening, and extension of the lesion into the duodenum.

Infiltrating Masses

Adenocarcinoma

The incidence of gastric cancer has dropped strikingly during the past four decades, and it continues to decrease. However, in Asia and in particular Japan, gastric cancer is one of the more common carcinomas and causes of mortality. There may be some slight decline in the rate in Japan, possibly associated with intensive screening programs.

Historically, adenocarcinoma, which manifests as a diffuse infiltrative process within the stomach, is described as a scirrhous type of lesion and is the most common cause of the linitis plastica configuration of the stomach seen on UGI studies. The diffuse infiltrative process results in desmoplastic changes in the wall of the stomach, rendering the stomach somewhat tubular, narrow, and rigid (see Fig. 2-12).

Lymphoma

Primary gastric lymphoma may have a multiplicity of presentations in the stomach. A marked increase in the fold pattern and infiltrative changes is the most common presentation (Fig. 2-47). This can be accompanied by ulceration. The stomach may be involved in part or in whole. Evaluation of radiographs may present difficulty in distinguishing between lymphoma and carcinoma. Fluoroscopic examination can be helpful in many cases of lymphoma because of the relative pliability of the stomach despite the apparent extent of disease. In many cases, degrees of peristalsis will also be retained. These findings relate to the overall lack of fibrosis and desmoplastic reaction associated with lymphoma but commonly seen with adenocarcinoma. The exception would be a Hodgkin's-type lymphoma.

Pseudolymphoma

Although pseudolymphoma or lymphoreticular hyperplasia of the stomach is a benign condition, it is virtually impossible to distinguish this benign process from

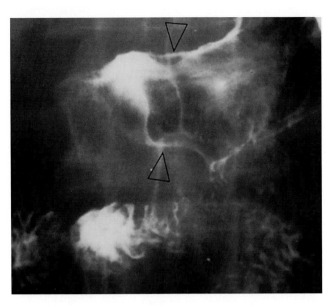

Fig. 2-47   Patient with lymphomatous infiltration of the distal stomach giving a narrow, tubular appearance without obstruction *(arrowheads)*.

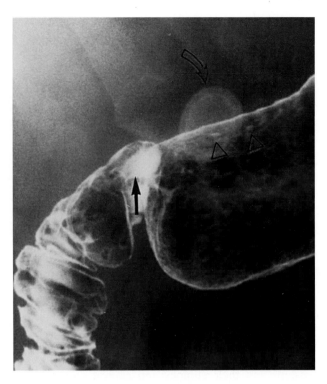

Fig. 2-48   Patient with chronic peptic disease and numerous tiny erosions *(arrowheads)*, as well as a 1.5-cm pyloric channel ulcer *(arrow)* and a laminated gallstone *(curved arrow)*.

malignant disease of the stomach, such as lymphoma or carcinoma. The spectrum of radiological problems presented by this disease includes gastric masses with associated ulceration and infiltrative disease of the stomach commonly with associated ulceration. The etiological origins of this process, also occasionally referred to as lymphofollicular gastritis, are not clear. It is believed by some to represent an unusual late stage of peptic ulceration of the stomach, whereas others have suggested that it is the least aggressive of the spectrum of lymphoma types. Focal lymphoreticular hyperplastic changes have been reported elsewhere in the bowel, often associated with ulcers. Microscopic examination of this lesion presents some difficulty to the pathologist in attempting to differentiate it from lymphoma. This is particularly the case on a frozen section.

Metastatic lesions

As previously discussed, metastatic lesions, particularly in the breast and lung, can present as both focal and diffuse infiltrative changes in the stomach. A local contiguous spread, such as from adjacent pancreatic malignancy, may on rare occasions give a similar appearance.

Leukemic infiltration

All types of leukemia may involve the GI tract. Indeed, autopsy studies suggest that virtually all patients have some degree of GI involvement. In the stomach, this generally is an infiltrative, diffuse process resulting in thickened irregular folds and is virtually indistinguishable from adenocarcinoma. There may be associated ulcerations and bleeding.

Gastric Erosions and Ulcers

A gastric erosion is a superficial mucosal defect, which unlike a gastric ulcer does not penetrate into the submucosa. These are virtually impossible to see on single-contrast examinations and can be detected relatively frequently using high-quality double-contrast technique. An integral part of the double-contrast technique consists of washing barium over the portions of the stomach most likely to harbor erosions and obtaining a barium pool sufficiently thin to demonstrate the erosions.

These erosions may be seen in any portion of the stomach but are most common within the antrum (Fig. 2-48). The distribution can be asymmetrical. There is a tendency for erosions to line up on folds. A small lucent halo around an erosion is commonly demonstrated and has been referred to as complete erosion. This halo represents a circular area of edema around the erosive defect. Erosions lacking this edematous halo have been referred to as incomplete erosions and are often difficult to demonstrate even on high-quality

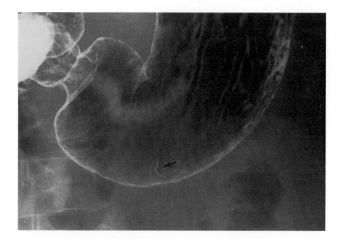

Fig. 2-49   Air-contrast UGI examination demonstrates short, superficial linear ulcer along the greater curvature of the stomach *(arrow)*.

double-contrast studies. Often, these are short, linear erosions (Fig. 2-49).

There is considerable controversy regarding gastric erosions and their etiology and clinical course. High-quality double-contrast evaluations of the stomach show that these lesions are much more common than previously thought.

The gastric mucosa, under normal circumstances, is protected from the acidic environment of the stomach by a surface layer of mucus in which secreted bicarbonate results in a pH gradient near neutral at the cellular level. In addition, prostaglandins within the gastric mucosa appear to play an important part in maintaining and supporting the epithelium in the presence of potentially harmful acid.

Gastric mucosal erosive changes may be acute or chronic. Erosive changes appear to be most common in patients with peptic disease and hyperacidity. It may be a manifestation of *H. pylori*–induced peptic ulcer disease in many patients. There is also a higher incidence of gastric erosions associated with excessive ingestion of alcohol or salicylates. Other medications, including indomethacin, reserpine, corticosteroids, ibuprofen, and potassium chloride, have also been implicated.

Gastric erosive changes are a common cause of UGI bleeding, and hemorrhagic erosive gastritis is thought to be responsible for 10% to 20% of upper tract bleeding.

Other causes that may result in gastric mucosal erosions include Crohn's disease and viral gastritis, such as cytomegalovirus or herpesvirus. Such lesions have also been described in Behçet's syndrome. There is also reason to suspect that a significant proportion of erosive gastritis, particularly of the chronic nature, may be idiopathic, thus distinctively different from that induced by peptic ulcer disease, aspirin, alcohol, other medications, or *H. pylori* gastritis.

A different manifestation of multiple superficial gastric erosions is related to patients who are undergoing acute, severe physiological or emotional stress. This has been described as a relatively common occurrence in patients with extensive burns in which the superficial ulcers have been referred to as Curling's ulcers. Cushing's ulcers are identical gastric superficial ulcers that have been described as a complication in patients with intracranial disease, severe head trauma, or postcraniotomy. These stress-type ulcers are almost always superficial, virtually never perforate, and in many patients are painless, with an incidence of GI bleeding in the range of 10% to 20%.

Malignant Versus Benign Gastric Ulceration

The widespread use of high-quality double-contrast technique in evaluation of the stomach has improved the ability of the radiologist to detect and classify ulcers as benign versus malignant. Various distinguishing features of gastric ulceration have been suggested to successfully classify gastric ulcers as benign versus malignant. The features listed in Table 2-1 can be helpful in making this differentiation. Some of the items will be more useful than others, but taken all together they can give the radiologist direction as to how to classify gastric ulcerations.

There are three radiological classifications of gastric ulcers—benign, malignant, and indeterminate. In general, it has been found that when ulcers contain well-defined radiological features of benignity, they are almost always benign, and ulcerations that blatantly display the features of malignancy are almost always malignant. There is, however, a large category in which there may be features of both benignity and malignancy demonstrated. In such an instance, the disposition to assign the ulcer to one category or another is unclear. Such ulcers are categorized as indeterminate in nature. In patients with radiologically malignant or indeterminate gastric ulcers, follow-up gastroscopy and biopsy are always indicated. In patients for whom radiological features of benignity are overwhelming, automatic gastroscopy and biopsy are probably poor uses of medical resources, personnel, and health care dollars.

- Location. Around 90% of all benign gastric ulcers are located in the antrum, and 75% of these are on the lesser curvature. Although most malignant ulcers occur in the antrum, various studies suggest that they occur here with less frequency than benign ulcers, and, in fact, malignant ulcers can be seen anywhere in the stomach. In particular, ulcers seen on the greater curvature or in parts of the stomach other than the antrum should be viewed with greater degrees of suspicion.

Table 2-1   Malignant versus benign ulceration: radiological distinguishing features

Feature	Benign	Malignant
Location	Mostly antrum, 75% lesser curvature	Most lesions in antrum but can occur anywhere
Convergence of folds	To edge of crater	Stop short of crater edge
Fold shape	Normal or uniformly swollen (edematous)	Amputated, fused, or clubbed folds that may fail to reach crater edge
Projections beyond expected confines of gastric wall	Yes	No
Position of ulcer mound or mass	Central	Eccentric
Ulcer shape	Round or linear	Irregular
Ulcer collar	Yes, well-defined	May be present but shaggy and irregular
Multiplicity	Increased frequency 10%-30%	Less frequent
Associated duodenal ulcer disease	Increased association 50%-60%	Less frequent
Carman's sign and Kirklin complex	No	Yes
Crescent sign	Yes	No
Response to therapy	Reduction of size in 4-6 weeks	No reduction in size, ulcer may enlarge

- Convergence of folds. In virtually all benign ulcers, gastric folds can be identified up to the edge of the ulcer crater (Fig. 2-50). It is extremely common for the rugal pattern to stop short of the crater margin of a malignant ulcer. This differentiation is one of the most important radiological differences between the types of ulcers.
- Fold shape. In benign ulcers, the adjacent fold pattern can be normal, or it may demonstrate the uniform or beaded widening secondary to edema and swelling. However, as previously stated, these folds will proceed to the edge of the ulcer crater. The malignant ulcer may demonstrate a variety of abnormal fold patterns in the adjacent mucosal surface. This can include amputated, fused, or clubbed folds, all of which are abnormal and often fail to reach the crater edge (Fig. 2-51). Fold configuration represents an important differentiating factor.
- Projections beyond expected confines of gastric wall. This has been an acceptable and reliable sign of differentiation for decades. Benign ulcers tend to excavate into the normal mucosal wall, giving a distinct impression of projecting beyond the adjacent mucosal boundaries. On the other hand, a malignant ulcer representing ulceration in a mass will quite frequently give the impression of ulceration that does not extend beyond the adjacent mucosal confines of the stomach. However, some care should be taken with the interpretation of this sign. A chronic gastric ulcer in which some degree of alternating healing and exacerbation has occurred can give a configuration identical to that of a malignant ulcer as a result of fibrosis, cicatrization, and contraction of the adjacent gastric wall.

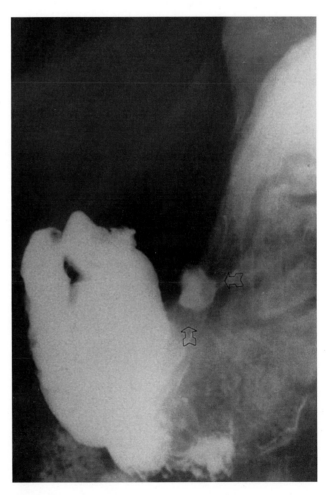

Fig. 2-50   A large benign ulcer is seen along the lesser curvature of the body of the stomach. Note the gastric folds coming up to the edge of the ulcer crater *(arrows).*

- Position of the ulcer on the mound or mass. Benign ulcers excite inflammatory and edematous changes in the adjacent tissues in a concentric distribution about the ulcer crater (Fig. 2-52). The appearance is therefore that of a centrally located ulcer on a raised mass or mound of edematous tissue. Conversely, the point of ulceration that occurs on a malignant tumor is not predictable and is often eccentric.
- Ulcer shape. Benign ulcers are generally round. Distinct linear ulcers will almost always be benign. Malignant ulcers can be occasionally round and well-defined but more often are found to be irregular with poor definition of the margins.
- Ulcer collar. A uniform ulcer collar about a centrally located ulcer is a good sign for benignity (Fig. 2-53). Undermining of the adjacent soft tissue and subsequent edematous changes result in the appearance of an ulcer collar. When the edematous changes are restricted to the overhanging mucosa about the crater margin, the configuration may, in profile, be that of a thin, well-demarcated lucent ulcer collar, known as a Hampton line. Ulcer collars may be present on malignant ulcers but they are generally thick, irregular, and shaggy in appearance.
- Multiplicity. Although this cannot be considered a strong sign for either benignity or malignancy, it does apparently have some statistical significance.

Literature reports have suggested an increased potential of benignity when multiple ulcers are present (Fig. 2-54).
- Associated duodenal ulcer disease. Associated duodenal ulcer disease is a statistically differentiating point that must be correlated with all other distinguishing features. The increased association between benign gastric ulcers and duodenal ulcers has been reported with considerable variance.

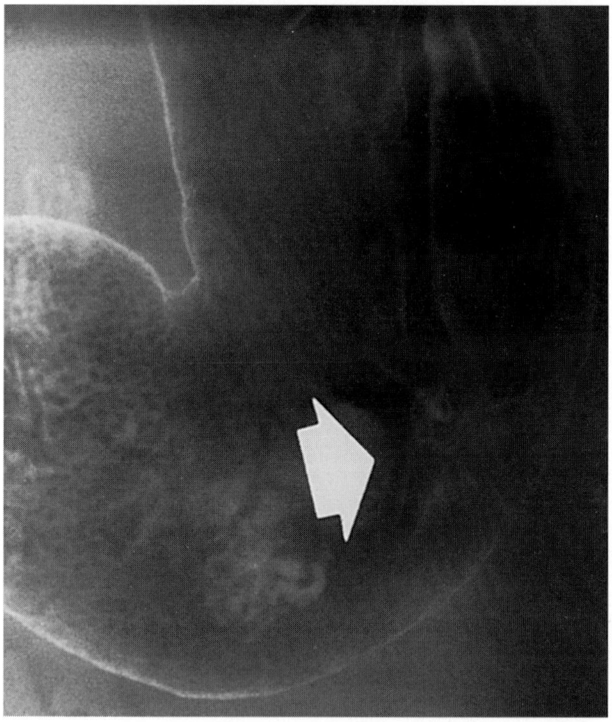

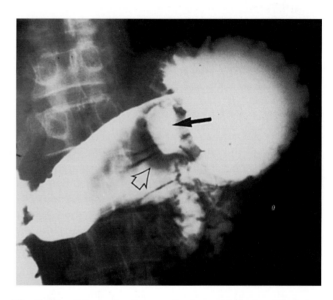

Fig. 2-52 A large, benign gastric ulcer with barium-filled ulcer crater is demonstrated *(arrow)*, as well as an edematous ulcer collar *(open arrow)*.

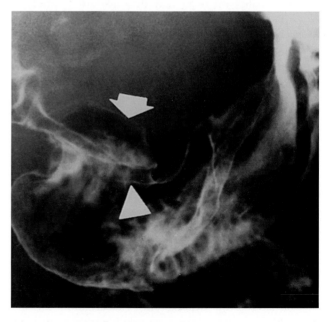

Fig. 2-53 A huge gastric ulcer is seen along the lesser curvature of the stomach *(arrow)*. A well-defined ulcer collar *(arrowhead)* is seen at the margin of the ulcer.

![Fig. 2-51](shallow gastric ulcer radiograph)

Fig. 2-51 A shallow gastric ulcer *(arrow)* is seen with associated adjacent clubbed and amputated folds indicative of malignant lesion.

- Carman's meniscus sign and Kirklin complex. First described by Carman in the late 1920s, Carman's sign (Box 2-7) is thought to be diagnostic of a particular type of ulcerated neoplasm. The ulcer is almost always located on the saddle portion of the stomach on the lesser curvature of the antrum and body. The malignant lesion will lack significant mass effect. The type of ulceration is usually large and flat, with raised edges. In single-contrast barium-filled examination of the stomach with compression of this saddle region, the heaped-up edges of the ulcer will approximate and entrap barium within the flat ulcer bed, giving a meniscoid configuration to the trapped barium within the ulcer, in which the inner margin is concave toward the lumen (Fig. 2-55).

  Where the heaped-up margins of the ulcer approximate and meet and entrap barium, as a result of compression, the lucent margin that surrounds the concavity of the ulcer represents the approximated heaped-up ulcer edges. This is called the Kirklin complex. Because of the special circumstances regarding the nature of the mass, configuration and location of the ulcer, and the need for the barium-filled stomach and compression views, this sign will rarely be identified on double-contrast views of the stomach.

- Crescent sign. Benign ulcers occurring along the greater curvature of the antrum or body and in which significant mucosal undermining has occurred may demonstrate the configuration of a crescent-shaped ulceration with its concavity directed away from the gastric lumen.
- Response to therapy. With adequate treatment, almost all benign gastric ulcers will undergo a reduction of size in a 4- to 6-week period. Expected deformity changes associated with scarring and cicatrization can also be identified. Alternatively, there will be no change in malignant ulcers or they will increase in size. This differentiating factor is significant, although it has been noted that on rare

Box 2-7	Recipe for the Carman Meniscus Sign: Necessary Ingredients

Flat tumor with heaped-up edges
Located on saddle area of lesser curve antrum of stomach
Seen in single-contrast examination or single-contrast phase of biphasic examination
Seen only with compression

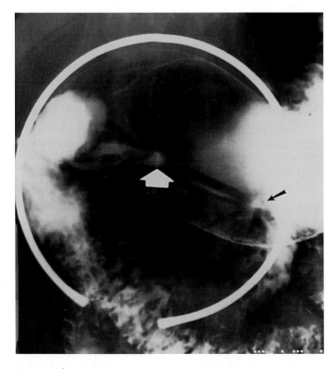

Fig. 2-54 Multiple, small gastric ulcers are demonstrated *(arrows)*.

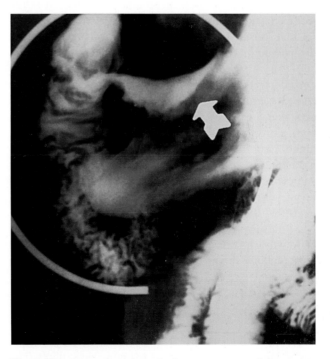

Fig. 2-55 Large ulcer along the lesser curvature of the antrum of the stomach, under compression, demonstrates concavity of the ulcer crater *(arrow)* along its luminal side. This is Carman's meniscus sign of malignancy.

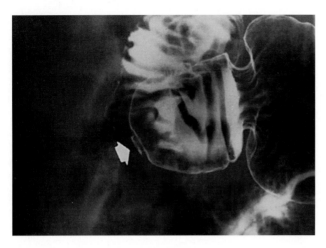

Fig. 2-56 Small, shallow protrusion along the greater curvature of the stomach *(arrow)* was diagnosed at UGI examination to be a shallow gastric ulcer. Note the absence of inflammatory changes about the area. Endoscopy showed no evidence of inflammation or ulceration and a small antral diverticulum.

occasions a malignant ulcer may undergo some degree of decrease in size with peptic ulcer treatment.

Miscellaneous

Diverticula

Fundal diverticula

The most common of diverticula encountered in the stomach arise from the cardiofundal region, usually seen on the posterior wall of the stomach. It is a true diverticulum, containing all the layers of the stomach, and can range in size from 1 to 10 cm. These are considered to be congenital and, for the most part, of no clinical significance. Reports of bleeding from gastric diverticula exist in the literature, citing incidences as high as 14%. However, this is probably considerably higher than the experience of most endoscopists and GI radiologists. Additionally, if a diverticulum becomes sufficiently large, impaired emptying and stasis may result, although these are rare complications.

Antral diverticula

Antral diverticula are unusual intramural projections of mucosa in the gastric wall. They are almost always located along the greater curvature of the antrum of the stomach. There has been an association with ectopic pancreatic tissue reported in approximately 10% to 15% of cases (Fig. 2-56).

Radiologically, the partial diverticulum on the greater curvature of the antrum has a "collar-button" appearance and is often misdiagnosed as a benign gastric ulcer. The persistent appearance, lack of inflammatory changes around the partial diverticulum, and lack of tenderness when compressing this region should help the radiologist avoid this mistake (Fig. 2-57).

Postoperative stomach

The most common types of gastric surgeries are the partial gastrectomy and gastrojejunostomy (Billroth II), antrectomy and gastroduodenostomy (Billroth I), diverting gastrojejunostomy, and gastric partitions for morbid obesity. Radiographic abnormalities seen in complications of gastric resection include the following.

Pseudomass

Pseudomass can be seen following Billroth I or Billroth II procedure, although it is more common in the latter. It represents the plication deformity that results when the divided end of the stomach is oversewn to restrict the size of the stoma (Fig. 2-58). The radiological problem presented in this situation is that of a masslike filling defect seen at or near the anastomotic site. It is generally more prominent on immediate postoperative examinations secondary to the edematous changes that persist in the region. On subsequent examinations it may seem less prominent and over a period of time may appear static in its configuration and size. Without a baseline postoperative examination, the deformity can easily simulate neoplastic recurrence.

Postoperative gastric bezoars

As previously discussed, bezoar is not an uncommon complication of gastric surgery (see Fig. 2-8). The bezoars encountered in this setting are almost always phytobezoars and can be asymptomatic. If the bezoar becomes sufficiently large, obstruction of the stoma, distention of the gastric remnant, and irritation and erosion of the mucosa can occur.

Gastric stump carcinoma

Although there continues to be some controversy regarding the incidence and occurrence of carcinoma in the gastric remnant, the postoperative stomach is at higher risk for carcinoma than the nonoperated stomach. These lesions are most commonly seen in patients 10 years after partial gastrectomy and, as previously discussed, may be due to chronic gastritis secondary to bile reflux (Fig. 2-59).

Chronic gastric remnant gastritis

One of the more common postoperative complications seen in the stomach is chronic gastritis. It is hypothesized that the lack of pyloric protection results in chronic reflux of bile and pancreatic secretions stimulating inflammatory changes in the gastric remnant. The common radiological appearance is of enlarged gastric rugae, although erosions and even ulcers have been associated with chronic gastritis.

Stomal ulceration

Recurrent ulceration after partial gastrectomy for peptic ulcer disease commonly appears on the jejunal side of the gastrojejunostomy and is known as a stomal or marginal ulcer (Fig. 2-60). When these ulcers are sufficiently large, they are difficult to miss. However, smaller marginal ulcers are readily missed on UGI studies and particularly on single-contrast examinations. The

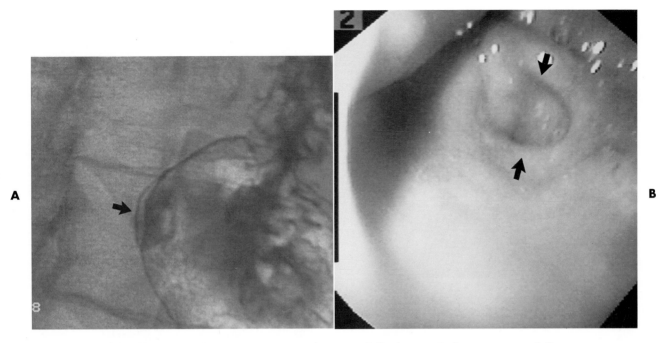

Fig. 2-57   Antral diverticulum. **A,** Digital image of distal stomach demonstrates a shallow excavation in antrum *(arrow)*. Note lack of edematous changes in the area. **B,** Endoscopic image of area demonstrates the margins of the antral diverticulum *(arrows)*. Note normal mucosa both in and around diverticulum.

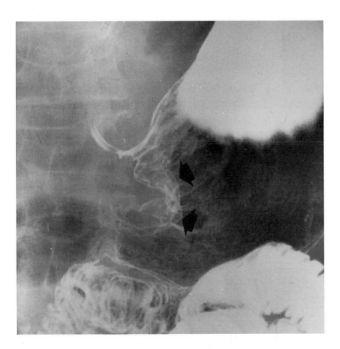

Fig. 2-58   This patient has had a Billroth II gastric resection. UGI examination shows large mass along the margin of the gastric stump *(arrows)*. Ominous as this appears, it represents nothing more than a prominent plication defect.

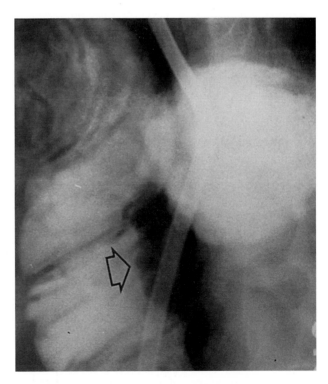

Fig. 2-59   UGI study in a patient with previous gastrectomy. The anastomosis is open. Along the margin of the efferent loop there is nodularity *(arrow)* that proved to be a recurrent adenocarcinoma.

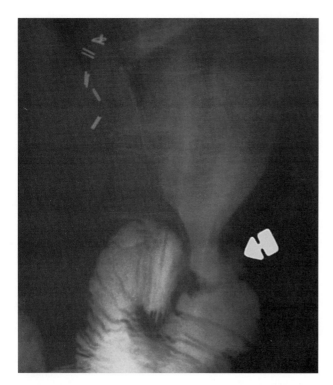

Fig. 2-60 Patient with previous gastrectomy and Billroth II resection presents with recurrent pain. UGI study demonstrates large stomal ulcer *(arrow)*.

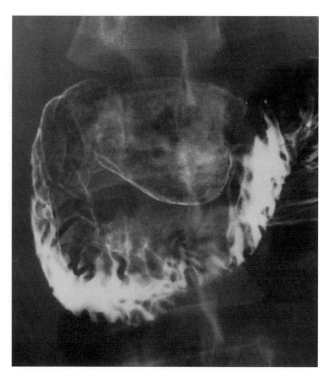

Fig. 2-61 Air-contrast view of normal duodenal bulb utilizing 0.1 mg IV glucagon.

presence of recurrent ulcers on the anastomotic margin is probably unrelated to chronic small bowel reflux and more likely suggests the possibility of inadequate gastric resection, the possible existence of an antral remnant inadvertently left behind, or even the presence of a pancreatic islet cell Zollinger-Ellison–type tumor. Additionally, some have suggested that an excessively long afferent loop may predispose to marginal ulcers.

Chronic gastroesophageal reflux

Patients with partial gastric resections will experience an increased incidence of gastroesophageal reflux. Indeed, any patient undergoing any surgery involving mobilization of the stomach may experience increased reflux and subsequent reflux esophagitis.

Jejunal gastric intussusception

Jejunal gastric intussusception is infrequent, but when it does occur it can occur as an acute or chronic recurrent process. The acute intussusception is often a surgical emergency with compromise of the blood supply in the intussuscepted small bowel loops. These patients will present with severe abdominal pain, nausea and vomiting, and evidence of UGI obstruction. Patients with the chronic recurring type may have no more symptoms than occasional vague upper abdominal discomfort. The intussusception may spontaneously decompress after several minutes.

A large intraremnant filling defect often suggestive of intussusception in its configuration and barium pattern

will be seen. In the chronic transient variety, the patient may have vague upper abdominal symptoms, and unless the intussusception is occurring at the time of examination, the diagnosis will probably not be considered.

Gastric wall emphysema

Gastric intramural pneumatosis is an unusual finding. The most common cause relates to the ingestion of corrosive acidic material with subsequent necrosis of the mucosa. In addition, it can be seen in the phlegmonous type of gastritis, in which the offending bacterial agent is a gas-producing organism. Air in the gastric wall has also been associated with gastric ulcers and instrumentation of the stomach secondary to endoscopy and placement of tubes.

DUODENUM

The evaluation of the duodenum is normally included as part of the UGI examination. It should include both air-contrast views and compression views, particularly of the duodenal bulb region. Hypotonic duodenography has also been helpful in evaluating this region. The desired result is usually achieved by 0.1 to 0.5 mg of IV glucagon (Fig. 2-61). Occasionally, the duodenum can be located in a posterior position directly behind the gastric antrum. Under such circumstances, profiling the duode-

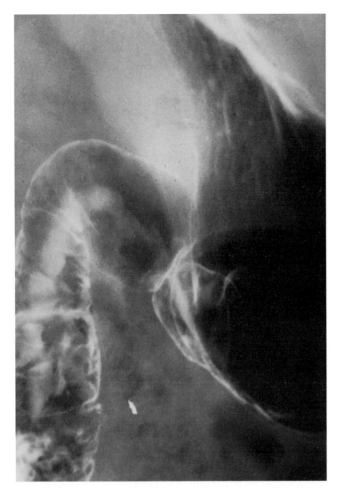

Fig. 2-62   Profiled gastric antrum and duodenal bulb in a posteriorly located duodenum.

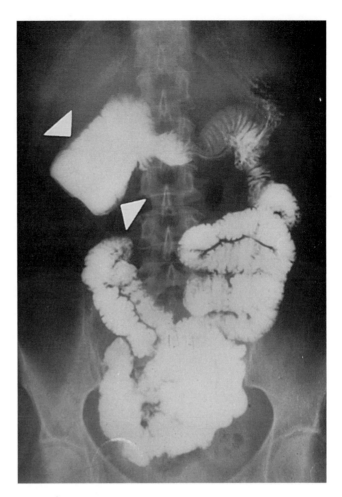

Fig. 2-63   Megaduodenum *(arrowheads)* in a patient with scleroderma.

nal bulb, particularly for air-contrast views, can be difficult. In the left lateral position, the air-filled bulb may be overlapped by portions of the antrum. Angulation of the x-ray tube during fluoroscopy, if this facility is available, may be helpful in separating the duodenal bulb from the antrum. When angulation is not available, a few simple maneuvers may be undertaken. The first is an attempt to evaluate the duodenum in the left oblique position while the patient is upright. The weight of the barium within the stomach may sufficiently pull the gastric antrum downward to allow visualization of the duodenum bulb, which tends to be fixed. Alternatively, with the patient recumbent and in the left lateral position, a bolster (inflated balloon or pillow) is placed in the patient's epigastrium and the patient is asked to roll downward toward the bolster and the table (LAO position). This maneuver will often displace the stomach away from the duodenum, permitting an unobstructed profile view of the air-filled duodenum and pyloric channel (Fig. 2-62).

Most of the radiological problems associated with the duodenum are also common to the remainder of the

small bowel. For this reason, discussion of these entities in this section will be quite limited and more detail will be found in Chapter 3.

Dilated (Nonobstructed) Lumen

Neuromuscular abnormalities account for most of the findings of a dilated flaccid duodenum during UGI examination. These include scleroderma, idiopathic intestinal pseudoobstruction, and diabetes mellitus. Patients on anticholinergic atropine-like medication may exhibit similar findings (Fig. 2-63).

In patients with nontropical sprue, dilatation of the small bowel is a common finding and may be seen within the duodenum as well. Most of the other findings associated with sprue tend to be confined to the more distal small bowel.

Occasionally, a dilated nonobstructed duodenal sweep may be seen in patients with severe acute illnesses, trauma, or burns. In these patients, distention of both the stomach and occasionally the duodenum may be encountered. Intraabdominal processes, which result

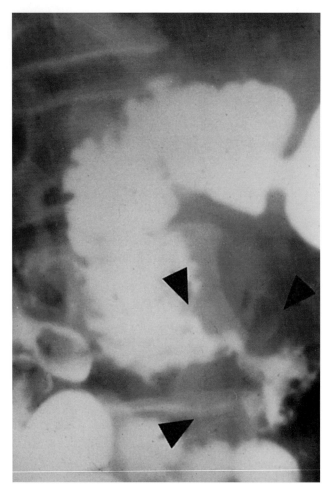

Fig. 2-64 Crohn's disease involving the duodenal sweep with resultant stricture *(arrowheads)*.

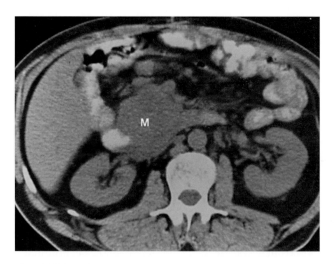

Fig. 2-65 CT through the pancreas demonstrates a large mass *(M)* invading the adjacent contrast-filled duodenal sweep.

in an adynamic ileus, can also involve the duodenum, causing dilatation. Although the esophagus is the main GI site of involvement in patients with Chagas' disease, the intramural plexi of the duodenum can also be damaged by the trypanosomes, resulting in diminished peristalsis and dilatation.

Dilated duodenum has been described in eating disorders, such as anorexia nervosa or postpartum cachexia.

Narrowed Lumen

More than 90% of peptic ulcer disease involving the duodenum affects the duodenal bulb. It can occur as an acute episode, recurrent disease, or chronic disease. In recurrent and chronic disease, duodenal bulb deformity is common, and a small, contracted narrow duodenal bulb will often be seen in patients with chronic peptic ulcer disease. This can occasionally result in obstruction and a dilated stomach.

Approximately 10% of duodenal ulcers are postbulbar in location. These are radiologically difficult to see. Quite often, the radiological findings are thickened, irregular folds, with an area of focal narrowing. However, Crohn's disease or tuberculosis involving the duodenum, although relatively uncommon, can give an identical appearance (Fig. 2-64). Inflammatory changes affecting adjacent pancreas or, less commonly, the gallbladder, can also result in postbulbar stricture. Malignancy arising from the pancreatic head can also invade any portion of the duodenal sweep, resulting in strictured narrowing (Fig. 2-65). This most commonly occurs in the descending and proximal transverse portion of the duodenum.

Annular pancreas is an unusual condition involving the descending duodenum. It represents an embryological abnormality of pancreatic development in which the ventral bud of the pancreas encircles the duodenum. This produces circumferential indentation of the descending duodenum by the surrounding pancreatic tissue. It is often diagnosed in infancy or childhood, although a significant number of these patients will not be identified until adolescence or adulthood. Occasionally, periduodenal fibrosis of the duodenal wall can develop at the site of the long-standing stricture resulting from the annular pancreatic tissue. For this reason, surgical relief of the annular extrinsic compression may not always be curative and, on occasion, a gastroenterostomy bypass may be indicated.

The intraluminal diverticulum of the duodenum, or "wind sock deformity," is a thin, intraluminal web or membrane (Fig. 2-66). The "wind sock" configuration occurs as a result of the web being stretched and billowed into the distal lumen by the prolonged and constant effect of peristaltic activity.

Bleeding into the duodenal wall, as a result of trauma or other causes, such as Henoch-Schönlein purpura, hemophilia, or anticoagulation therapy, can present as discrete intramural mass, diffuse infiltrative changes with thickened fold pattern, or a combination, with associated narrowing.

The superior mesenteric artery syndrome is a condition in which duodenal obstruction occurs as a result of narrowing of the angle between the aorta and the superior mesenteric artery at the point where the duodenum passes between them. This is most commonly seen in burn patients, patients in body casts, or patients who have experienced acute severe illness with substantial weight loss. It is thought that the loss of retroperitoneal fat results in a narrowing of the angle between the vessels. Another condition that can result in duodenal narrowing and potential obstruction is midgut volvulus, seen in patients with incomplete rotation of the midgut. The volvulus can occur as a result of fibrous bands overlying the proximal portion of the duodenum, around which the midgut can rotate (Ladd's bands) and

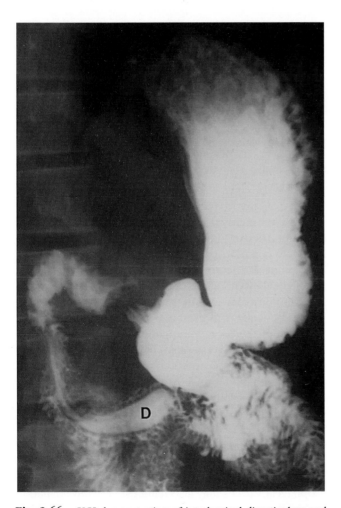

Fig. 2-66   UGI demonstration of intraluminal diverticulum and "wind sock" configuration (D).

twist. Volvulus can also occur as a result of rotation of the midgut about a markedly abbreviated small bowel mesentery that may occur as a result of incomplete rotation.

Aorticoduodenal fistulas are usually complications of prosthetic aortic Dacron grafts. However, they originally were described as complications of aortic abdominal aneurysms. The distal portion of the duodenum, in contact with the graft or aneurysm, will break down as a result of focal pressure or erosion of the aorta dissecting into the duodenal wall. The condition is potentially fatal. Contrast examination of the distal duodenum can show several possible findings. These include mass effect, luminal narrowing, ulceration, and even tracking of contrast along the outside of the graft. Complete obstruction of the intestinal lumen in the neonate (duodenal atresia) results from failure of cannulization of the duodenum during early intrauterine life. The incidence is higher in infants with Down's syndrome, and quite often these patients present within several hours after birth with the classic "double-bubble" sign, representing an air-filled and distended stomach and duodenal bulb. Another congenital cause of duodenal narrowing is duodenal duplication. Although this is quite rare, it can result in a large periduodenal mass impressing and narrowing the duodenum. The duplicated segment may also be continuous with the main lumen.

Adenocarcinoma of the duodenum, although rare, occurs most commonly in the distal half of the duodenum and in most instances has the typical apple-core configuration (Fig. 2-67). Metastatic disease to the duodenum is also uncommon but can occur as an encircling obstructing mass, quite often in the distal portion of the duodenal sweep (Fig. 2-68).

Thickened Folds

The most common causes of thickened duodenal folds, particularly in the more proximal duodenum, are peptic ulcer disease and pancreatitis. The changes are a result of edema, both from direct inflammatory changes involving the duodenum and indirect changes involving the pancreatic head.

In acute pancreatitis, the changes may be limited to the medial inner curve of the duodenal sweep. There may be thickening and tethering of folds that can result in the "reverse figure 3" sign (also seen with pancreatic carcinoma) described on the UGI examination (Fig. 2-69).

Patients with Zollinger-Ellison syndrome will always have fold prominence within the duodenum as a result of the marked amount of gastric acid secretion stimulated by pancreatic gastrinoma. A small number of patients with this uncommon disease will have the offending gastrinoma located within the duodenum.

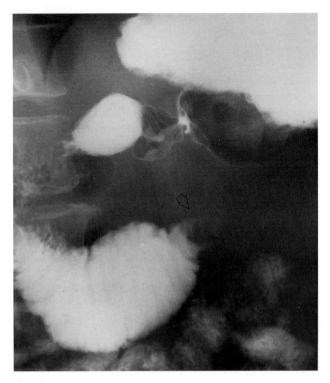

Fig. 2-67 Primary adenocarcinoma of the duodenum with annular narrowing and obstruction *(arrows)*.

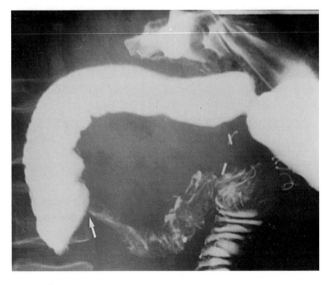

Fig. 2-68 Metastatic disease involving the duodenal sweep *(arrow)*, eccentrically narrowing the lumen.

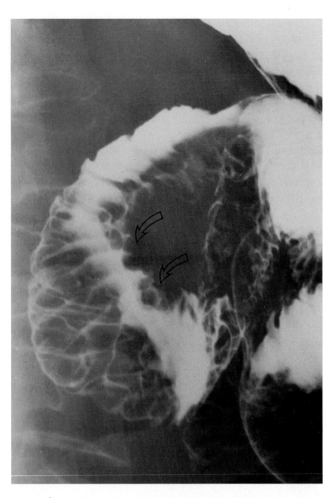

Fig. 2-69 UGI study in patient with acute severe pancreatitis resulting in marked thickening of duodenal folds and the "reverse figure 3" configuration on the inner margin *(arrows)*.

Crohn's disease of the duodenum most commonly is seen as thickened folds (Fig. 2-70).

Parasitic infection in the small bowel commonly involves the duodenum and results in thick, irregular folds. *Ascaris lumbricoides* commonly involves the distal small bowel. However, both *Strongyloides stercoralis* and intestinal hookworm, *Ancylostoma duode-* *nale,* have a marked preference for the proximal small bowel, particularly the duodenum. *Giardia lamblia* is a relatively common protozoan parasite that involves the duodenum and jejunum with resultant fold thickening and irregularity (Fig. 2-71). Both hypersecretion and hypermotility may also be seen in patients with giardiasis. Additionally, the presence of lymphoid hyperplasia has been observed in some patients with giardiasis.

Fold thickening can also be observed in patients with eosinophilic gastroenteritis. These patients often present with abdominal pain, nausea, vomiting, and eosinophilia on their peripheral blood smear. Fold thickening usually involves the gastric antrum and duodenum. Whipple's disease involves the proximal small bowel with thickened and irregular folds in the duodenum and proximal jejunum.

Occasionally, patients with portal hypertension and esophageal varices may also manifest varicoid formation within the proximal duodenum. This is seen as thickened and smooth serpiginous folds. Frequently, the

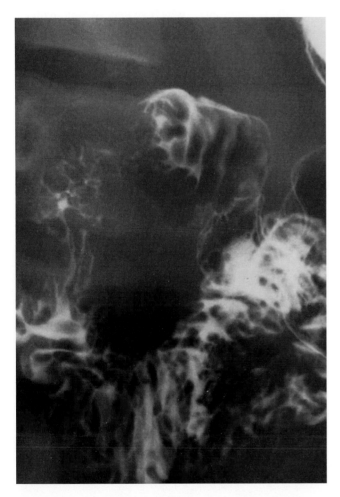

Fig. 2-70 Thickening of folds in the duodenal bulb and postbulbar region secondary to Crohn's disease.

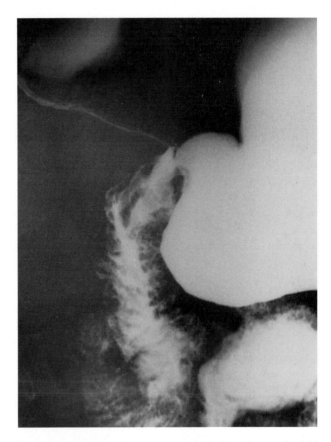

Fig. 2-71 Patient with giardiasis with thickened, irregular folds with fine nodularity.

presence of duodenal varices is an indication of portal vein occlusion. Duodenal intramural bleeding may also manifest as thickened regular folds with the classic "stack of coins" appearance.

Lymphomas may have multiple physical manifestations within the small bowel, among which is diffuse fold thickening. Its presence in the duodenum is very uncommon, and, when present, like lymphomas elsewhere in the gut, it almost never obstructs. Patients in chronic renal failure or on chronic dialysis will commonly demonstrate thickened folds within the duodenum. There is also an increased incidence of peptic ulcer disease within such patients, although the persistent thickened folds are probably not peptic in origin. Uniform thickening of folds within the duodenum, and indeed within both the jejunum and ileum, can occur in both primary and secondary amyloidosis.

Filling Defects

Flexural pseudopolyp

One of the most common and troublesome of duodenal filling defects is the flexural pseudopolyp (Fig. 2-72). This phenomenon is usually seen in thin patients with a sharp, acute angle between the apex of the duodenal bulb and the descending duodenum. Because of the acuteness of the angle, mucosa can pile up on the medial inner aspect of the duodenum at the level of the apex of the bulb. This results in a filling defect that can easily be diagnosed as a nonexistent polypoid mass. Demonstration of this mass in a thin individual with a sharp bulbar duodenal angle should alert radiologists to the possibility of a flexural pseudotumor. This can be confirmed by evaluating the area in question with the patient in different positions, particularly supine positions that may open the bulbar duodenal angle and change the configuration of the filling defect.

Pancreatic rests

Pancreatic rests or ectopic pancreatic tissue within the duodenum can result in a well-defined filling defect (Fig. 2-73). These are not neoplastic lesions and are of embryonic origin. They are smooth, can be round or lobulated, and usually measure 1 to 2 cm in diameter. They more commonly present as solitary filling defects in the duodenal bulb or second portion of the duodenum. They can also be seen in the gastric antrum. A characteristic radiological finding is the central collection of barium (dimple) that may be confused with a small ulcer on the surface of a neoplastic polypoid lesion.

Mesenchymal tumors

Mesenchymal benign tumors, such as stromal cell tumors (leiomyomas) and lipomas, are the most common benign lesions of the duodenum. They are usually solitary and submucosal in origin and have a smooth surface. These can ulcerate on the surface, although this is uncommon in the duodenum. The duodenal variety is usually smaller than those seen elsewhere in the bowel. Neurofibroma and hemangioma can also occur within the duodenum but are rare.

Adenoma

Duodenal adenomas are uncommon. When present, they are seen radiologically as mucosal polypoid lesions usually no more than 1 cm in diameter. The exception is the villous adenoma, which when symptomatic is commonly 2 to 3 cm in size (Fig. 2-74). Patients may present with either GI bleeding or symptoms related to intussusception. These lesions have a high potential for malignant degeneration.

Carcinoid/APUDoma

Similarly, carcinoid tumors arising from argentaffin cells within the mucosa can be seen in the duodenum

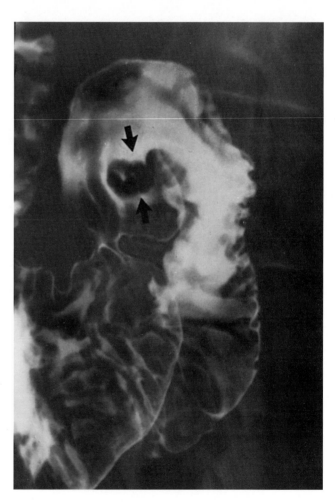

Fig. 2-72 Polypoid filling defect in the duodenal bulb *(arrows)* that proved to be a flexural pseudotumor. No polyps were identified at endoscopy.

and particularly in the peripapillary region of the second portion of the duodenum. The radiological appearance is variable and may appear as discrete smooth polyps or as irregular infiltrating processes. A variant of this, the APUDoma, can arise from amine precursor uptake and decarboxylation (APUD) cells. These tumors are histologically similar to ileal carcinoid tumors and are frequently associated with multiple endocrine neoplasia (MEN) syndromes.

Various polypoid syndromes may also have polyps within the duodenum. This includes familial polyposis, Peutz-Jeghers syndrome, and Cronkhite-Canada syndrome, as well as Cowden's disease.

Brunner's gland hyperplasia and Brunner's gland adenoma

Multiple filling defects in the duodenal bulb are also a presentation of Brunner's gland hyperplasia (Fig. 2-75). This process can also extend into the second portion of the duodenum. The etiology of this condition is unclear. Normal function of the Brunner's glands, which produce alkaline secretion to protect the sensitive duodenal mucosa from damaging effects of gastric acid, does not appear to be impaired. A variation of this is the Brunner's gland adenoma or hamartoma, which is a rare lesion caused by focal overgrowth of the tissue elements of the Brunner's glands in the proximal duodenum (Fig. 2-76). They are usually seen as smooth polypoid masses, often about 1 cm in size.

Lymphoid hyperplasia

Benign lymphoid hyperplasia of the duodenum with multiple small filling defects may be a normal finding in children, although in adults the condition has been

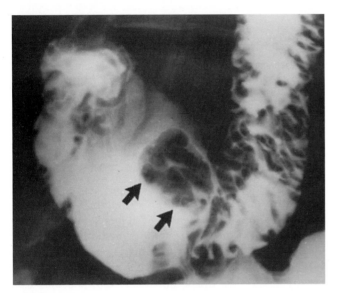

Fig. 2-73   A lobulated filling defect *(arrows)* is seen in the duodenal bulb with a small, central barium collection (dimple) representing a pancreatic rest.

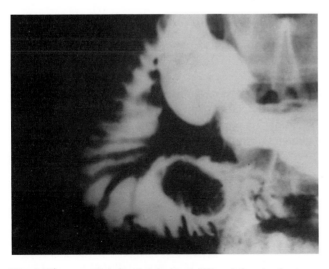

Fig. 2-74   A well-defined, lobulated filling defect in the transverse portion of the duodenum representing a villous adenoma.

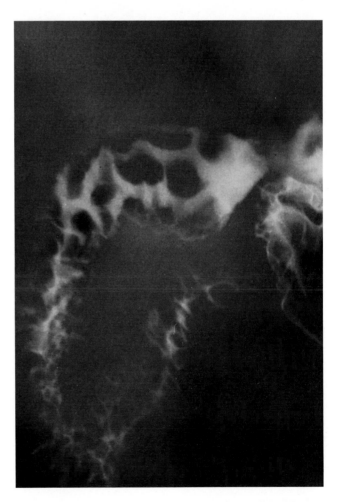

Fig. 2-75   Multiple, large, and rounded nodular filling defects in the duodenal bulb and postbulbar region representing Brunner's gland hyperplasia.

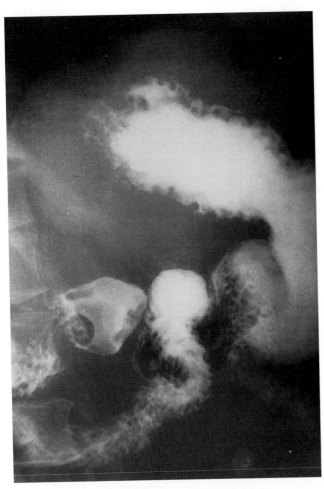

Fig. 2-76 A solitary filling defect near the apex of the duodenal bulb suggests the possibility of a flexural pseudotumor. However, this was found to be a Brunner's gland adenoma.

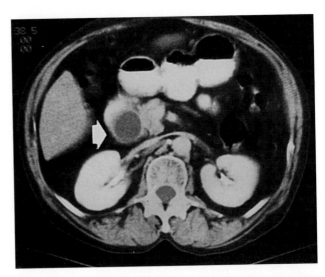

Fig. 2-77 Large cystic dilatation in the common bile duct representing a choledochal cyst *(arrow)* impressing the duodenum.

associated with hypogammaglobulinemia and the concomitant presence of giardiasis.

Choledochocele

Occasionally, a round, smooth defect arising in the region of the papilla is seen and is a result of choledochocele formation. This is a variation of the choledochal cyst (Fig. 2-77).

Kaposi's sarcoma

Kaposi's sarcoma is a relatively common lesion seen in AIDS patients. The major sites of involvement include the stomach and small bowel, although lesions may be demonstrated within the duodenum. The appearance is that of multiple polypoid lesions frequently ulcerated on the surface. Hematogenous metastatic disease, particularly breast or melanoma, may have a similar appearance.

Papillitis

Abnormalities of the papilla of Vater may also manifest as a duodenal filling defect. Most commonly this is papillitis, resulting from inflammation and an enlargement of the major papilla, usually resulting from traumatic stone passage or peripapillary fibrotic changes.

Heterotopic gastric mucosa

An uncommon cause of multiple plaquelike filling defects in the duodenal bulb is heterotopic gastric mucosa (Fig. 2-78). These filling defects can be of varying size and configuration and form a mosaic pattern usually in the base of the duodenal bulb, and they can easily be missed on single-contrast examination. The exact clinical significance of this condition is unclear. There appears to be no malignant potential.

Extrinsic Processes

Pancreatic disease

The most common extrinsic process involving the duodenal sweep is a result of pancreatic disease in the head of the pancreas. This can be inflammatory, with diffuse enlargement of the pancreas or pseudocyst formation. Also, pancreatic neoplasms, either benign or malignant, can impress the duodenum.

Kidney and adrenal gland diseases

Disease processes arising from the right kidney or adrenal gland, if sufficiently large, can impress the outer aspect of the descending portion of the duodenal sweep (Fig. 2-79).

Enlarged common bile duct, gallbladder, and liver

Abnormalities arising in the liver and biliary system can also, on occasion, result in extrinsic impression of

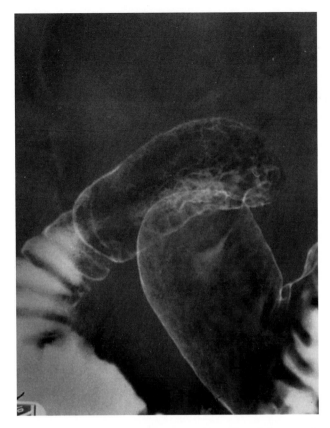

Fig. 2-78 Multiple, irregular, plaquelike filling defects at the base of the duodenal bulb representing heterotopic gastric mucosa.

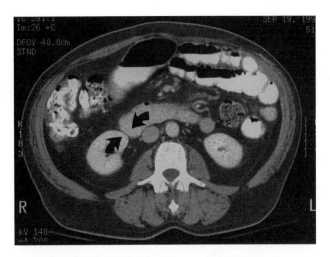

Fig. 2-79 Relationship of the right kidney and the proximal duodenal sweep. CT section through this region shows intimate relationship between contrast-filled duodenum and anterior-medial aspect of the kidney *(curved arrows)*.

the duodenum. This includes an enlarged gallbladder, whether it be from obstructive causes or passive dilatation. An enlarged common bile duct can occasionally impress the duodenal sweep at the level of the apex of the bulb (Fig. 2-80).

Other causes

Large choledochal cysts can also result in a significant duodenal impression. Retroperitoneal lymph node masses in the peripancreatic region can also lead to an extrinsic impression on the duodenal sweep (Fig. 2-81).

Duodenal Ulceration

Peptic ulcer disease

Duodenal peptic ulcer disease is a common entity and accounts for a sizeable portion of the health care costs expended on GI diseases. The relationship between *H. pylori* and peptic ulcer disease has been discussed earlier in the chapter. It is estimated that between 10% and 15% of North American men have suffered from duodenal ulcer disease at some time in their life. The

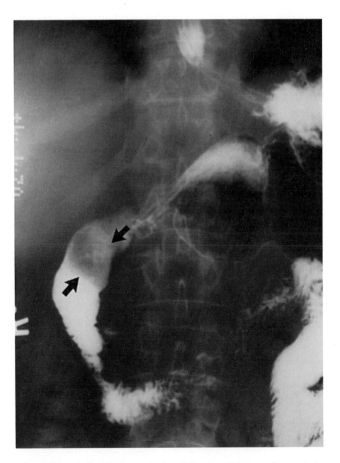

Fig. 2-80 Obstruction of the biliary system and extrinsic impression of the postbulbar duodenum *(arrows)* by a dilated common bile duct.

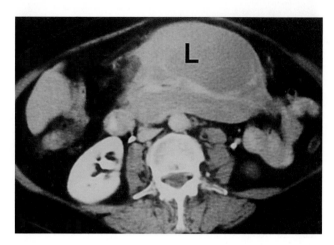

Fig. 2-81   Large, retroperitoneal lymph node mass (L) sand-wiching and compressing the retroperitoneal portion of the duodenal sweep.

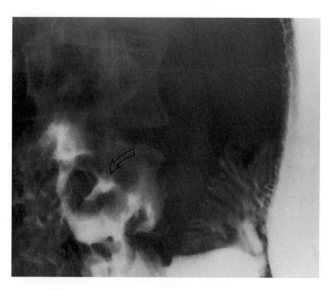

Fig. 2-82   Typical appearance of duodenal bulb ulcer with central ulcer crater (curved arrow) and surrounding edema.

incidence is less for women. The disease is a direct effect of the corrosive effect of gastric acid on the duodenal mucosa and the breakdown of normal protective anti-acid mechanisms within the duodenal bulb. Various risk factors are also thought to play an important role in the possible etiological origins of the disease. These include *H. pylori,* alcohol, and certain types of drugs, such as aspirin and other NSAIDs that also have a direct corrosive effect.

The presence of duodenal ulcer disease is probably not an isolated phenomenon and is simply a manifestation of one facet of the spectrum of peptic ulcer disease involving the distal esophagus, gastric antrum, and duodenal bulb. Careful evaluation of the stomach of patients with duodenal ulcer disease will almost always demonstrate gastritis. The incidence of peptic esophagitis in these patients is also increased.

Radiological diagnosis traditionally has been based upon a persistent barium collection seen within the duodenal bulb (Fig. 2-82). However, the advent of widespread use of endoscopy resulted in numerous assertions that the radiological evaluation of the duodenum for peptic ulcer disease was quite insensitive. The ability of the radiologist to demonstrate duodenal ulceration can be significantly improved if the examination of the duodenal bulb includes both good air-contrast views, as well as single-contrast views with compression (Fig. 2-83). Occasionally, a good portion, if not all, of the duodenal bulb may be ulcerated, resulting in a "giant duodenal ulcer" (Fig. 2-84). These ulcers may assume triangular configuration of the duodenal bulb and, as a result, be missed during UGI study. Certain factors should alert the radiologist to the possibility of a giant duodenal ulcer (Box 2-8). These include the unusual

persistence of barium within the duodenal bulb, little or no discernible fold pattern within the bulb, and postbulbar narrowing or spasm (Fig. 2-85).

Other causes

Duodenal ulcerations or erosions may be seen in a variety of other conditions, including the Zollinger-Ellison syndrome, Crohn's disease of the duodenum, tuberculosis of the small bowel, as well as ulceration resulting from viral diseases.

Duodenal Diverticulosis

Duodenal diverticula are seen on approximately 5% of routine UGI studies. They represent serosal and mucosal herniations through the muscular wall and are not true diverticula (Fig. 2-86). They usually occur in the second portion of the duodenum along the inner margin of the duodenal C-loop within 1 to 2 cm of the major papilla. Duodenal diverticula are usually only incidental findings. Complications, such as hemorrhage, infection, or enterolith formation, have been reported. On occasion, the papilla of Vater may empty directly into a duodenal diverticulum, resulting in the potential of difficult cannulation and possible perforation during endoscopic retrograde cholangiopancreatography.

Duodenal Positional Abnormalities

Midgut malrotation

Midgut malrotation is a result of incomplete rotation of the midgut during intrauterine life. Although this can predispose to midgut volvulus in children, it is more often seen as degrees of incomplete rotation and often as

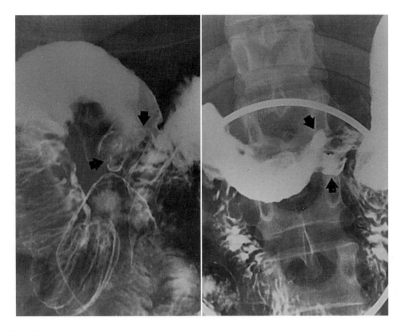

Fig. 2-83   Air-contrast views *(left)* suggest possibility of ulcer craters in the form of "ring shadows" *(arrows)*. Single-contrast compression views of the same area *(right)* demonstrate two well-defined ulcer craters *(arrows)*.

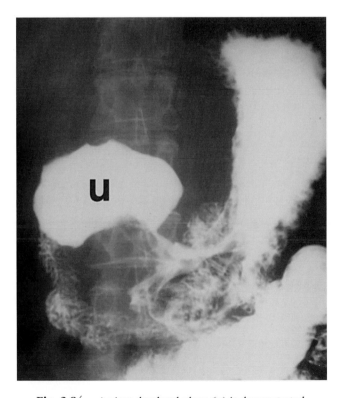

Fig. 2-84   A giant duodenal ulcer *(u)* is demonstrated.

Box 2-8   A Subtle Giant: The Giant Duodenal Ulcer

RADIOLOGICAL SIGNS

Little, if any, fold pattern in duodenal bulb
No change in configuration of bulb
Always with postbulbar narrowing
Barium retained, especially on delayed images

spine. The position of the cecum is quite variable, but in complete malrotation it is located largely in the left abdomen.

Displacement of C-loop by extrinsic mass

Any large mass in the upper abdomen can displace the C-loop of the duodenum. The most common are masses arising from the pancreas, stomach, kidney, or adrenals.

Paraduodenal hernias

Paraduodenal hernias occur when there is incomplete fixation of the posterior peritoneum and potential spaces develop. Bowel loops can be sequestered in these potential spaces. If the paraduodenal hernia is on the right, the ligament of Treitz and the entire C-loop may be displaced. Left-sided paraduodenal hernias are 2 to 3 times more common. These conditions may be associated with vague upper abdominal symptoms or can be found as an incidental finding on an UGI study (Fig. 2-87).

an incidental finding. The location of the ligament of Treitz (marking the duodenal-jejunal junction) is key to making this diagnosis. The ligament is located inferiorly and medially to its expected position. In cases of complete malrotation it is located to the right of the

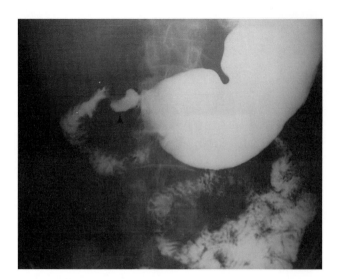

Fig. 2-85 A large, somewhat triangular barium collection *(arrowhead)* looks like a deformed duodenal bulb. However, note (1) absence of folds in "duodenal bulb"; (2) postbulbar narrowing; and (3) persistence of barium in "bulb" on delayed films. These three signs are very suggestive of a giant duodenal ulcer, which this proved to be.

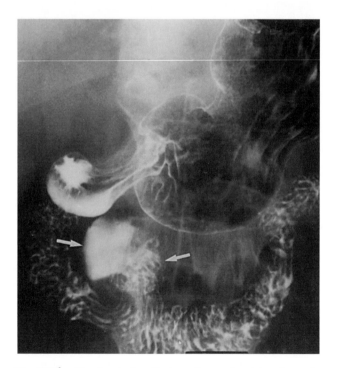

Fig. 2-86 Duodenal diverticulum *(arrows)* arising from the medial aspect of the transverse duodenum.

Intrathoracic stomachs

Displacement and distortion of the duodenal sweep can also be seen in patients with exceedingly large hiatal hernias, in which most of the stomach is intrathoracic in position. The ligament of Treitz may be pulled medially.

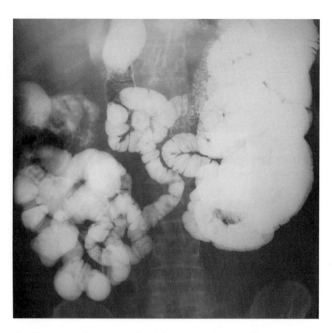

Fig. 2-87 Left paraduodenal hernia. Patient with vague upper abdominal complaints. UGI study and small bowel follow-though disclose sequestration of small bowel loops in the left upper quadrant. Only a few loops of ileum are seen before cecum is reached.

Lesser sac hernias

Lesser sac hernias are uncommon and result when loops of bowel pass through the foramen of Winslow (epiploic foramen) and become sequestered in the lesser sac behind the stomach.

SUGGESTED READINGS

Balfe DM, Koehler RE, Karstaedt N, et al: Computed tomography of gastric neoplasms, *Radiology* 140:431-436, 1981.

Balthazar EJ, Rosenberg H, Davidian MM: Scirrhous carcinoma of the pyloric channel and distal antrum, *AJR* 134:669-673, 1980.

Blaser MJ: Gastric Campylobacter-like organisms, gastritis, and peptic ulcer disease, *Gastroenterology* 93:371-383, 1987.

Bothen NF, Eklof O: Diverticula and duplications (enterogenous cysts) of the stomach and duodenum, *AJR* 96:375-381, 1966.

Buchholz PR, Haisten AS: Phytobezoars following gastric surgery for duodenal ulcer, *Surg Clin North Am* 52:341-352, 1972.

Butz WC: Giant hypertrophic gastritis, *Gastroenterology* 39: 183-190, 1960.

Camblos JF: Acute volvulus of the stomach, *Am Surg* 35:505-509, 1969.

Choi SH, Sheehan FR, Pickren JW: Metastatic involvement of the stomach by breast cancer, *Cancer* 17:791-797, 1964.

Chuang VP, Wallace S, Stroehlein JR, et al: Hepatic artery infusion chemotherapy: gastroduodenal complications, *AJR* 137:347-350, 1981.

Clements JL, Jinkins JR, Torres WE, et al: Antral mucosal diaphragms in adults, *AJR* 113:1105-1111, 1979.

Cohen S, Laufer I, Snape WJ, et al: The gastrointestinal manifestations of scleroderma: pathogenesis and management, *Gastroenterology* 79:155-166, 1980.

Cohen Y, Heun SW: Phytobezoar after gastrectomy, *Br J Surg* 58:236-237, 1971.

Cotton PB, Shorvon PJ: Analysis of endoscopy and radiography in the diagnosis, follow-up and treatment of peptic ulcer disease, *Clin Gastroenterol* 13:383-403, 1984.

Davenport HW: Salicylate damage to the gastric mucosal barrier, *N Engl J Med* 276:1307-1312, 1967.

Delikaris P, Golematis B, Missitziz J, et al: Smooth muscle neoplasms of the stomach, *South Med J* 76:440-442, 1983.

Dodd GD, Sheft D: Diverticulum of the greater curvature of the stomach: a roentgenologic curiosity, *AJR* 107:102-104, 1969.

Dooley CP, Cohen H: The clinical significance of Campylobacter pylori, *Ann Intern Med* 108:70-79, 1988.

Edelman MJ, March TL: Eosinophilic gastroenteritis, *AJR* 91:773-778, 1964.

Farman J, Faegenburg D, Dallemand S, et al: Crohn's disease of the stomach: the "ram's horn" sign, *AJR* 123:242-251, 1975.

Feczko PJ, Halpert RD, Ackerman LV: Gastric polyps: radiological evaluation and clinical significance, *Radiology* 155:581-584, 1985.

Feliciano DV, Van Heerden JA: Pyloric antral mucosal webs, *Mayo Clin Proc* 52:650-653, 1977.

Felson B, Berkmen YM, Anastacio MH: Gastric mucosal diaphragm, *Radiology* 92:513-517, 1969.

Gelfand DW, Moskowitz M: Massive gastric dilatation complicating hypotonic duodenography, *Radiology* 97:637-639, 1970.

Gerson DE, Lewicki AM: Intrathoracic stomach: when does it obstruct? *Radiology* 119:257-264, 1976.

Ghahremani GG: Nonobstructive mucosal diaphragms or rings of the gastric antrum in adults, *AJR* 121:236-247, 1974.

Goldberg HI: Radiographic evaluation of peptic ulcer disease, *J Clin Gastroenterol* 3(suppl 2):57-65, 1981.

Goldner FH, Boyce HW: Relationship of bile in the stomach to gastritis, *Gastrointest Endosc* 22:197-199, 1976.

Goldstein HM, Cohen LE, Hagen R, et al: Gastric bezoars: a frequent complication in the postoperative ulcer patient, *Radiology* 107:341-344, 1973.

Goldstein SS, Lewis JH, Rothstein R: Intestinal obstruction due to bezoars, *Am J Gastroenterol* 79:313-318, 1984.

Gonzalez G, Kennedy T: Crohn's disease of the stomach, *Radiology* 113:27-29, 1974.

Goodwin CS, Armstrong JA, Marshall BJ: Campylobacter pyloridis, gastritis and peptic ulceration, *J Clin Pathol* 39:353-365, 1986.

Hricak H, Thoeni RF, Margulis AR, et al: Extension of gastric lymphoma into the esophagus and duodenum, *Radiology* 135:309-312, 1980.

Hyson EA, Burrell M, Toffler R: Drug-induced gastrointestinal disease, *Gastrointest Radiol* 2:183-212, 1977.

Ishikura H, Sato F, Naka H, et al: Inflammatory fibroid polyp of the stomach, *Acta Pathol Jpn* 36:327-335, 1986.

Ivey KJ: Drugs, gastritis, and peptic ulcer, *J Clin Gastroenterol* 3(suppl 2):29-34, 1981.

Jacobs DS: Primary gastric lymphoma and pseudolymphoma, *Am J Clin Pathol* 40:379-394, 1963.

Joffe N: Some unusual roentgenologic findings associated with marked gastric dilatation, *AJR* 119:291-299, 1973.

Johnson OA, Hoskins DW, Todd J, et al: Crohn's disease of the stomach, *Gastroenterology* 50:571-577, 1966.

Jolobe OM, Montgomery RD: Changing clinical pattern of gastric ulcer: are anti-inflammatory drugs involved? *Digestion* 29:164-170, 1984.

Kilman WJ, Berk RN: The spectrum of radiological features of aberrant pancreatic rests involving the stomach, *Radiology* 123:291-296, 1977.

Kobayashi S, Prolla JC, Kirsner JB: Late gastric carcinoma developing after surgery for benign conditions: endoscopic and histologic studies of the anastomosis and diagnostic problems, *Am J Dig Dis* 15:905-912, 1970.

Kressel HY: Peptic disease of the stomach and duodenum. In Margulis AR, Burhenne HJ, editors: *Alimentry tract radiology,* ed 3, St Louis, 1983, Mosby.

Laufer I, Hamilton J, Mullens JE: Demonstration of superficial gastric erosions by double contrast radiography, *Gastroenterology* 68:387-391, 1975.

Levine MS, Creteur V, Kressel HY, et al: Benign gastric ulcers: diagnosis and follow-up with double contrast radiography *Radiology* 164:9-13, 1987.

Llancza PP, Salt WB: Gastric volvulus: more common than previously thought? *Postgrad Med* 80:279-288, 1986.

Loo FD, Palmer DW, Soergel KH, et al: Gastric emptying in patients with diabetes mellitus, *Gastroenterology* 86:485-494, 1984.

Lucas CE, Sugawa C, Riddle J, et al: Natural history and surgical dilemma of "stress" gastric bleeding, *Arch Surg* 102:266-273, 1971.

Marks IN, Bank S, Werbeloff L, et al: The natural history of corrosive gastritis: report of five cases, *Am J Dig Dis* 6:509-524, 1963.

Martel W, Abell MR, Allan TNK: Lymphoreticular hyperplasia of the stomach (pseudolymphoma), *AJR* 127:261-265, 1976.

Menuck LS: Gastric lymphoma, a radiologic diagnosis, *Gastrointest Radiol* 1:157-161, 1976.

Menuck LS, Amberg JR: Metastatic disease involving the stomach, *Am J Dig Dis* 20:903-913, 1975.

Menuck L: Plain film findings of gastric volvulus herniating into the chest, *AJR* 126:1169-1174, 1976.

Muhletaler CA, Gerlock AJ, Desoto L, et al: Gastro duodenal lesions of ingested acids: radiographic findings, *AJR* 135:1247-1252, 1980.

Neimark S, Rogers AI: Gastric polyps: a review, *Am J Gastroenterol* 77:585-587, 1982.

Nelson SW: Some interesting and unusual manifestations of Crohn's disease (regional enteritis) of the stomach, duodenum, and small intestine, *AJR* 107:86-101, 1969.

Olmstead WW, Cooper PH, Madewell JE: Involvement of the gastric antrum in Ménétrier's disease, *AJR* 126:524-529, 1976.

Ominsky SH, Moss AA: The postoperative stomach: a comparative study of double-contrast barium examinations and endoscopy, *Gastrointest Radiol* 4:17-21, 1979.

Op den Orth JO, Dekker WL: Gastric adenomas, *Radiology* 141:289-293, 1981.

Ott DJ, Chen YM, Gelfand DW, et al: Radiographic accuracy in gastric ulcer: comparison of single-contrast and multiphasic examination, *AJR* 147:697-700, 1986.

Ott DJ, Munitz HA, Gelfand DW, et al: The sensitivity of radiography of the postoperative stomach, *Radiology* 144: 741-743, 1982.

Overholt BF, Jeffries GH: Hypertrophic hypersecreting protein-losing gastropathy, *Gastroenterology* 58:80-87, 1970.

Patterson CP, Combs MJ, Marshall BJ: Helicobacter pylori and peptic ulcer disease: evolution to revolution to resolution, *AJR* 168:1415-1420, 1997.

Pearson S: Aberrant pancreas, *Arch Surg* 63:168-184, 1951.

Perez CA, Dorfman RF: Benign lymphoid hyperplasia of the stomach and duodenum, *Radiology* 87:505-510, 1966.

Pillari G, Weinreb J, Vernace F, et al: CT of gastric masses: image patterns and a note on potential pitfalls, *Gastrointest Radiol* 8:11-17, 1983.

Poppel MH: Gastric intussusceptions, *Radiology* 78:608-620, 1962.

Pruitt BA, Goodwin CW: Stress ulcer disease in the burned patient, *World J Surg* 5:209-222, 1981.

Raotma H, Angervall L, Dahl I, et al: Clinical and morphological studies of giant hypertrophic gastritis (Ménétrier's disease), *Acta Med Scand* 195:247-252, 1974.

Reese DF, Hodgson JR, Dockerty MB: Giant hypertrophy of the gastric mucosa (Ménétrier's disease): a correlation of the roentgenographic, pathologic and clinical findings, *AJR* 88:619-626, 1962.

Scatarige JC, Fishman EK, Jones B, et al: Gastric leiomyosarcoma: CT observations, *J Comput Assist Tomogr* 9:320-327, 1985.

Scharschmidt BF: The natural history of hypertrophic gastropathy, *Am J Med* 63:644-652, 1977.

Schuman BM, Waldbaum JR, Hiltz SW, et al: Carcinoma of the gastric remnant in the U.S. population, *Gastrointest Endosc* 30:71-73, 1984.

Sohn JS, Levine MS, Furth EE, et al: Helicobacter pylori gastritis: radiographic findings, *Radiology* 195:763-767, 1995.

Thoeni RF, Gedgaudas RK: Ectopic pancreas: usual and unusual features, *Gastrointest Radiol* 5:37-42, 1980.

Thompson G, Somers S, Stevenson GW: Benign gastric ulcer: a reliable radiologic diagnosis? *AJR* 141:331-333, 1983.

Thompson WM, Kelvin FM, Gedgaudas RK, et al: Radiologic investigation of peptic ulcer disease, *Radiol Clin North Am* 20:701-720, 1982.

Tomasulo J: Gastric polyps: histologic types and their relationship to gastric carcinoma, *Cancer* 18:721-726, 1965.

Treichel J, Gerstenberg E, Palme G, et al: Diagnosis of partial diverticula, *Radiology* 119:13-18, 1976.

Turner CJ, Lipitz LR, Pastore RA: Antral gastritis, *Radiology* 113:305-312, 1974.

Wallace RG, Howard WB: Acute superior mesenteric artery syndrome in the severely burned patient, *Radiology* 94:307-310, 1970.

Weinstein WM: Gastritis. In Sleisenger MH, Fordtran JS, editors: *Gastrointestinal disease: pathophysiology, diagnosis, management,* Philadelphia, 1983, WB Saunders.

EXAMINATION TECHNIQUES

The mesenteric small bowel extends from the ligament of Treitz to the ileocecal valve and consists of the jejunum and ileum, which are entirely intraperitoneal and are attached posteriorly to a mesentery.

Plain films of the abdomen are often the first radiological examination obtained in evaluating suspected small bowel disease, particularly obstruction or adynamic ileus. Their role is confined mainly to the emergency or postoperative patient. The standard supine film (kidneys, ureters, and bladder) can be supplemented with erect or lateral decubitus films to detect air-fluid levels or free intraperitoneal air.

A wide variety of fluoroscopic procedures using barium are available for studying the mesenteric small bowel. Nonintubation methods include the small bowel follow-through examination (performed in conjunction with an upper gastrointestinal series) and the dedicated small bowel study (in which only the small bowel is examined) (Fig. 3-1). Both methods use an approximately 40% weight/volume barium suspension. A dedicated small bowel study should include intermittent fluoroscopy with palpation and spot-filming of suspect areas, along with routine overhead films.

Intubation methods (small bowel enema or enteroclysis) are performed by injecting barium directly through a tube (12 to 14F) placed fluoroscopically into the jejunum. These procedures include single-contrast techniques (using barium alone) and double-contrast techniques (using air or methylcellulose in addition to barium) (Fig. 3-2). This method employs a denser barium, typically 50% to 80% weight/volume, depending on the method used. Careful graded compression under fluoroscopy is imperative in both nonintubation and intubation examinations to unfold and separate overlapping small bowel loops. The drawbacks to the intubation methods include higher radiation dose because of fluoroscopy, discomfort to the patient (some patients require mild sedation), and complications related to the intubation or reflux of contrast with aspiration. However, this method also has an increased yield in detecting subtle mucosal pathology or mass lesions.

A peroral pneumocolon is sometimes used to improve visualization of the distal small bowel. This procedure is performed during a small bowel follow-through examination or small bowel meal. When barium has reached the terminal ileum or cecum, air is insufflated into the rectum. Intravenous glucagon is usually given to promote reflux of air from the colon through the ileocecal valve. This distends the distal small bowel lumen and creates a double-contrast appearance. The distal small bowel can also be examined by retrograde injection of barium, either through a preexisting ileostomy or through the colon with reflux across the ileocecal valve.

Water-soluble contrast material can be used to confirm the position of jejunostomy tubes (or other percutaneously placed small bowel catheters) because barium injected into the peritoneal cavity through an incorrectly positioned tube may cause peritonitis. Water-soluble contrast material, however, is not useful for routine evaluation of the small bowel because the hyperosmolar contrast material draws fluid into the bowel lumen, causing progressive dilution of the contrast material and rendering the study nondiagnostic. In cases of suspected small bowel obstruction, hyperosmolar water-soluble contrast material is contraindicated because it causes worsening of the luminal distention.

Computed tomography (CT) is useful for studying many forms of small bowel disease (Fig. 3-3). Its excellent evaluation of the bowel wall and extrinsic processes is complementary to conventional contrast studies, which are better for demonstrating motility and mucosal abnormalities. The rapid scanning times now widely available with CT, particularly spiral CT, prevent

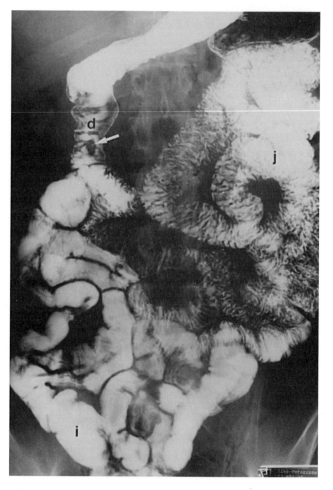

Fig. 3-1   Normal small bowel follow-through examination demonstrates fold patterns of duodenum (d), jejunum (j), and ileum (i). An ovoid filling defect in the mid-descending duodenum (arrow) represents the normal ampulla seen en face.

image degradation by peristalsis of bowel loops. Adequate bowel opacification is essential for optimal display of small bowel abnormalities on CT. Four 8-oz cups of dilute barium or dilute water-soluble contrast material are administered over a 45-minute period beginning 1 hour before scanning.

Ultrasound may detect distended fluid-filled loops of small bowel in cases of obstruction and a thickened bowel wall resulting from inflammatory or neoplastic disease. The usefulness of ultrasound is limited, however, because of deflection of sound waves by air within the small bowel lumen. However, since ultrasound is often one of the first modalities used in evaluating patients with acute abdominal complaints, it may detect unsuspected small bowel pathology before other studies.

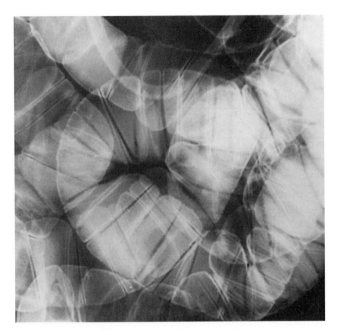

Fig. 3-2   Spot film from a double-contrast enteroclysis examination demonstrates jejunal fold pattern.

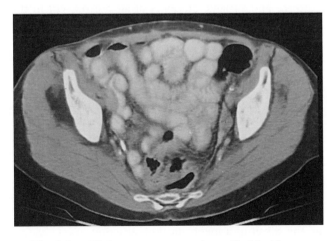

Fig. 3-3   CT demonstrates normal opacified ileal loops.

The most commonly used nuclear imaging technique pertaining to the small bowel is the Meckel's scan (for detecting ectopic gastric mucosa in Meckel's diverticula), which uses technetium pertechnetate, which is excreted by gastric mucosa. Another frequent use of nuclear studies is the gastrointestinal (GI) bleeding scan, using radioactive sulfur colloid or labeled red blood cells. Occasionally, radionuclides that detect inflammatory conditions are used in evaluating the small bowels of patients with Crohn's disease and other inflammatory conditions.

Angiography is used primarily for demonstrating and treating vascular thrombosis and hemorrhage involving the small bowel, in both the acute and the chronic states. It is unique in that treatment of these small bowel conditions can be performed in selected circumstances.

Various drugs have an effect on small bowel motility, and these can sometimes be employed to assist in small bowel evaluation. Metoclopramide has a dual effect on the intestinal tract. First, it aids in increasing gastric emptying, helping deliver barium to the small bowel faster. Next, it increases small bowel peristalsis. It can be given intravenously for immediate effect, or given orally, which usually requires 30 minutes for action. It is primarily used during intubation examination of the small bowel. A variety of drugs decrease small bowel motility. The most commonly used is glucagon. Even doses smaller than 1 mg can have a profound hypotonic effect on the small intestine, and this usually lasts for 15 to 30 minutes. It must be given intramuscularly or intravenously. It should also be noted that anticholinergics such as morphine compounds, atropine, and diphenoxylate will also affect small bowel transit.

RADIOLOGICAL EVALUATION

As noted above, the radiologist has a variety of modalities available to evaluate for possible small bowel disease. It is beyond the scope of this book to indicate which methods are most efficacious for evaluating a particular small bowel condition, whether suspected or real. Currently there is some controversy concerning these different methods, and each has its own proponents. In choosing what study to perform, other factors enter into the decision, particularly what equipment may be available (CT) and the particular skill or comfort level of the radiologist with a given technique. Perhaps the most important factor is the clinician managing the patient. Often the clinicians have a particular approach to a clinical situation with which they feel comfortable, and radiologists must communicate with clinicians regarding what they believe is the best modality to use.

Regardless of the imaging methods, there are several features of the small bowel that are consistent with all

Box 3-1 The Rule of "3s": Abnormal Small Bowel Measurements

Small bowel diameter—3 cm or greater
Small bowel folds—3 mm or greater
Small bowel wall thickness—3 mm or greater
Difference between air-fluid levels in a single loop of bowel—3 cm or greater (usually indicates mechanical obstruction rather than adynamic ileus)

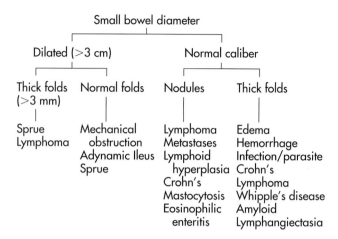

Fig. 3-4   Basic algorithm for small bowel disease. Many diseases have a variable appearance.

examination types and will be referred to frequently throughout the chapter.

- Diameter. The maximum normal diameter of the small bowel is 3 cm. With intubation methods, this is frequently exceeded, and differences in bowel diameter, rather than the actual size, become more important for evaluation.
- Fold thickness. The folds of the small bowel (valvulae conniventes) are typically 1.5 to 2 mm in size. When the size of the valvulae begins to reach or exceed 3 mm over a segment of bowel and is fairly consistent during the study, it should be considered abnormal.
- Bowel wall thickness. The distance between two loops of bowel is the width of two bowel walls. Since each bowel wall is usually less than 1.5 mm in diameter, the distance between bowel loops should not exceed 3 mm. This must be measured at adjacent loops of bowel that are adequately distended.
- Differential air-fluid levels. This is evaluated on upright abdominal radiographs and indicates the difference in air-fluid levels in a single loop of bowel. When this difference exceeds 3 cm, the likelihood of a mechanical obstruction increases.
- Secretions. Typically there is no discernible fluid in the small bowel. If excess fluid is encountered, seen as dilution of the barium column, then this should be considered abnormal.
- Transit time. There is such a great variation in transit time that this criterion is almost meaningless.

One rule of thumb to use in evaluating the small bowel is the rule of "3s." In reviewing the criteria above, it is apparent that most small bowel measurements are considered abnormal once they reach "3" or greater (Box 3-1).

Radiologists frequently like to use an algorithmic approach in evaluating an organ in which a multitude of diseases may occur, such as the small bowel. We have included one for your convenience (Fig. 3-4). However, it should be noted that many diseases do not lend

themselves to simple classification. Also, some diseases such as lymphoma or Crohn's disease can present in a variety of appearances. Because of this, it is not recommended that one adhere too closely to this approach.

DILATED SMALL BOWEL

Mechanical Obstruction Resulting in Distention

Adhesions

Dilatation of the small bowel occurs in a wide variety of conditions, some associated with mechanical obstruction and others in which no obstructing lesion is present. The most common obstructing lesion causing distention of the mesenteric small bowel is an adhesion or band, usually resulting from previous abdominal surgery. Supine plain films typically demonstrate distended air-filled loops of small bowel, identified by the linear folds traversing the circumference of the bowel lumen (valvulae conniventes or plicae circulares) (Fig. 3-5). Distended loops may lie in a tiered or stepladder pattern, and variable amounts of air are present in the colon, depending on the level, grade, and duration of the obstruction. Distended small bowel loops containing mostly fluid (with little or no air) usually appear as a gasless abdomen on supine films.

On erect or lateral decubitus films, the small amounts of air rise within the dilated fluid-filled loops to form a series of bubbles or short air-fluid levels (string of pearls). When more air is present, air-fluid levels are longer and often appear at different heights within the same bowel loop (differential levels). Differential air-fluid levels can be seen in both mechanical obstruction and adynamic ileus. However, when the separation of the air-fluid levels exceeds 3 cm, then it is more likely to be the result of a mechanical obstruction.

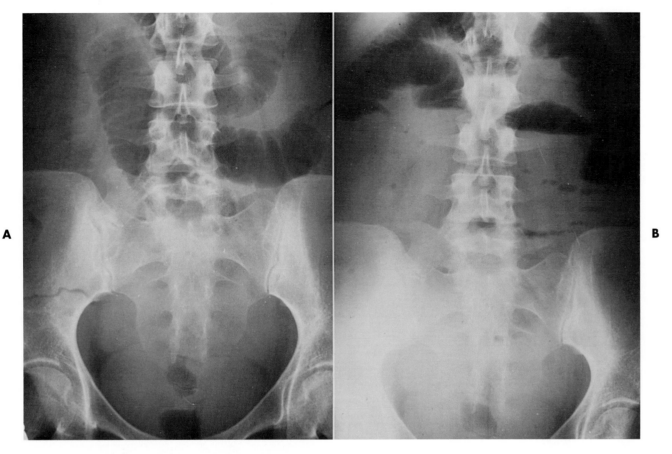

Fig. 3-5 **A,** Supine film demonstrates multiple dilated small bowel loops in a patient with small bowel obstruction secondary to adhesions. **B,** Upright film shows associated air-fluid levels.

Although small bowel obstruction resulting from an adhesion may spontaneously resolve, continued or worsening symptoms may lead to barium studies to delineate the level, cause, and severity of the obstruction. In an incomplete small bowel obstruction, a transition zone can be detected between the dilated loops proximal to the obstruction and the normal caliber loops distal to it. An adhesion appears as a well-defined linear impression crossing the bowel lumen at the site of obstruction. Entrapment of a loop of bowel by one or more adhesions may result in a closed-loop obstruction.

CT is also useful for evaluating suspected small bowel obstruction. In addition to possibly determining the site of obstruction, CT can provide information about intramural and extraintestinal disease, which may indicate the cause of obstruction.

Hernias

External and internal hernias containing small bowel may be associated with obstruction and proximal distention and, like adhesive bands, sometimes cause closed-loop obstruction. Inguinal hernias are common and may contain a variable length of ileum. Paraumbilical hernias, incisional hernias involving the anterior or lateral abdominal wall, and spigelian hernias (caused by weakness at the lateral aspects of the rectus abdominis muscles) may all contain loops of small bowel. Other unusual external hernias include femoral, obturator, sciatic, peristomal, and lumbar types.

Internal hernias usually represent defects in the mesentery or peritoneum and include paraduodenal, pericecal, and intersigmoid hernias (Fig 3-6). Small bowel loops rarely extend into the lesser sac through the foramen of Winslow.

On contrast studies, hernias containing small bowel may be indicated by abnormal location or clustering of loops (Fig. 3-7). Smooth extrinsic compression on the loops as they enter and exit the hernia is also a useful finding on contrast studies. Supplementary examination in the lateral position is usually necessary to detect herniation through the anterior abdominal wall because this is easily obscured on frontal films. CT is often useful in displaying the abnormal location of herniated loops of bowel and may also define other hernia contents, including colon and omentum (Fig. 3-8).

Volvulus

Small bowel volvulus occurs when a loop of bowel twists around its mesenteric axis. Primary volvulus is seen mostly in children as a result of intestinal malrotation, whereas secondary volvulus occurs in adults and is associated with preexisting factors, including adhesions, internal hernias, and tumors. Torsion of a bowel loop causes constriction of its mesenteric vascular supply and often results in ischemia or infarction if not treated promptly. Plain films and barium studies are frequently nonspecific, but CT is useful in demonstrating dilated loops of small bowel radially distributed around the twisted edematous mesentery (Fig. 3-9).

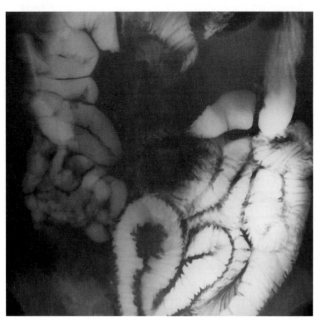

Fig. 3-6   Note small bowel loops in the right upper quadrant with displacement of the duodenum. This patient has a paraduodenal hernia.

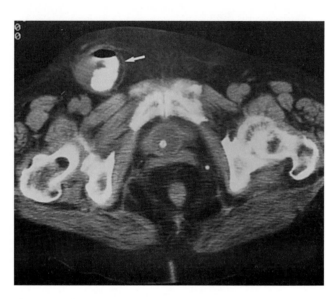

Fig. 3-8   CT shows an opacified loop of bowel in a right inguinal hernia *(arrow)*.

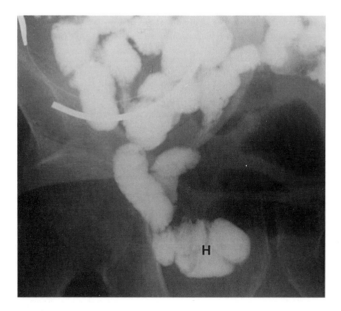

Fig. 3-7   A loop of distal ileum *(H)* overlying the right pubic bone lies in an inguinal hernia.

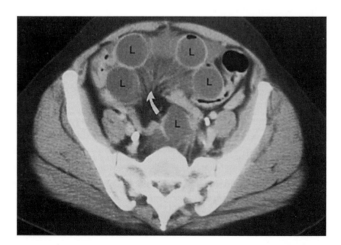

Fig. 3-9   CT demonstrates fluid-filled small bowel loops *(L)* around edematous mesentery *(curved arrow)*. (From Goodman P, Raval B: CT diagnosis of acquired small bowel volvulus, *Am Surg* 56:628, 1990.)

Intussusception

Intussusception represents invagination or telescoping of a bowel loop to form an inner loop (intussusceptum) enclosed within an outer loop (intussuscipiens). The inner loop and its associated mesentery may become edematous and cause a small bowel obstruction. In adults, small bowel intussusception is usually caused by a tumor or other mass acting as a lead point, and symptoms are often sporadic. On barium examination, small bowel intussusception typically demonstrates a coil-spring appearance, denoting barium trapped between the inner and outer loops of bowel (Fig. 3-10). CT shows the inner loop and its mesentery surrounded by the outer loop and may identify the lead mass (Fig. 3-11).

Neoplasms

Various intrinsic neoplasms, both primary and metastatic, can occlude the small bowel lumen (Fig. 3-12).

Nonneoplastic strictures

Intrinsic inflammatory, infectious, and ischemic processes can lead to stricture formation with distention of proximal small bowel loops. Postoperative anastomotic strictures may also cause proximal obstruction.

Intraluminal masses

Intraluminal masses may cause small bowel obstruction by occluding the lumen. These masses most commonly lodge at the ileocecal valve and include impacted foreign bodies and gallstones (gallstone ileus).

In meconium ileus equivalent, inspissated fecal material obstructs the distal ileum in children or adults with cystic fibrosis. This complication may be prevented by routine ingestion of pancreatic enzyme supplements.

Extrinsic masses

Likewise, extrinsic inflammatory and neoplastic masses can compress and obstruct adjacent small bowel loops. This is less important in the mesenteric small bowel than in the duodenum, which is fixed and in close proximity to many organs including the pancreas, right kidney, gallbladder, and liver.

Colonic lesions

Colonic lesions, particularly carcinoma of the proximal colon, may produce distended loops of small bowel with little or no air in the colon. This mimics a distal small bowel obstruction but is easily evaluated with a barium enema.

Distention without Obstruction (Adynamic Ileus)

Sprue

Small bowel distention can also occur in the absence of a mechanical obstruction. Nontropical sprue (celiac disease), a reversible condition caused by malabsorption of dietary gluten, typically produces dilatation of proximal small bowel loops because of hypersecretion of fluid. Flocculation, segmentation, and a moulage (fea-

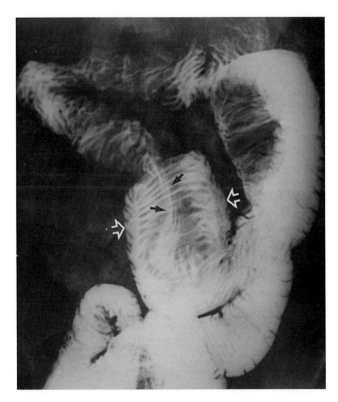

Fig. 3-10   Small bowel intussusception demonstrates intussusceptum *(arrows)* and intussuscipiens *(open arrows)*.

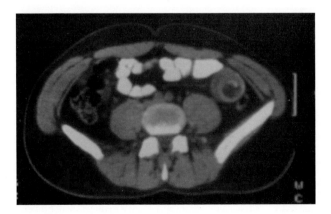

Fig. 3-11   On the left side of the abdomen there is a large intraluminal mass with associated rings about it. This is consistent with a tumor producing intussusception.

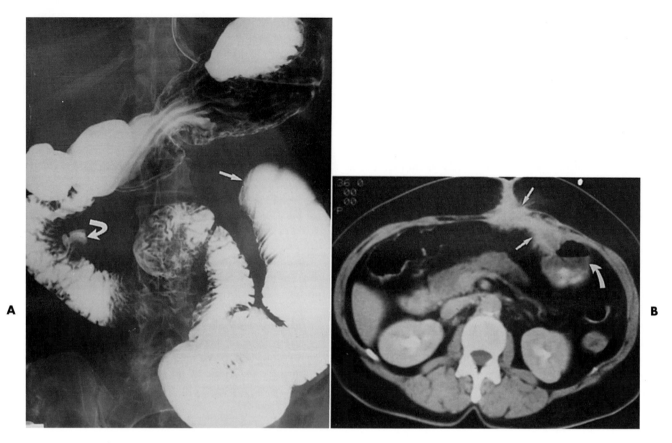

Fig. 3-12 **A,** Complete jejunal obstruction *(arrow)* with proximal dilatation. A duodenal diverticulum is also noted *(curved arrow)*. **B,** CT shows an irregular soft tissue mass *(arrows)* in the anterior abdominal wall adjacent to a distended bowel loop *(curved arrow)*. This represents metastatic colon carcinoma.

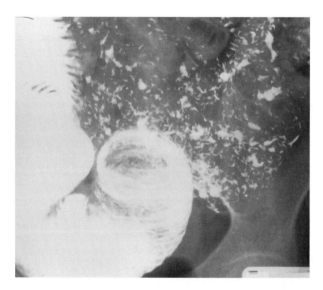

Fig. 3-13 Classic coil-spring appearance in distal small bowel in patient with sprue. These intussusceptions in sprue are usually transient.

tureless or castlike) appearance of the barium column were once considered classic features of sprue but are less often demonstrated with the improved barium suspensions now widely available. An increase in separation of jejunal folds is suggestive of sprue and is best demonstrated with enteroclysis technique. Sprue is associated with an increased incidence of small bowel intussusception, which occurs without a lead mass and is typically transitory and asymptomatic (Fig. 3-13). Other complications of sprue include small bowel ulcerations or strictures (ulcerative enteritis), lymphoma, adenocarcinoma of the proximal small bowel, squamous cell carcinoma of the esophagus, hyposplenism, and a rare condition known as cavitating lymph node syndrome (Box 3-2).

Tropical sprue occurs in certain tropical locations and radiographically appears similar to nontropical sprue. However, unlike nontropical sprue, the tropical form is associated with severe vitamin B_{12} and folic acid deficiencies and megaloblastic anemia. Tropical sprue responds to folic acid or antibiotic therapy but not to a gluten-free diet.

Lactose intolerance and other hypersecretory states

Lactose intolerance is a common cause of malabsorption in adults that results from acquired deficiency of the enzyme lactase in the small bowel. Following a lactose-containing meal, hypersecretion of fluid into the small bowel causes luminal distention and symptoms of bloating and cramps. Lactose intolerance is easily treated by either eliminating dairy products from the diet or supplementing the diet with commercially available lactase enzymes. Other hypersecretory states including Zollinger-Ellison syndrome and cryptosporidial enteritis may likewise cause small bowel distention as a result of increased fluid content.

Neuromuscular and motility abnormalities

Various neuromuscular and motility abnormalities can affect the small bowel and lead to luminal distention. The best known of these is scleroderma (progressive systemic sclerosis), in which smooth muscle atrophies and is replaced by fibrous tissue (Fig. 3-14). In the mesenteric small bowel, smooth asymmetric sacculations (pseudodiverticula) are sometimes seen. Crowding of folds (hidebound bowel) is a characteristic finding of scleroderma involving the small bowel. Spinal cord injuries can also result in bowel dilatation, often on a chronic basis.

Chagas' disease, a parasitic infection common in Brazil, can cause distention of the duodenum and mesenteric small bowel by destroying the neural plexus. Associated abnormalities are often seen in the esophagus, colon, and heart.

Peritonitis or severe abdominal pain

Peritonitis, severe abdominal pain, and recent abdominal surgery are important causes of adynamic ileus, a condition characterized by decreased peristalsis of the bowel. Supine abdominal films reveal distention of small bowel, colon, or both, and upright films typically show air-fluid levels to be at equal heights within the same bowel loop (nondifferential levels). Localized abdominal

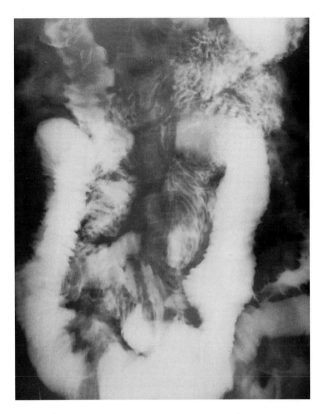

Fig. 3-14 Diffuse mild dilatation of the small bowel as seen in scleroderma.

pain caused by conditions such as appendicitis, cholecystitis, or pancreatitis may be associated with focal bowel dilatation and air-fluid levels (sentinel loops).

Other causes

Other causes of adynamic ileus include drugs (anticholinergics, morphine), metabolic disorders resulting in electrolyte imbalance, and previous vagotomy. Idiopathic pseudoobstruction is a chronic form of adynamic ileus of unknown etiology. Ischemia resulting from thromboembolic disease, vasculitis, or low-flow states may decrease small bowel motility and increase distention. Associated fold thickening caused by intramural edema or hemorrhage may also be present.

NARROWED SMALL BOWEL

Narrowing Resulting from Intrinsic Abnormality

Narrowing of the small bowel lumen can result from numerous intrinsic and extrinsic processes.

Crohn's disease

Crohn's disease (regional enteritis) is usually confined to the terminal ileum but may involve any portion of the small bowel. Early in the disease, spasm and edema associated with ulcerations can cause luminal narrowing, and later in the disease, continued inflammation and fibrosis often lead to stricture formation (Figs. 3-15 and 3-16). Skip lesions consisting of narrowed segments of small bowel separated by normal or dilated segments are sometimes noted. These can produce bizarre radiographic findings although clinically the patient may not be that symptomatic.

Neoplasms

Primary neoplasms of the small bowel, including adenocarcinoma, lymphoma, leiomyosarcoma, and carcinoid tumor, can cause focal narrowing of the lumen (Fig. 3-17). Primary tumors do this by infiltration of the bowel wall, which is more typically seen with carcinoma. Lymphomas and sarcomas may either narrow or dilate the lumen. Carcinoid tumors narrow the lumen by their associated desmoplastic response, producing fibrosis and kinking. Metastatic spread to the small bowel through contiguous, peritoneal, or hematogenous routes can also lead to one or more areas of narrowing.

Zollinger-Ellison syndrome

Involvement of the distal duodenum and proximal jejunum is uncommon in peptic ulcer disease but sometimes occurs in severe ulcer diathesis, as seen in Zollinger-Ellison syndrome, because of the increased acidity in the proximal small bowel.

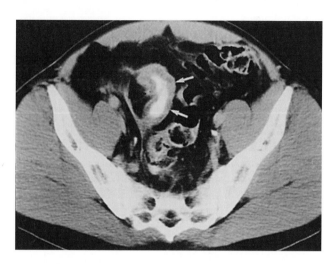

Fig. 3-16   CT shows thickened wall *(arrows)* of distal ileum in a patient with Crohn's disease.

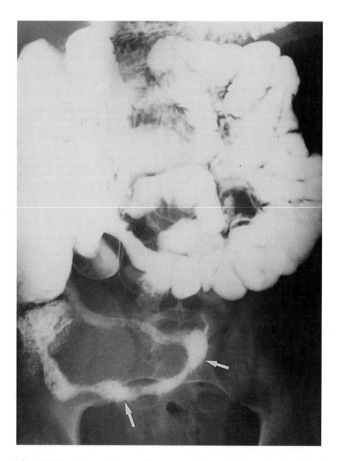

Fig. 3-15   Narrowing and mucosal irregularity of the distal ileum *(arrows)* associated with separation of bowel loops in a patient with Crohn's disease.

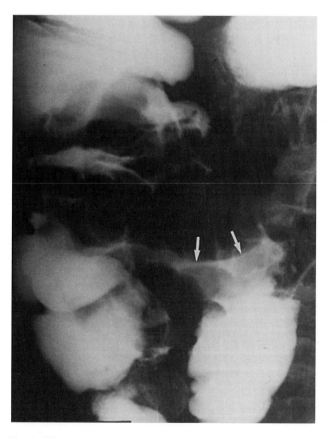

Fig. 3-17   Large polypoid mass in the ileocecal region causing narrowing of the terminal ileum *(arrows)* represents non-Hodgkin's lymphoma.

Graft-versus-host disease

Graft-versus-host disease is a potential complication of bone marrow transplantation in immunocompromised patients and represents rejection of the patient's own tissues by the donor bone marrow lymphocytes. Diffuse narrowing of the small bowel with effacement of folds has been compared with the appearance of ribbon or toothpaste.

Ischemia and radiation

Small bowel ischemia can cause luminal narrowing secondary to spasm, intramural edema or hemorrhage, or stricture formation. Similar findings are sometimes seen following radiation and are caused by endarteritis and subsequent small bowel ischemia (Fig. 3-18).

Drug-induced narrowing

Various drugs have been associated with small bowel narrowing because of their local toxic effects. These include potassium chloride tablets and floxuridine and other related chemotherapeutic agents.

Postoperative narrowing

Narrowing at surgical anastomoses is usually related to edema in the immediate postoperative period and fibrosis with stricture formation later on.

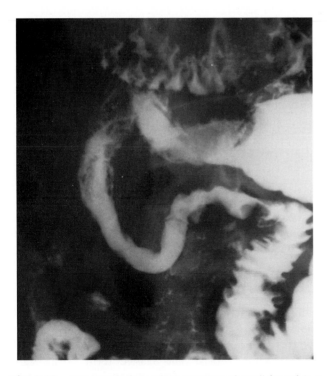

Fig. 3-18 Narrowed, featureless segment of small bowel is a sequela of ischemia.

Volvulus and intussusception

In small bowel volvulus, narrowing results from torsion of a loop of bowel, whereas in intussusception, edema of the intussuscepted loop and its mesentery causes narrowing.

Infection

Several infectious agents can cause small bowel narrowing. The protozoan *Giardia lamblia* may cause narrowing secondary to thickening of folds in the duodenum and proximal jejunum. The roundworm *Strongyloides stercoralis* causes similar findings and also may cause tubular narrowing of the bowel lumen resulting from spasm or stricture formation (Table 3-1).

Tuberculosis of the small bowel caused by *Mycobacterium tuberculosis* may result from drinking unpasteurized milk or swallowing infected sputum. The ileocecal region is most often involved, with narrowing sometimes causing marked distortion of this area. Small intestinal tuberculosis may be difficult to distinguish from Crohn's disease. Other infections in which fold thickening and luminal narrowing are usually localized to the distal ileum include *Campylobacter fetus jejuni, Yersinia enterocolitica,* and *Salmonella typhi* (typhoid fever). *Anisakis,* a small roundworm transmitted by eating raw fish, has been reported to cause narrowing of the jejunum or ileum secondary to spasm and ulceration.

Cytomegalovirus (CMV) enteritis occurs with increased frequency in immunocompromised patients, especially those with acquired immunodeficiency syndrome (AIDS). This can cause diffuse small bowel narrowing, ulcerations, and effacement of folds. Associated esophagitis, gastritis, or colitis may also be present in patients with disseminated CMV infection.

Narrowing Resulting from Extrinsic Abnormality

Adhesions

Extrinsic narrowing of the small bowel is usually related to an adhesion and probably ranks as the primary cause of small bowel obstruction. This usually results from prior surgery or inflammatory conditions of the abdomen, with fibrous bands of tissue developing in the peritoneal cavity as a result (Fig. 3-19). Adhesions are rarely detected by any of the imaging methods, and their presence is inferred from the clinical history as well as lack of other findings on radiographic studies.

Hernias

Hernias are a frequent cause of small bowel obstruction as well. The actual hernia itself does not produce the problem. Instead, the size of the opening into the hernia will have significant effect on any bowel loops passing through it. The smaller the opening, the more

Table 3-1   Infectious and parasitic diseases of the small bowel

	Scientific name	Origin	Area of involvement
BACTERIA			
Yersinia	*Yersinia enterocolitica*	Water	Terminal ileum
Tuberculosis	*Mycobacterium tuberculosis*	Milk, pulmonary	Distal small bowel
	Mycobacterium avium-intracellulare	Soil	Entire small bowel
Dysentery	*Salmonella typhosa*	Water, food	Distal small bowel
	Shigella dysenteriae	Water, food	Distal small bowel
Helicobacter	*Helicobacter fetus jejuni*	Ingested	Distal small bowel
VIRUS			
Herpes	Herpes simplex	Person	Distal small bowel
CMV	Cytomegalovirus species	Person	Entire small bowel
AIDS	Acquired human immunodeficiency virus	Person	Entire small bowel
FUNGUS			
Blastomycosis	*Paracoccidioides brasiliensis*	Soil	Distal small bowel
Histoplasmosis	*Histoplasma capsulatum*	Pulmonary	Entire small bowel
Candida	*Candida albicans*	Ingested	Entire small bowel
PROTOZOAN			
Cryptosporidiosis	*Cryptosporidia enteritis*	Water	Proximal small bowel
	Isospora belli	Water	Proximal small bowel
Giardiasis	*Giardia lamblia*	Water	Proximal small bowel
Amoebiasis	*Entomeoba histolytica*	Water	Proximal small bowel

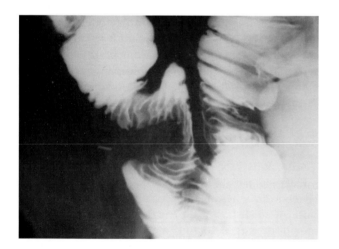

Fig. 3-19   The distal small bowel is narrowed and kinked due to adhesions.

likely that loops of bowel entering it will be affected. The bowel lumen, and possibly vascular supply, becomes more easily compromised by a small opening, resulting in obstruction.

Serosal metastases and other extrinsic masses

Various extrinsic masses can also compress and narrow the small bowel lumen. The most common of these are serosal metastases. The primary tumor may arise within the abdomen, most commonly seen with ovarian or gastric cancer. Even extraabdominal tumors such as breast or lung can produce intraperitoneal deposits of tumor, thus causing multifocal areas of narrowing. Whenever multiple areas of obstruction are encountered, metastatic tumor should be a primary consideration. Other abdominal masses, such as cysts and mesenchymal tumors, can also produce narrowing of the small bowel by extrinsic compression (Fig. 3-20).

NARROWED TERMINAL ILEUM

The category of a narrowed terminal ileum deserves a separate discussion in that it is one of the more common abnormalities encountered during small bowel examinations.

Crohn's Disease

In most practices, Crohn's disease is by far the most common cause of terminal ileal narrowing. This can be due to either active disease with ulceration, or chronic disease with fibrosis. The classic term "string-sign," originally applied to Crohn's disease, refers to a narrowed terminal ileum with displacement of the adjacent bowel loops (Box 3-3).

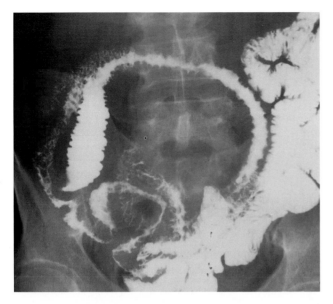

Fig. 3-20   Extensive narrowing of distal small bowel is secondary to extensive mesenteric involvement by lymphoma.

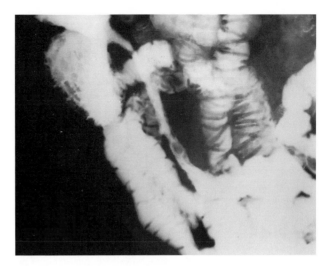

Fig. 3-21   Narrowed and ulcerated terminal ileum and cecum. Although this is due to tuberculosis, the changes are identical to Crohn's disease.

Box 3-3 **Complications of Crohn's Disease**
Strictures and obstruction
Fistulas and sinus tracts
Perforation and abscesses
Malignancy (adenocarcinoma, rarely lymphoma)

It should be noted that backwash ileitis from ulcerative colitis never produces narrowing of the terminal ileum, even after healing.

Infection

The next most common cause for narrowing of the terminal ileum is usually some type of infectious process. Tuberculosis can produce changes in the terminal ileum that are identical to Crohn's disease (Fig. 3-21). This disease is usually encountered in large cities, in which there is a large immigrant population, or in a person who travels overseas. Another infectious process that also frequently appears like this is *Yersinia*. This is bacterial infection that sporadically can infect the terminal ileum. It produces self-limited inflammatory changes in the terminal ileum that usually resolve over a few weeks or months. Many other infections of the bowel can involve the terminal ileum and produce inflammatory changes with narrowing. However, these often involve the rest of the small bowel and typically are not isolated to just the terminal ileum.

Neoplasms

Lymphoma is more frequent in the distal small bowel and is the most common neoplastic process to involve the terminal ileum. It can infiltrate through the bowel wall, producing narrowing and irregularity or nodularity of the folds (Fig. 3-22). Carcinoid also occurs in that region. The narrowing it produces is related to the desmoplastic changes that occur in the adjacent mesentery. The ileum is also a common area for metastases, particularly from serosal spread of intraabdominal tumors (Fig. 3-23). This is related to the flow of ascitic fluid in the abdomen. Both ovarian and upper abdominal tumors have been known to produce marked narrowing of the terminal ileum. Tumors of the cecum or ileocecal valve can extend in a retrograde fashion to involve the terminal ileum. Rarely, primary carcinoma of the small bowel could occur in the region.

Extrinsic Masses

The pelvis and right lower quadrant are frequent sites for abscesses or intraabdominal masses or tumors. Since the terminal ileum is on a relatively short mesentery, it is not as free to move as the rest of the intestines, and the terminal ileum may become secondarily involved by these adjacent processes. When the terminal ileum abuts an abscess, such as can be encountered with a periappendiceal abscess, the terminal ileum narrows and becomes spastic. These changes may mimic Crohn's disease or other inflammatory processes. Terminal ileal narrowing can also be seen in mesenteric panniculitis and pseudomyxoma peritonei.

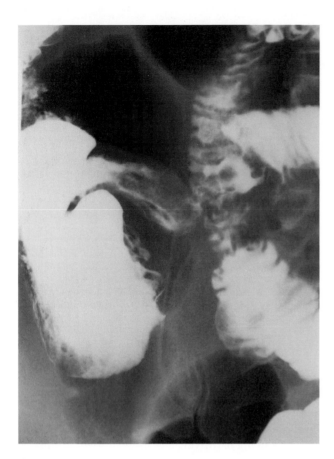

Fig. 3-22   Short segment of terminal ileal narrowing from lymphoma.

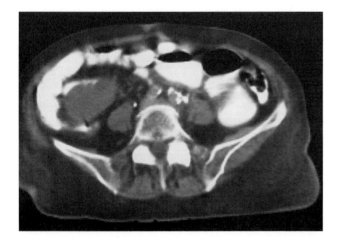

Fig. 3-23   CT demonstrates a large serosal mass compressing the terminal ileum. This is metastatic ovarian carcinoma.

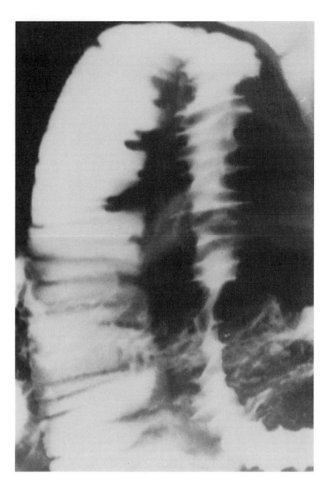

Fig. 3-24   Thickened folds and luminal narrowing represent segmental small bowel hemorrhage secondary to oral contraceptive medication.

THICKENED FOLDS

Fold thickening is characteristic of a variety of abnormalities affecting the small bowel. In some conditions, folds appear uniformly or regularly thickened, whereas in other conditions, thickening is nodular or irregular. Fold thickening can also be focal or diffuse, depending on the underlying disease or the extent or severity of that disease. These features provide a pattern-based approach to the differential diagnosis of thickened small bowel folds.

Uniformly Thickened Folds

Intramural hemorrhage

Uniformly thickened small bowel folds are typical of intramural hemorrhage. In these conditions, blood or transudate infiltrates into the submucosal layer of the bowel wall. As the folds become thicker, the space between adjacent folds becomes shorter, with the overall appearance likened to a stack of coins (Fig. 3-24).

Small bowel hemorrhage is caused by various insults including hemophilia, mesenteric ischemia or infarction, vasculitis, coagulopathy, anticoagulant medications, and trauma. Unusual disease entities such as Henoch-Schönlein purpura and idiopathic thrombocytopenic purpura can have this appearance. The changes typically involve a short segment of bowel and rarely involve the entire bowel. This segmental involvement along with the appropriate clinical history helps differentiate it from edema.

Edema

Edema of the small bowel may complicate mesenteric ischemia or infarction, congestive heart failure, and hypoproteinemia (resulting from hepatic, renal, or GI disease). It is probably most frequently seen in patients with end-stage liver disease, because of a combination of hypoproteinemia and portal venous congestion. Angioneurotic edema is an unusual cause of small bowel edema. In this disease, a genetic defect in the complement inactivation system can trigger episodes of small bowel edema, as well as hives and life-threatening laryngeal edema. Between attacks of angioneurotic edema, patients are asymptomatic and the small bowel folds appear normal.

Lymphangiectasia represents dilatation of intestinal lymphatic channels, resulting in inadequate lymph drainage. There can also be an associated hypoproteinemia. The disease may be congenital or acquired and typically demonstrates diffuse thickening of small bowel folds (Fig. 3-25). Other causes of small bowel edema that are associated with nonuniform or nodular fold thickening are discussed later in this section.

Radiation

Radiation to the abdomen or pelvis can lead to endarteritis in small bowel loops within the radiation port. Like other forms of ischemia, radiation enteritis causes uniform thickening of small bowel folds.

Eosinophilic enteritis

Eosinophilic enteritis is characterized by eosinophilic infiltration of the GI tract. This disease most often affects the stomach or small bowel and may be transmural or confined to the mucosa, muscularis, or serosa. With primary mucosal involvement of the small bowel, folds often appear thickened. The thickening may be uniform or nodular, focal or diffuse. Associated fold thickening or luminal narrowing of the gastric antrum and proximal duodenum may also occur. Although peripheral eosinophilia and a history of allergy suggests the diagnosis of eosinophilic enteritis, these factors are absent in approximately 25% and 50% of patients, respectively.

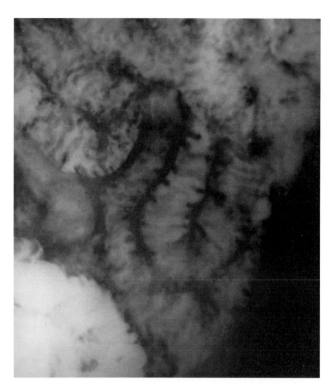

Fig. 3-25 Diffuse small bowel fold thickening as seen in lymphangiectasia.

Abetalipoproteinemia

Abetalipoproteinemia is a rare genetic disease in which abnormal lipid metabolism leads to fat malabsorption, cerebellar degeneration, and acanthocytosis (pointed-shaped red blood cells). Deposits of fat in epithelial cells of the duodenum and jejunum produce uniform or nodular thickening of folds. Similar findings have been noted in small bowel xanthomatosis, an extremely rare condition in which lipid-laden macrophages infiltrate the bowel wall.

Nodular or Irregularly Thickened Folds (Focal and Diffuse)

In contrast to the straight thickened folds typical of intramural hemorrhage, nodular or irregular fold thickening is featured in numerous diseases affecting the small bowel. In some, involvement is primarily focal or segmental, whereas in others, the small bowel is diffusely abnormal.

Whipple's disease

Whipple's disease causes nodular thickened folds in the duodenum and proximal jejunum (Fig. 3-26). Macrophages containing abundant periodic acid–Schiff (PAS) positive material are found throughout the lamina propria layer of the bowel wall, and characteristic rod-shaped gram-positive bacilli have been identified within these cells. Whipple's disease occurs mostly in middle-aged men; presenting symptoms include diarrhea, arthralgias, fever, and adenopathy. The pleura, pericardium, and central nervous system may also be involved. Although long-term treatment with antibiotics is often curative, an infectious etiology for this disease remains controversial (Box 3-4).

Infection

Numerous organisms can affect the small bowel and many cause nodular fold thickening. These include bacteria, viruses, protozoa, worms, and fungi (see Table 3-1). Overall, the changes they produce in the small bowel are similar, and it is typically impossible to distinguish the different organisms by their radiographic appearance, except for a select few. Sometimes the distribution of the abnormalities can help in narrowing the possibilities. The parasites *Strongyloides* and *Giardia* usually are localized to the duodenum and proximal jejunum (Fig. 3-27). A similar appearance has been described in hookworm infestation (ancylostomiasis).

Focal involvement of the distal ileum is suggestive of tuberculosis, typhoid fever, and *Yersinia* or *Campylobacter* enteritis.

In AIDS, otherwise unusual types of small bowel infections occur frequently, with most causing focal or

---

Box 3-4   Whipple's Disease

Occurs predominantly in middle-aged males
Clinical symptoms include diarrhea, arthralgias, fevers, neurologic symptoms
Glycoprotein-laden macrophages in bowel wall (PAS stain positive)
Bacilli also evident in bowel wall
May also affect heart valves, central nervous system, and joint capsules
Potentially fatal, but responds dramatically to antibiotics

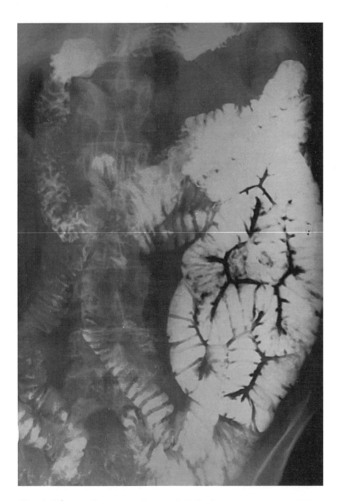

Fig. 3-26 Diffuse small bowel fold thickening represents Whipple's disease.

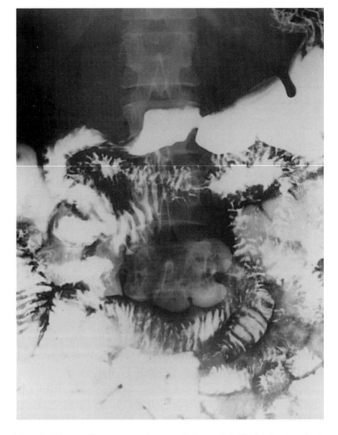

Fig. 3-27 Diffuse, irregular small bowel fold thickening in a patient with giardiasis.

diffuse thickening and nodularity of folds. Etiologies include CMV, *Mycobacterium avium-intracellulare* (MAI), *Cryptosporidium,* and *Isospora belli* (Fig. 3-28; Box 3-5).

Thickened folds in eosinophilic enteritis and abetalipoproteinemia can appear straight or nodular. Involvement in eosinophilic enteritis may be focal or diffuse, whereas in abetalipoproteinemia, the ileum is usually spared.

Crohn's disease

Crohn's disease of the small bowel may demonstrate coarsely thickened folds. This represents edema or inflammation. Although it is typically in the terminal ileum, other portions of the bowel may be involved, even with sparing of the terminal ileum. Associated findings include ulcerations, eccentric involvement, and skip lesions.

Lymphoma

Nodular thickened folds are one of the manifestations of small bowel lymphoma, of which there are many. The infiltration of malignant lymphocytes into the mucosal and submucosal layers of the bowel wall may be focal or diffuse.

Mastocytosis

Mastocytosis is an uncommon disease characterized by the proliferation of histamine-secreting mast cells. Although often localized to the skin (urticaria pigmentosa), the disease may also involve lymph nodes, liver, spleen, and bone (osteoblastic lesions). GI tract involvement produces fold thickening and nodularity throughout the small bowel and occasionally in the distal stomach. Episodes of flushing, pruritus, headache, and diarrhea may occur following the release of histamine from the mast cells (Fig. 3-29).

Box 3-5   Manifestations of AIDS in the Small Bowel

Thickened folds	—Usually a manifestation of infection, occasionally Kaposi's
Masses	—Malignancy, either lymphoma or Kaposi's sarcoma
Bull's-eye lesions	—Metastatic Kaposi's sarcoma
Adenopathy	—Neoplastic, either lymphoma or Kaposi's
	—Infectious, *Mycobacterium avium-intracellulare*

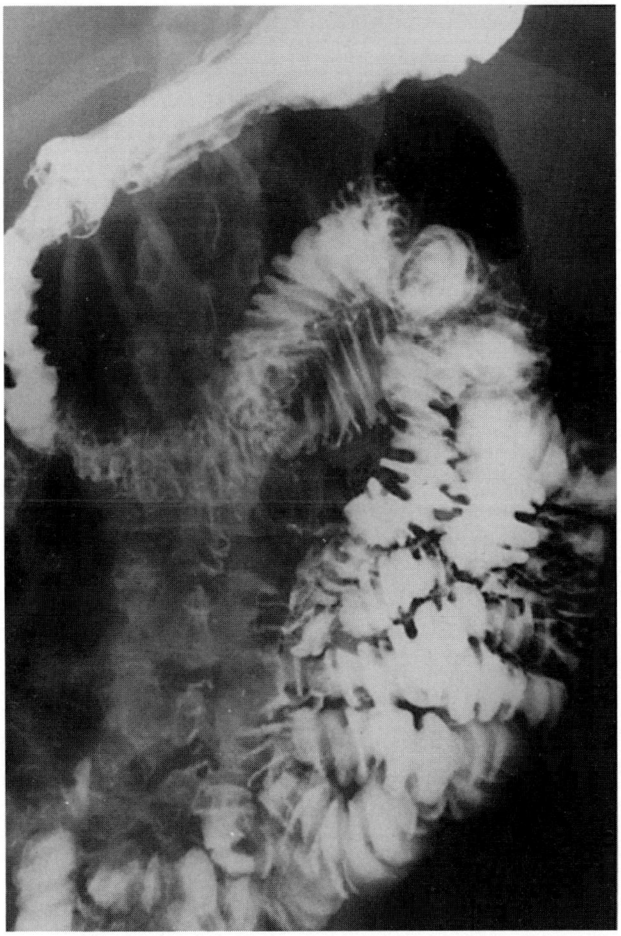

Fig. 3-28   Diffuse small bowel fold thickening caused by MAI in a patient with AIDS.

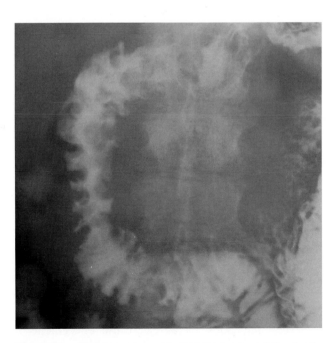

Fig. 3-29   Nodular, asymmetric fold thickening of the duodenum from mastocytosis.

Eosinophilic enteritis and graft-versus-host disease

Both eosinophilic enteritis and graft-versus-host disease can cause a similar alteration of the small bowel fold pattern. These changes are typically more diffuse.

Amyloidosis

Amyloidosis is a systemic disease in which extracellular deposits of amyloid occur throughout the body, including the GI tract. Small bowel folds may appear diffusely thickened and nodular. This disease most often occurs in patients with underlying multiple myeloma or chronic inflammatory conditions but sometimes may be primary in nature.

Edema

Small bowel edema, though typically causing uniform fold thickening, is sometimes associated with coarsened or nodular thickened folds. In Zollinger-Ellison syndrome, the markedly elevated levels of gastric acid result in severe inflammation and edema of the proximal duodenum and may even cause similar findings in the distal duodenum and proximal jejunum. Nodular thickened folds are also seen in edematous small bowel adjacent to an inflammatory mass. This can involve the jejunum (pancreatitis) or ileum (appendicitis, tuboovarian abscess).

Waldenström's macroglobulinemia

Waldenström's macroglobulinemia, a rare disease caused by proliferation of immunoglobulin M–producing plasma cells, may involve the small bowel. This results in diffuse fold thickening and tiny mucosal nodules.

DIMINISHED OR EFFACED FOLDS

Loss of the normal small bowel fold pattern results in a tubular appearance that may be focal or diffuse. This is not always the result of actual loss of the folds, but in some conditions the folds become so thickened that no barium can penetrate between the valvulae, and the folds no longer become discernible. This is often associated with thickening and rigidity of the bowel wall. It may be preceded by focal or diffuse fold thickening and can actually be considered at the end of the spectrum of small bowel fold thickening. When there is complete absence of any folds, this is often termed a moulage pattern.

Infection

Several infectious agents can cause effacement of small bowel folds and narrowing of the lumen. In CMV enteritis and cryptosporidiosis, small bowel involvement is typically diffuse, whereas in strongyloidiasis, disease

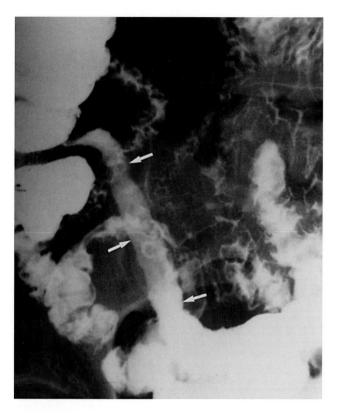

Fig. 3-30   Tubular distal ileum *(arrows)* resulting from CMV enteritis in a patient with AIDS.

is localized to the duodenum and proximal jejunum (Fig. 3-30).

Graft-Versus-Host Disease

In graft-versus-host disease, donor lymphocytes from a bone marrow transplant attack host tissues. The GI tract is usually affected, and a tubular appearance of the small bowel is frequently noted (Fig. 3-31) secondary to infiltration and edema of the bowel wall. This is a good example of when the apparent loss of fold pattern is actually due to severe fold thickening, not allowing any barium to pass in between the folds.

Sprue

Sprue (celiac disease) is associated with a decrease in the number of folds per inch in the duodenum and proximal jejunum. Occasionally, folds may be absent, resulting in a tubular-shaped lumen. However, unlike most other causes of diminished small bowel folds, sprue may produce luminal dilatation rather than narrowing.

Crohn's Disease

In Crohn's disease, small bowel loops may appear featureless and narrowed secondary to edema or fibrosis.

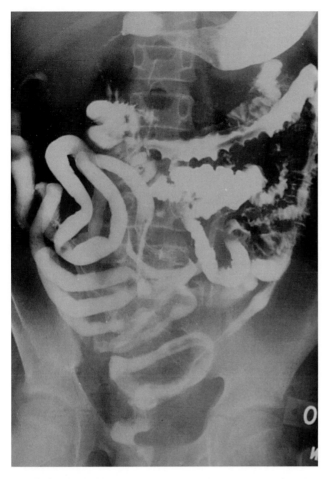

Fig. 3-31   Diffuse effacement of small and large bowel folds in a child with graft-versus-host disease.

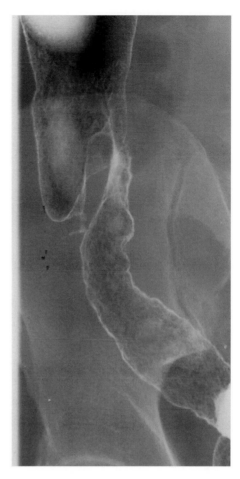

Fig. 3-32   Featureless terminal ileum and cecum from long-standing ulcerative colitis.

The length of bowel involved is variable, but the condition is often seen in long-standing disease (Fig. 3-32).

Scleroderma

Scleroderma results in fibrotic changes in the bowel wall. Usually the fold pattern is actually more prominent because of crowding of the valvulae. However, in severe end-stage disease, the small bowel loops become somewhat featureless with a diminished fold pattern.

Other Causes

Small bowel ischemia or infarction sometimes causes effacement of the fold pattern. Dilatation or narrowing of the lumen and scalloping of the bowel wall (thumbprinting) may also be noted. Similar findings in radiation enteritis reflect the underlying endarteritis and subsequent ischemia.

Toxic chemicals, introduced either by direct ingestion (potassium chloride tablets) or by vascular infusion (floxuridine and related chemotherapeutic agents), can reduce or eliminate small bowel folds.

A tubular-appearing small bowel may result from infiltration of the bowel wall. This has been described in amyloidosis, lymphoma, and other infiltrative diseases.

Featureless dilatation of the terminal ileum (backwash ileitis) sometimes occurs in patients with chronic ulcerative pancolitis. A similar finding can also result from long-term cathartic abuse (cathartic colon). In both conditions, the ileocecal valve is patulous.

TINY NODULES

Discrete tiny nodules in the small bowel are sometimes associated with thickened folds. This pattern is seen in Whipple's disease, mastocytosis, Waldenström's macroglobulinemia, and small bowel infection (*Yersinia* enteritis, MAI, disseminated histoplasmosis).

Tiny nodules can also be seen in the absence of fold thickening. In nodular lymphoid follicular pattern, prominent lymphoid follicles in the small bowel wall appear as tiny round uniform nodules (Fig. 3-33). This is often termed lymphoid hyperplasia, but it is not really a pathologic condition, nor is it always associated with a

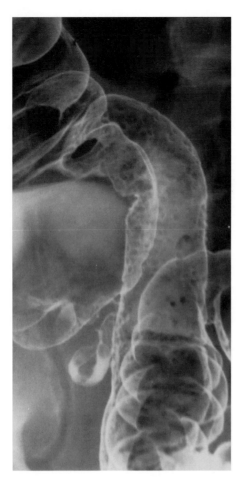

Fig. 3-33 Multiple small uniform nodules in the terminal ileum of a 17-year-old patient represent nodular lymphoid hyperplasia.

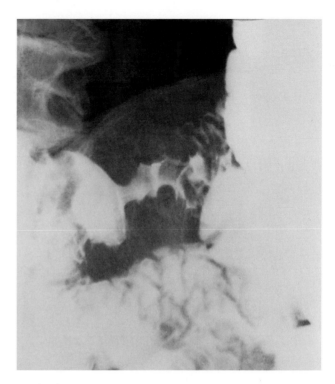

Fig. 3-34 Annular lesion of small bowel from primary adenocarcinoma.

disease. This is a normal finding in children and young adults, especially in the terminal ileum where lymphoid tissue is most abundant. It is even encountered as a normal finding in older adults with no underlying disease. The small bowel folds appear normal in these patients. However, fold thickening is often present in older patients with diffuse nodular lymphoid hyperplasia associated with immunoglobulin deficiency or giardiasis of the small bowel.

SOLITARY MURAL MASSES

Malignant Tumors

Adenocarcinoma

Adenocarcinoma, though the most common primary malignant neoplasm of the duodenum, occurs with decreasing frequency from proximal jejunum to distal ileum. It arises in the mucosal layer and typically infiltrates the bowel wall to cause a short annular narrowing with mucosal destruction, circumferential wall thickening, and overhanging margins (Fig. 3-34). If encountered in its early stages, small bowel adenocarcinoma appears as a polypoid intraluminal mass. Clinical symptoms associated with adenocarcinoma include obstruction, bleeding, and abdominal pain. Since it often does not produce early symptoms, obstruction is the most frequent presentation. An increased incidence of adenocarcinoma has been noted in the duodenum and proximal jejunum in patients with celiac disease and in the ileum in patients with Crohn's disease (Table 3-2).

Leiomyosarcoma

Leiomyosarcoma of the small bowel arises in the muscular or submucosal layer and grows either away from the lumen (exoenteric) or toward it (endoenteric) (Table 3-2). Leiomyosarcomas are more common in the jejunum and ileum than in the duodenum and account for approximately 9% of primary malignant neoplasms of the small bowel.

Exoenteric lesions often produce few symptoms until they have attained a large size and have outgrown their blood supply. Central necrosis and cavitation of the tumor lead to ulceration and hemorrhage into the adjacent bowel lumen. Contrast studies may show either extrinsic compression of bowel loops by the large intramural mass or an irregular collection of barium within the necrotic portion of the tumor itself. CT is useful in demonstrating both the enhancing peripheral

Table 3-2 Neoplasms of the small bowel

Type	Location	Characteristics
MALIGNANT		
Adenocarcinoma	Usually jejunum	Mass or annular lesion
Lymphoma	Usually ileum but can occur anywhere	Variable appearance from solitary to multiple nodules, strictures or dilatation, mesenteric masses
Carcinoid	Usually ileum	Nodule or mass, bowel kinking and mass effect; variable malignancy; can be multiple
Leiomyosarcoma	Anywhere	Mass, often extending extraluminal
Metastases	Anywhere	Single or multiple intraluminal polyps, mural masses, intussusception, ulceration
BENIGN		
Leiomyoma	Usually jejunum	Solitary mass; variable ulceration
Adenoma	Usually ileum	Solitary intraluminal polyp; may intussuscept
Lipoma	Usually ileum	Same as adenoma
Neurofibroma	Usually ileum	Luminal or submucosal polyp
Hemangioma	Anywhere	Sessile polyps, phleboliths

component and the necrotic or gas-containing central component of the lesion.

The endoenteric form of small bowel leiomyosarcoma usually appears as a compressible intraluminal mass. This may cause bleeding, intussusception, or obstruction. Leiomyosarcomas may be difficult to distinguish from leiomyomas both radiographically and histologically. Metastases usually occur through hematogenous spread to the liver or lungs.

Lymphoma

Lymphoma affects the small bowel more often than any other portion of the GI tract. This usually represents secondary involvement by non-Hodgkin's lymphoma and occurs with greatest frequency in the distal ileum because of the predominance of lymphoid tissue there (Box 3-6).

Small bowel lymphoma has a variety of radiographic appearances including fold thickening or effacement, luminal narrowing, aneurysmal dilatation, diffuse nodularity, and extrinsic compression by mesenteric masses (Fig. 3-35). Solitary or multiple focal mural masses can also be seen. With continued enlargement, these masses may become exoenteric, undergoing excavation and ulceration, or endoenteric, producing an intraluminal polypoid mass with the potential for intussusception.

Non-Hodgkin's lymphoma of the small bowel is a recognized complication of celiac disease. It also occurs with increased frequency in patients with immunodeficiency as a result of AIDS or immunosuppression resulting from antirejection medications following organ transplantation. In Mediterranean lymphoma, diffuse

Box 3-6 Lymphoma

Non-Hodgkin's lymphoma (Hodgkin's type is rare)
More common in distal small bowel (ileum)

Variable appearance:	Mass or polyp
	Multiple polyps (polyposis)
	Infiltrative (aneurysmal dilatation)
	Endoexoenteric
	Mesenteric (adenopathy)
Predisposing conditions:	Sprue
	Immunosuppression (AIDS, transplant recipients)

small bowel involvement results in severe intestinal malabsorption.

Carcinoid tumor

Carcinoid tumor is the most common primary neoplasm of the small bowel (Box 3-7). It arises from argentaffin cells in the crypts of Lieberkühn and occurs most commonly in the distal ileum. Carcinoid tumors less than 1 cm in diameter usually cause no symptoms and rarely metastasize. A carcinoid tumor may be noted incidentally on contrast studies as a smooth, round submucosal mass.

As the tumor enlarges, it may extend into the overlying mucosa and lead to ulceration or intussusception. Outward extension into the muscular and serosal layers may induce a local desmoplastic reaction consisting of

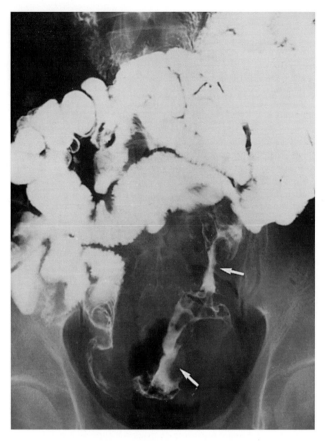

Fig. 3-35 Distorted, irregular ileal loop *(arrows)* represents non-Hodgkin's lymphoma.

angulation, tethering of folds, and partial obstruction. This represents the local effects of serotonin, which is produced by the tumor from the dietary amino acid tryptophan. Carcinoid tumors measuring 1 to 2 cm in diameter metastasize in about 50% of cases, and those larger than 2 cm metastasize in about 90% of cases. Regional metastases are usually located in the mesentery or lymph nodes and are commonly larger than the primary tumor. On CT, these lesions may demonstrate a stellate appearance or dystrophic calcifications (Fig. 3-36).

Metastasis

Liver metastases from carcinoid tumor are usually hypervascular and may cause carcinoid syndrome, characterized by episodic cutaneous flushing, wheezing, and diarrhea. The liver normally degrades serotonin into 5-hydroxyindoleacetic acid (5-HIAA) and thereby prevents it from entering the systemic circulation. However, in the presence of liver metastases, serotonin may pass through the right heart into the lungs, producing carcinoid syndrome and damaging the right heart valves before being broken down in the lungs to 5-HIAA. Bone metastases from carcinoid tumor are typically osteoblastic.

Metastatic disease to the small bowel occurs through hematogenous, peritoneal, contiguous, or lymphatic spread and can cause a variety of radiographic findings. Although metastases are often multiple, solitary lesions are sometimes demonstrated.

Benign Tumors

Mesenchymal tumor

Benign tumors arising in mesenchymal tissues of the small bowel wall include leiomyoma, lipoma, neurofibroma, and hemangioma, in order of descending frequency. The most common of these is leiomyoma, a hypervascular nonencapsulated smooth muscle tumor

---

Box 3-7 Carcinoid Tumor

Amine precursor uptake and decarboxylation tumor, may be found anywhere in gastrointestinal or genitourinary tract or bronchi

Location—appendix most common, then small bowel (typically ileum)

All potentially malignant, >2 cm most likely to metastasize

Hormonally active—secrete serotonin

Serotonin is converted in liver and lungs to 5-HIAA, which is elevated in urine

May provoke a desmoplastic reaction in small bowel

Usually asymptomatic

Carcinoid syndrome: Occurs with liver metastases (95%)

Intestinal hypermotility—diarrhea and cramping

Vasomotor—flushing

Bronchoconstriction—wheezing

Endocardial fibrosis—right-sided heart valves

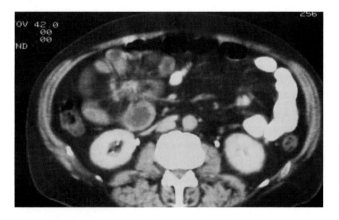

Fig. 3-36 CT shows a radiating appearance of the mesenteric vessels secondary to the desmoplastic reaction seen in carcinoid.

(Fig. 3-37). Leiomyoma, like its malignant counterpart leiomyosarcoma, can undergo endoenteric or exoenteric growth with resultant complications of intussusception or tumor necrosis and ulceration, respectively.

Lipoma, an encapsulated fatty tumor, is characterized fluoroscopically by its softness and compressibility during palpation. Continued stretching of the tumor by bowel peristalsis may form a pedunculated intraluminal mass that can ulcerate or act as a lead point for intussusception (Fig. 3-38).

Neurofibroma and other neural tumors are unusual solitary mural masses in the small bowel. Occasionally, they may be multiple in nature, particularly if the patient suffers from neurofibromatosis.

Hemangioma represents a focal proliferation of vascular channels. Though phleboliths are uncommonly demonstrated, their presence in association with a submucosal mass is indicative of a hemangioma.

Adenoma

Adenomas, benign mucosal tumors arising in glandular epithelium, may appear sessile or pedunculated. They are actually the second most common small bowel tumor encountered, after leiomyoma. They may develop anywhere in the small bowel, but are more common in the ileum.

Carcinoid tumor and inflammatory fibroid polyp

Carcinoid tumor of the small bowel demonstrates variable malignant potential.

Inflammatory fibroid polyp (eosinophilic granuloma) is composed primarily of connective tissue and appears as a smooth submucosal mass in the small bowel, stomach, or colon. Although eosinophilic infiltration of

the mass is characteristic, the focal nature of the mass and the absence of associated peripheral eosinophilia differentiate it from eosinophilic gastroenteritis. Complications of inflammatory fibroid polyp include ulceration and intussusception.

Other Masses

Endometrioma

Endometrioma of the small bowel represents a focal deposit of ectopic endometrial tissue on the serosal surface of the distal ileum. The etiology of endometriosis is uncertain, and proposed theories include reflux of endometrial tissue through the fallopian tubes, hematogenous or lymphatic spread, and metaplasia of celomic epithelium. Small bowel involvement is uncommon and

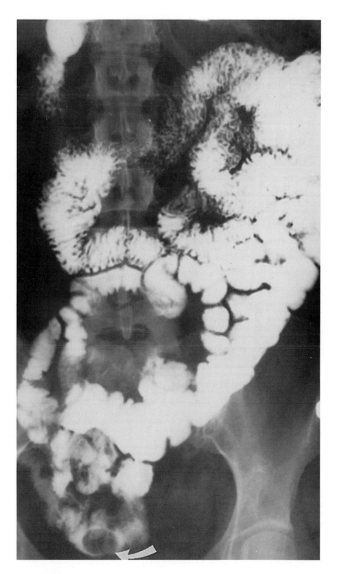

Fig. 3-38 Ovoid mass *(curved arrow)* in the distal ileum represents a lipoma.

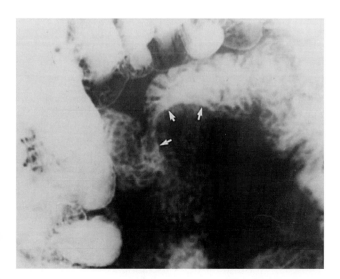

Fig. 3-37 Submucosal mass *(arrows)* represents a jejunal leiomyoma.

Table 3-3 Polyposis syndromes affecting the small bowel

Title	Type	Other features
Peutz-Jeghers syndrome	Hamartomas	Polyps throughout GI tract; mucocutaneous pigmentation
Cronkhite-Canada syndrome	Hamartomas	Alopecia, nail dystrophy, protein malabsorption
Juvenile polyposis	Hamartomas	Colon polyps, as well
Neurofibromatosis	Neurofibromas	Cutaneous fibromas and café au lait spots
Gardner's syndrome	Adenomas	Colonic polyps, osteomas, desmoid tumors
Familial polyposis	Adenomas	Typically colon tumors. Rarely small bowel tumors but without Gardner's stigmata

may appear as a focal mass with associated serosal tethering resulting from repeated episodes of intramural hemorrhage and subsequent fibrosis.

Duplication cyst

Duplication cyst is an embryologic abnormality that can occur anywhere in the small bowel. These cysts are tubular or round and may communicate with the adjacent bowel lumen. Although often discovered in childhood, duplication cysts are occasionally recognized incidentally in adults as a smooth intramural mass seen on contrast examination.

Hematoma

Unlike duodenal hematoma, focal hematoma of the mesenteric small bowel rarely causes a focal masslike appearance, possibly because of the tamponading effect of the circumferential serosal layer there.

Inverted Meckel's diverticulum

An inverted Meckel's diverticulum can also appear as a smooth, round or oval mass on contrast studies. When this occurs, the possibility of its presenting as an intussusception increases.

MULTIPLE MURAL MASSES

Many of the lesions that can occur as solitary mural masses can also occur as multiple mural masses. These lesions were described in greater detail in the previous section (Table 3-3).

Malignant Tumors

Metastasis

Metastasis to the small bowel can occur through peritoneal, hematogenous, lymphatic, or contiguous spread. Lesions are often multiple and may show variability in size secondary to repeated episodes of seeding (Fig. 3-39). Hematogenous dissemination can affect any segment of the small bowel. This occurs most

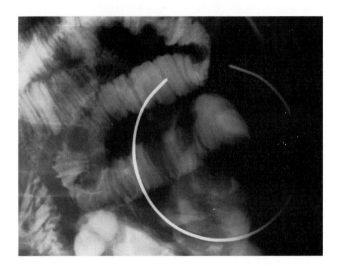

Fig. 3-39 Multiple small bowel nodules from metastatic lung carcinoma.

frequently in malignant melanoma and less often in breast or lung carcinoma. Metastatic melanoma typically produces submucosal nodules that may contain a central ulceration (target lesions). With further growth, these lesions may become primarily exoenteric (with subsequent necrosis and ulceration) or endoenteric (with subsequent intussusception). Small bowel metastases from breast carcinoma rarely result in focal scirrhous-type narrowing similar to that seen more commonly in the stomach.

Peritoneal spread through ascitic fluid leads to seeding of tumor on the serosal surface of the small bowel. Peritoneal fluid accumulates in the mesenteric reflections of the small bowel, especially at the ileocecal region because of its relatively dependent position. Serosal metastases most often occur secondary to GI or gynecological malignancies, particularly ovarian carcinoma. In addition to the nodular masses representing serosal tumor implants, associated fibrous reaction may cause tethering of folds and angulation of bowel loops (Fig. 3-40). CT is useful for demonstrating associated findings of peritoneal tumor spread including ascites, peritoneal implants, mesenteric infiltration, and omental cakes.

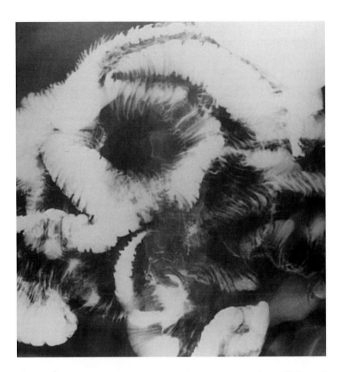

Fig. 3-40 Diffuse distortion and angulation of small bowel loops caused by peritoneal spread of colon carcinoma.

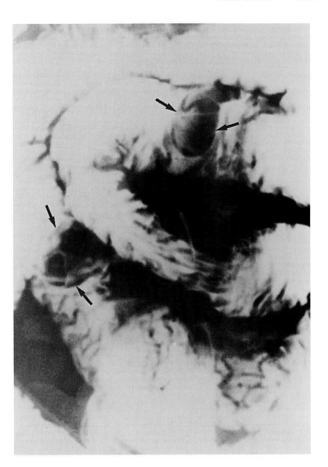

Fig. 3-41 Submucosal masses *(arrows)* represent non-Hodgkin's lymphoma in a patient with AIDS.

Direct or contiguous spread of tumor may involve the mesenteric small bowel, as seen in invasion of the distal ileum by pelvic or cecal tumors. Lymphatic spread has been reported to involve the distal ileum following ileocolic anastomosis for colon carcinoma.

Kaposi's sarcoma
Kaposi's sarcoma is a vascular tumor of the skin that can also affect visceral organs including the GI and respiratory tracts. Although once a rare disease, Kaposi's sarcoma is a common neoplasm in AIDS, particularly in homosexual men with AIDS. Submucosal nodules of Kaposi's sarcoma in the small bowel often resemble hematogenous metastases. Like metastatic malignant melanoma, Kaposi's sarcoma nodules may contain a central ulceration and at times act as a lead point for small bowel intussusception.

Lymphoma
Non-Hodgkin's lymphoma of the small bowel can produce multiple, discrete mural masses or diffuse nodularity. This most often involves the ileum as a result of the normal abundance of lymphoid tissue there (Fig. 3-41).

Carcinoid tumor
Carcinoid tumors of the small bowel are multiple in approximately one third of cases.

Benign Tumors

Hamartoma
Multiple hamartomas of the small bowel occur in several polyposis syndromes including Peutz-Jeghers, Cronkhite-Canada, juvenile polyposis, and Cowden's syndromes. Peutz-Jeghers syndrome is an autosomal-dominant disease characterized by mucocutaneous pigmentation and multiple small bowel polyps that may cause transient intussusception (Fig. 3-42). Cronkhite-Canada syndrome consists of multiple GI polyps, ectodermal abnormalities, and intestinal malabsorption. Gastrointestinal juvenile polyposis may involve any portion of the gastrointestinal tract. In Cowden's syndrome, GI polyps are associated with tumors of the breast, thyroid, and skin.

Adenoma
Multiple small bowel adenomas can occur in Gardner's syndrome. This autosomal-dominant disease is

characterized by diffuse adenomatous polyps of the colon and subsequent development of colon carcinoma. Extraintestinal tumors, including osteomas of the facial bones, sebaceous cysts, and desmoid tumors of the mesentery, also occur. The polyps that occur in the small bowel can be adenomatous and thus have a malignant potential, unlike the other polyposis symptoms described, which have no malignant potential. Patients with Gardner's syndrome have an increased incidence of ampullary carcinoma.

Mesenchymal tumor

Benign mesenchymal tumors of the small bowel, though usually solitary, may be multiple. This is especially true in neurofibromatosis, a genetic disease in which neural tumors can involve the skin, visceral organs, or central nervous system. Multiple neurofibromas of the small bowel in neurofibromatosis typically occur along the antimesenteric border. Small bowel lipomatosis is a rare condition characterized by multiple lipomas of the small bowel.

Carcinoid tumors exhibit variable malignant potential and are multiple in approximately one third of cases.

Other Masses

Postinflammatory polyps

Postinflammatory polyps of the small bowel are similar to those seen in the colon in the healing stages of

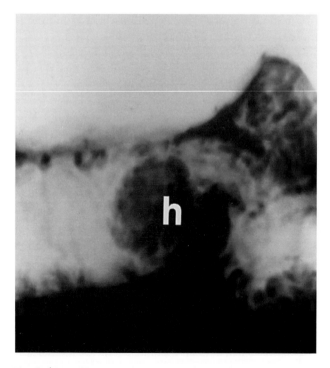

Fig. 3-42 Polypoid mass (*h*) in the jejunum represents a hamartoma in a patient with Peutz-Jeghers disease.

inflammatory bowel disease. In the small bowel, these are typically well-defined, round polyps of varying size and most often involve the terminal ileum. They may be secondary to Crohn's disease or, rarely, ulcerative pancolitis with backwash ileitis. The small branching (filiform) polyps are less commonly seen in the small bowel.

Pneumatosis cystoides intestinalis

Pneumatosis cystoides intestinalis is a disorder of variable etiology in which multiple subserosal cystic collections of gas indent the lumen of the small bowel or colon. The radiolucent appearance of the mural masses on plain films or CT is characteristic of this benign form of intestinal pneumatosis.

Varices

Varices of the mesenteric small bowel are unusual but can produce smooth submucosal masses similar to those seen in esophageal or gastric varices.

OTHER INTRALUMINAL ABNORMALITIES

Intraluminal masses in the small bowel include worms, bezoars, tubes, ingested foreign bodies, and calculi. Other lesions, such as pedunculated tumors and inverted diverticula, may simulate intraluminal masses.

Worms

The most common worm encountered in the small bowel is *Ascaris lumbricoides*. This roundworm is seen frequently, especially in tropical areas of the world. On contrast studies, ascaris appears as a long tubular intraluminal filling defect. A thin white line sometimes shown to bisect the length of the worm represents ingested barium in the worm's own GI tract (Fig. 3-43). Ascaris worms can be solitary or multiple, and when especially numerous, may cause a small bowel obstruction.

Tapeworms also can produce linear intraluminal filling defects on contrast examinations. These flatworms are usually much longer than ascaris worms and never demonstrate a thin white line bisecting their length because they do not have a continuous GI tract (Table 3-4).

Bezoars

Bezoars are uncommon in the small bowel. Phytobezoars (concretions of vegetable matter) usually result from ingestion of a large amount of high-fiber foods, such as citrus fruit. An increased incidence of small bowel phytobezoars has also been reported in patients with previous gastric outlet surgery and recent ingestion of persimmons. Phytobezoars can cause an obstruction anywhere in the jejunum or ileum and may resemble a villous tumor on contrast studies as a result of barium filling numerous interstices.

Other Foreign Bodies

Ingested foreign bodies sometimes become obstructed at the ileocecal valve because of physiological narrowing there. Prune pits have a characteristic biconvex shape. Radiopaque objects, such as coins, keys, and screws, are sometimes seen in the small bowel of psychiatric patients and are easily identified on abdominal plain films (Fig. 3-44). Ingested packets of heroin, cocaine, and other illegal drugs may appear on abdominal plain films as round or oval opacities, sometimes surrounded by a thin crescent of air (double condom sign). These drug packets may cause mechanical bowel obstruction or drug intoxication when leakage or rupture of a packet occurs.

Various iatrogenically placed feeding or drainage catheters may become dislodged and pass into the small bowel, where they appear as tubular filling defects. These include surgical or endoscopic gastrostomy and jejunostomy tubes. Balloon-tip catheters may demonstrate the inflated balloon as well as the tubular portion

Table 3-4 Intestinal worms in the small bowel			
Type	**Scientific name**	**Origin**	**Area of involvement**
Hookworm	*Necator americanus*	Soil	Proximal small bowel
	Ancylostoma duodenale	Soil	Proximal small bowel
Tapeworm	*Taenia saginata*	Beef	Entire small bowel
	Taenia solium	Pork	Entire small bowel
	Diphyllobothrium latum	Fish	Entire small bowel
Roundworm	*Ascaris lumbricoides*	Water	Entire small bowel
Strongyliasis	*Strongyloides stercoralis*	Water	Entire small bowel
Anisakiasis	*Anisakis* species	Raw fish	Entire small bowel

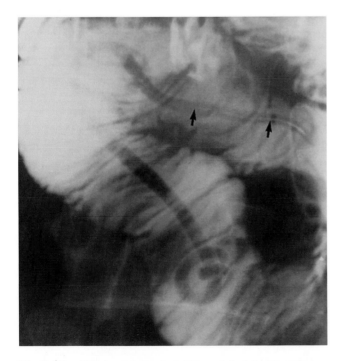

Fig. 3-43   Tubular intraluminal filling defect in the jejunum represents an ascaris worm. The thin white line bisecting part of the length of the worm *(arrows)* indicates barium in the worm's GI tract. (From Goodman P: Diagnostic radiology case number 16, *Intern Med* 12:46, 1991.)

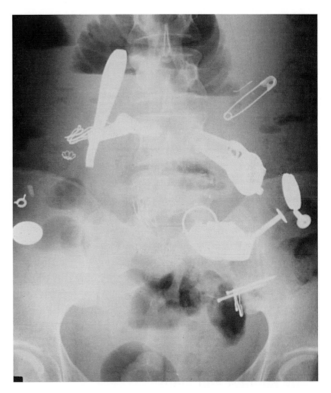

Fig. 3-44   Small bowel obstruction in a psychiatric patient who has ingested multiple metallic objects.

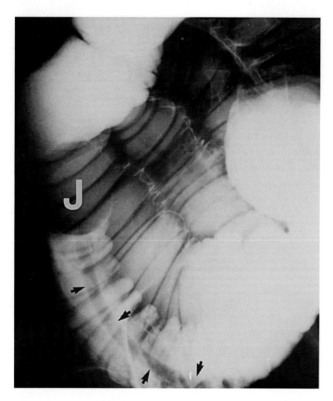

Fig. 3-45 Small bowel obstruction caused by migration of a jejunostomy tube *(arrows)* and impaction of the balloon tip *(J)*.

of the catheter (Fig. 3-45). The Garren-Edwards gastric bubble, an intragastric balloon once used to treat morbid obesity, has also been reported to spontaneously deflate and migrate into the small bowel, where it can cause obstruction.

Gallstone

Erosion of a gallstone into the duodenum can lead to gallstone ileus, a mechanical obstruction caused by impaction of the gallstone in the small bowel, usually at the ileocecal valve. The ectopic gallstone is visible on plain films in approximately 25% of cases. On contrast studies, it may appear as a round or oval filling defect in the distal small bowel. Associated findings include distal small bowel obstruction and air in the biliary tree (caused by reflux of air through the biliary-enteric fistula). A similar case has been reported in which a renal staghorn calculus eroded into the duodenum and subsequently became impacted at the ileocecal valve.

Air Bubbles and Stool

Air bubbles anywhere in the small bowel and fecal debris refluxed across the ileocecal valve into the distal ileum also appear as intraluminal filling defects. Rarely,

in patients with gastrointestinal bleeding or after surgical procedures, a blood clot may be seen within the lumen. Characteristically they conform to the dimensions of the bowel.

Inverted Diverticulum

Any diverticulum may invert and appear almost entirely intraluminal. Classically this is seen in the duodenum but is also rarely encountered in the rest of the small bowel, particularly with inverted Meckel's diverticula.

EXTRINSIC PROCESSES

Adhesions

Extrinsic compression of small bowel loops may result from adhesive bands. Although they are extremely common, they are rarely demonstrated by imaging methods.

Organomegaly and Adenopathy

Focal or diffuse enlargement of abdominal or pelvic organs and distention of other hollow viscera may compress or displace adjacent small bowel. These extrinsic masses cause a spectrum of radiographic appearances depending on their size, location, and relationship to the peritoneal cavity (Fig. 3-46). Although the mass effect typically is smooth, an extrinsic inflammatory or neoplastic mass may evoke serosal tethering or fold thickening. Marked adenopathy caused by inflammatory, infectious, or neoplastic disease can cause similar findings.

Metastatic Disease

As discussed previously, peritoneal metastases can occur from both abdominal (gastric, ovarian, pancreatic) and extraabdominal tumors such as breast, lung, and melanoma. Metastases are probably the most common cause of multiple extrinsic masses affecting the small bowel.

Aortic Aneurysm

An abdominal aortic aneurysm causing extrinsic compression of small bowel may be recognized by curvilinear calcifications outlining the aneurysm or by a pulsatile appearance on fluoroscopy.

Other Masses

Mesenteric masses (cysts, tumors, and abscesses) typically cause focal displacement of bowel loops.

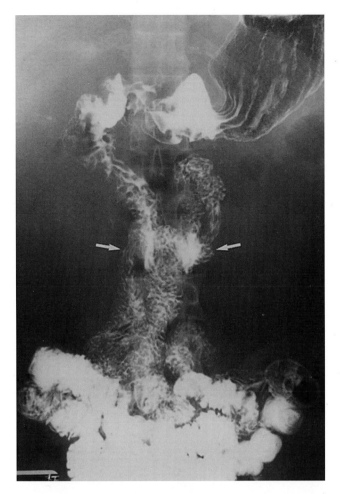

Fig. 3-46 Medial displacement of mid–small bowel loops *(arrows)* resulting from bilateral huge polycystic kidneys.

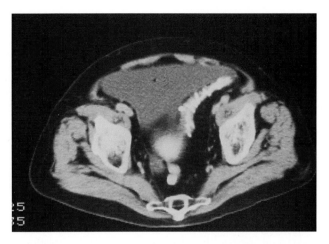

Fig. 3-47 CT demonstrates an extensive soft-tissue mass spreading through the lower abdomen in this patient with pseudomyxoma peritonei.

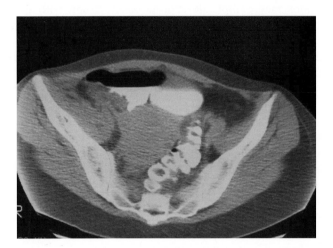

Fig. 3-48 Abdominal masses (desmoids) can be seen in Gardner's syndrome.

Mesenteric extension of leiomyosarcomas or other exoenteric masses arising from the bowel wall can also compress or displace adjacent bowel. Diffuse inflammation or infiltration of the mesentery may produce separation of bowel loops throughout the abdomen and pelvis. Focal peritoneal abscesses can produce localized mass effect and inflammation of nearby small bowel.

When a mucinous adenocarcinoma of the abdomen ruptures, it seeds the lower abdomen with tumor implants. These can continue to produce mucin, which usually fills the lower abdominal cavity with a mixture of gelatinous fluid and tumor cells. This can result in numerous extrinsic impressions or displacement of the bowel (Fig. 3-47). Retractile mesenteritis is a rare disease that produces fatty and fibrotic thickening of portions of the mesentery. This consists of a combination of inflammation, fibrosis, and fatty infiltration. When inflammation is the predominant pathologic feature of this process, it is often termed mesenteric panniculitis. These processes usually involve the distal small bowel mesentery, but can sometimes affect the sigmoid mesentery as well. Desmoid tumors are fibrous mesenchymal tumors involving the mesentery and peritoneal cavity (Fig. 3-48). These are seen in Gardner's polyposis syndrome.

Ascites

In the presence of diffuse ascites, supine films demonstrate small bowel loops floating together in the central portion of the abdomen. Sometimes the ascites may be loculated and appear as localized masses. This is occasionally seen in patients on peritoneal dialysis for renal failure.

Fatty Mesenteric Infiltration

Obese patients may sometimes have quite pronounced fatty changes in their mesentery, which result in separation and displacement of small bowel loops. In these patients, the mesenteric fat is diffuse in nature. Pelvic lipomatosis produces more focal fatty or fibrotic changes in the pelvic region. Although it usually involves the rectum, it can produce displacement or compression of small bowel loops in the pelvis. More localized fatty infiltration can be seen in patients with Crohn's disease or isolated lipodystrophy of the mesentery.

ULCERATIONS

Nonneoplastic

Zollinger-Ellison syndrome

Marked gastric hyperacidity as seen in Zollinger-Ellison syndrome can produce an ulcer diathesis affecting the proximal duodenum and less commonly the distal duodenum and proximal jejunum. Marginal ulcerations may complicate subtotal gastrectomy with gastrojejunal anastomosis. These ulcers occur most often in patients with underlying severe peptic ulcer disease and are usually located in the efferent loop just distal to the anastomotic site.

Crohn's disease

Ulcerations as a result of Crohn's disease can affect any portion of the small bowel and demonstrate a variety of radiographic appearances. Aphthoid ulcers are small, round, and uniform and consist of a central ulceration surrounded by a radiolucent rim of edema (Fig. 3-49). Deeper transverse and longitudinal ulcerations may combine to form a cobblestone pattern in which residual islands of preserved mucosa are separated by the crisscrossing transmural ulcers (Fig. 3-50).

Infection

Small bowel infections may also cause ulceration. GI tuberculosis most often involves the ileocecal area, where it can cause ulcers and appear radiographically similar to Crohn's disease. CMV enteritis in AIDS may result in ileal ulceration and subsequent perforation. Ileal ulcerations are also seen in enteritis caused by *Salmonella* (typhoid fever), *Yersinia,* and *Campylobacter* organisms. Parasitic infection by the *Strongyloides* and *Anisakis* roundworms may also cause ulcers in the small bowel.

Behçet's disease

Behçet's disease is a rare systemic vasculitis in which ulcerations occur in the mouth, genitalia, eyes, and GI

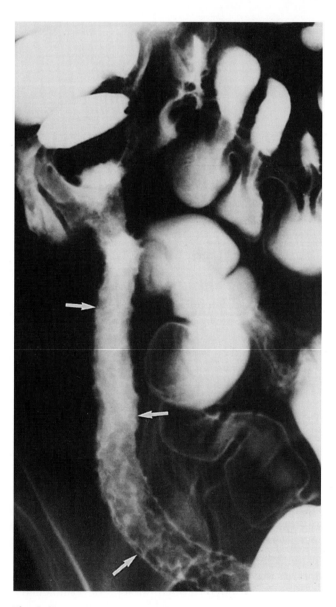

Fig. 3-50   Diffuse ulceration of the neoterminal ileum *(arrows)* represents recurrent Crohn's disease.

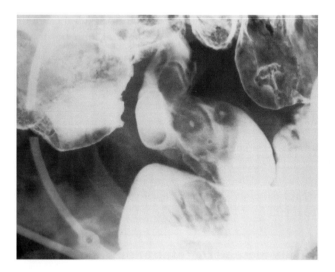

Fig. 3-49   Two distinct aphthous ulcers of the terminal ileum in Crohn's disease.

tract. Ileal ulcerations in this disease may appear either aphthoid or linear. Because of this, it will mimic the radiographic appearance of Crohn's disease.

Other causes

Ulcerative ileojejunitis is an uncommon condition, either idiopathic or secondary to sprue, in which ulcerations in the small bowel may lead to fibrosis and focal stricture formation. Small bowel ulcerations can also result from mucosal irritation by ingested enteric-coated potassium chloride tablets.

Neoplastic

Benign mesenchymal tumors

In addition to the many inflammatory causes of small bowel ulceration, various neoplastic masses in the small bowel can ulcerate. Benign mesenchymal tumors, including leiomyomas and lipomas, sometimes bleed because of ulceration of the overlying mucosa (Fig. 3-51). This is one of their most frequent presenting symptoms, as they will often remain asymptomatic.

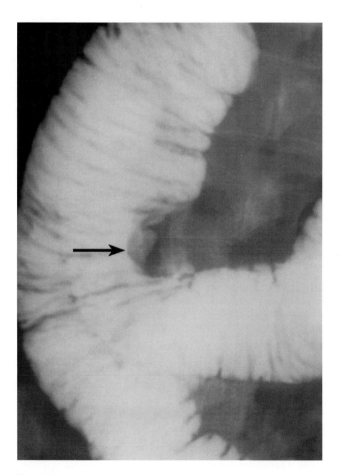

Fig. 3-51 Polyp with central ulceration *(arrow)* was a surgically proven leiomyoma.

Metastases

Ulcerating metastases to the small bowel most often result from hematogenous spread of malignant melanoma and less commonly breast or lung carcinoma. These masses vary in size and number and may radiographically resemble bull's-eye targets because of the central location of the ulcers.

Kaposi's sarcoma

Kaposi's sarcoma can produce similar ulcerated masses in the duodenum and less commonly in the mesenteric small bowel.

Malignant mesenchymal tumors

Leiomyosarcomas and other less common primary malignant mesenchymal tumors of the small bowel may undergo extensive necrosis and subsequent ulceration. Contrast studies and CT in these lesions demonstrate contrast material filling the large, irregular excavated portion of the mass.

Lymphoma, adenocarcinoma, and carcinoid tumor

Lymphoma, adenocarcinoma, and hematogenous metastases may cause a similar appearance because of infiltration of the bowel wall and resultant ulceration. Carcinoid tumors, which demonstrate variable malignant potential, may rarely cause similar findings, but ulceration is not a major feature.

FISTULAS AND SINUS TRACTS

Small bowel sinus tracts and fistulas may result from extension of preexisting small bowel ulcerations. Fistulas are connections between two mucosal-lined organs, such as between two loops of bowel or between the bowel and skin. Sinus tracts are confined areas of perforation that end blindly, often in inflammatory tissue, and do not connect to other organs.

Sinus tracts and fistulas are common features of severe Crohn's disease and may form between small bowel and adjacent colon, urinary bladder, abdominal wall, or other loops of small bowel (Fig. 3-52). Similar findings can be seen in intestinal tuberculosis, and the two cannot be distinguished by their radiographic features. Small bowel fistulas sometimes occur as a late complication of radiation therapy to the abdomen or pelvis. Fistulas forming from radiation therapy are the sequela of multiple processes, including ischemia and necrosis of bowel loops and matting of bowel loops from fibrosis and adhesions.

Postoperative sinus tracts and fistulas (enterocutaneous and enteroenteric) may result from a variety of factors. Often they are simply the result of a breakdown

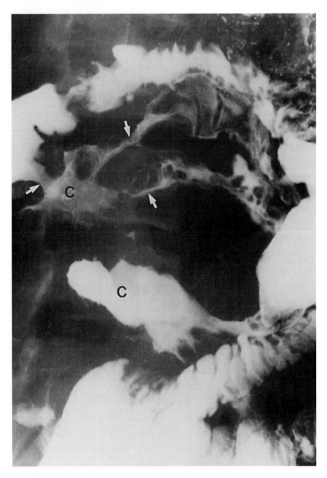

Fig. 3-52 Multiple enteric fistulae *(arrows)* and irregular barium collections *(C)* in a patient with Crohn's disease.

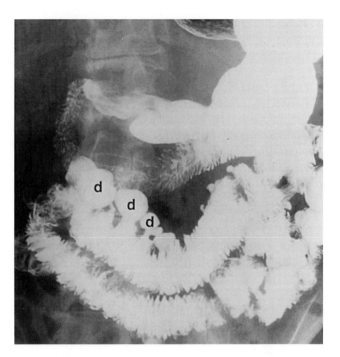

Fig. 3-53 Multiple jejunal diverticula *(d)*.

or interruption at an enteric anastomosis. Sometimes they result from ischemia and necrosis of a portion of bowel whose blood supply may have been compromised at surgery. This commonly occurs in surgery because of trauma or abdominal inflammatory processes.

Involvement of the small bowel by extrinsic processes can lead to the formation of sinus tracts or fistulas. Inflammatory masses of the gallbladder, pancreas, kidney, colon, or pelvic organs may become adherent to an adjacent loop of small bowel and erode into it.

Various neoplastic masses can form fistulous connections involving the small bowel. Primary tumors of the small bowel may invade adjacent bowel loops or other viscera, most commonly occurring with lymphoma. More typically seen are tumors from the colon or stomach with direct extension into the small bowel secondarily producing a fistula. Serosal metastases may also be a source of fistulas involving the small bowel, but fistulas are rarely due to hematogenous metastases.

DIVERTICULA

Jejunal and Ileal Diverticula

Jejunal and ileal diverticula are less common than duodenal diverticula. They occur along the mesenteric aspect of the bowel wall where penetrating blood vessels have produced focal defects in the muscular layer. Jejunal diverticula may be multiple and large (Fig. 3-53). Their main concern clinically is that they may develop bacterial overgrowth from stasis of bowel contents, leading to malabsorption and anemia. Ileal diverticula, though often multiple, are usually small and located in the terminal portion of the ileum (Fig. 3-54). Diverticulitis, enterolith formation, hemorrhage, and perforation are rare complications of jejunal and ileal diverticula. When ileal diverticula do become inflamed, the condition can mimic appendicitis.

Meckel's Diverticulum

Meckel's diverticulum is a congenital abnormality seen in up to 3% of the population (Box 3-8). Partial persistence of the omphalomesenteric duct results in a diverticulum along the antimesenteric aspect of the ileum, usually within 100 cm of the ileocecal valve. Meckel's diverticulum contains all layers of the bowel wall. Typically, they remain asymptomatic throughout

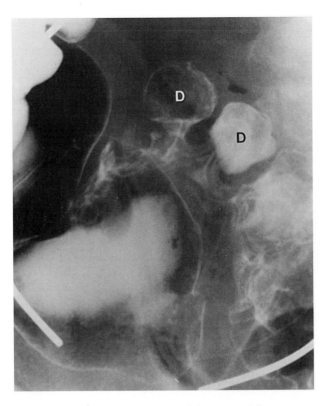

Fig. 3-54   Diverticula *(D)* of the terminal ileum.

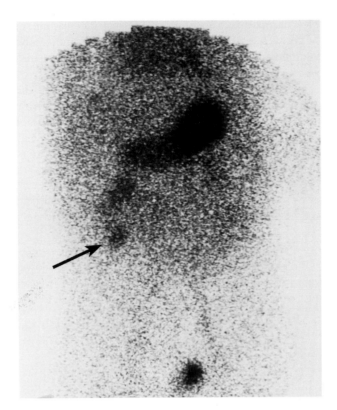

Fig. 3-55   Meckel's diverticulum is detected by increased uptake of the radiotracer by the ectopic gastric mucosa *(arrow)*.

Box 3-8   Meckel's Diverticulum

Occurs in up to 3% of the population
True diverticulum has all layers of bowel wall
Most are asymptomatic
Ectopic gastric mucosa in 20% to 30%—detectable by
    Tc-99m pertechnetate
Clinical problems: Bleeding
                     Intussusception
                     Enteroliths

life. However, less than half of the Meckel's diverticula will have gastric mucosa, which can be functional and produce acid. This causes ulceration in the adjacent ileum resulting in gastrointestinal bleeding. It is this ectopic gastric mucosa that accounts for its positive uptake on a technetium pertechnetate scan (Fig. 3-55). Occasionally it first presents during adulthood, usually secondary to obstruction, because the diverticulum may invaginate and be the lead point for intussusception. Diverticulitis, enterolith formation, perforation, and

neoplastic transformation are less commonly seen manifestations of Meckel's diverticulum.

Careful fluoroscopy using graded compression is often necessary to demonstrate a Meckel's diverticulum on small bowel follow-through examination because it may otherwise be obscured by overlapping bowel loops (Fig. 3-56). Enteroclysis has proven useful for revealing Meckel's diverticula and demonstrating the characteristic triradiate fold pattern at the junction of the diverticulum and the adjacent segment of ileum. A Meckel's scan using radioactive technetium-99m pertechnetate is sensitive for detecting diverticula that contain ectopic gastric mucosa.

Pseudodiverticula

Various abnormalities in the mesenteric small bowel may mimic diverticula. Any process that produces asymmetric inflammation and/or fibrosis can result in asymmetric sacculations or pseudodiverticula (Fig. 3-57). Classically, Crohn's disease can be an asymmetric inflammatory process that may produce asymmetric fibrosis of the bowel wall with subsequent pseudosacculations (Figs. 3-58). The fibrosis that is seen in scleroderma may also produce unusual sacculations of the bowel wall. Surgically created blind loops and communicating congenital duplications of the small bowel can also resemble diverticula.

In lymphoma, focal aneurysmal dilatation of the lumen, either fusiform or asymmetric, may result from destruction of the autonomic neural plexus by tumor infiltration. Focal saccular dilatation of the ileum may also be seen in ileal dysgenesis, a rare condition of uncertain etiology.

PNEUMATOSIS INTESTINALIS

Idiopathic Causes

Pneumatosis intestinalis indicates air in the bowel wall. This is idiopathic in approximately 15% of cases and secondary to various underlying diseases in the remaining 85%. Patients with idiopathic pneumatosis are asymptomatic, and the air collections are cystic in appearance. In secondary pneumatosis, the air collections are linear, and the patients usually have signs or symptoms of GI or pulmonary disease (Fig. 3-59).

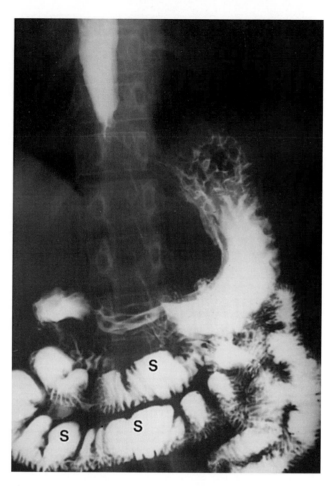

Fig. 3-57 Multiple eccentric sacculations *(S)* in the jejunum in a patient with scleroderma. Note the retained barium in the distal esophagus.

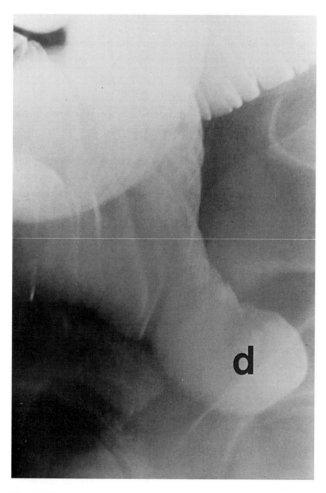

Fig. 3-56 A Meckel's diverticulum *(d)* extends from the distal ileum.

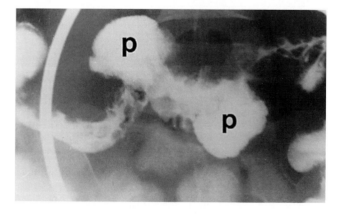

Fig. 3-58 Pseudosacculations *(p)* in the small bowel in a patient with Crohn's disease.

Ischemia/Infarction

Small bowel ischemia or infarction can cause mucosal necrosis and extension of luminal air into the bowel wall (Fig. 3-60). Air in the mesenteric and portal veins or pneumoperitoneum may follow with a high incidence of morbidity and mortality.

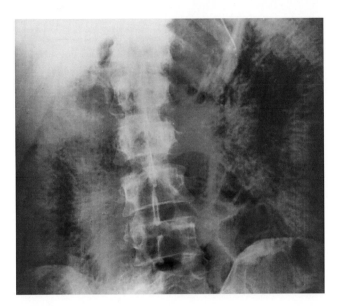

Fig. 3-59 Diffuse linear collections of air in the small bowel wall represent pneumatosis intestinalis.

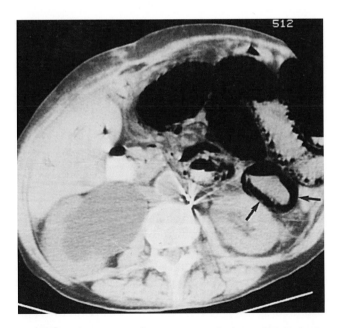

Fig. 3-60 CT shows extensive intramural air *(arrows)* surrounding intraluminal fluid in a patient with small bowel infarction.

Infection and Inflammation (Noninfectious)

Infectious and noninfectious enteritis may also cause pneumatosis because of luminal air passing into the bowel wall through mucosal ulcerations. Other factors, including luminal distention proximal to strictures and infection of the bowel wall by gas-forming organisms, may also play a role in the development of pneumatosis in these cases.

Other Causes

Pneumatosis has been reported following focal perforation of a small bowel diverticulum and iatrogenic trauma caused by indwelling catheters or previous enteric anastomoses. Scleroderma, celiac disease, and other related conditions are rarely complicated by pneumatosis of the small bowel.

Obstructive pulmonary disease can produce pneumatosis secondary to alveolar rupture and subsequent passage of air along interstitial pathways to the mediastinum and, through defects in the diaphragm, to the retroperitoneum, mesentery, and bowel wall.

Pneumatosis has also been reported in patients receiving steroids but may actually be related to the patients' underlying disease rather than to the steroids themselves.

POSTOPERATIVE SMALL BOWEL

Resection

Segmental resection of small bowel with end-to-end anastomosis is a commonly performed procedure in cases of small bowel infarction, perforation, or stenosis. The most frequent complication of this procedure is development of adhesions. In Crohn's disease, segmental small bowel resection is usually avoided whenever possible because of the high incidence of recurrent disease or fistulas at the margins of resection.

Anastomoses

Various enteric anastomoses to the stomach, colon, biliary tree, and pancreas have been described. In Billroth II subtotal gastrectomy, afferent and efferent loops of small bowel are anastomosed to the greater curvature of the gastric remnant. The afferent loop has a closed end and consists of the duodenum and a variable length of proximal jejunum. Current surgical construction of the anastomosis favors emptying of the stomach into the efferent loop, thereby avoiding distention of the afferent loop (afferent loop syndrome). A Roux-en-Y anastomosis can be performed simultaneously, connecting the afferent loop to the efferent loop beyond the gastrojejunostomy site. This prevents bile in the duodenum from refluxing into the gastric remnant where it may cause severe bile reflux gastritis.

Following the Billroth II procedure, several complications involving the small bowel may occur. Marginal ulcerations representing peptic ulceration of the jejunal mucosa typically involve the efferent loop just distal to the gastrojejunal anastomosis. In afferent loop syndrome, continued distention of the afferent loop may lead to bacterial overgrowth. Gastrojejunal and jejunogastric intussusception are unusual complications resulting from antegrade or retrograde intussusception at the anastomotic site.

In cases of gastric outlet obstruction, gastrojejunostomy can be used to bypass narrowing of the distal stomach, pylorus, or duodenum. Gastrojejunostomy is also performed in gastric bypass procedures for morbid obesity. Staples form a small gastric pouch that is then anastomosed side-to-side with a loop of proximal jejunum. Important complications of this procedure include anastomotic leakage and obstruction.

Intestinal Bypass

Intestinal bypass procedures were once used for treating morbid obesity but have now been abandoned because of the high incidence of complications (Fig. 3-61). Because of the decreased length of functioning small bowel, malabsorption occurred with subsequent development of gallstones, renal oxalate stones, and liver disease. Bacterial overgrowth also occurred in the lengthy bypassed segment (blind loop syndrome).

Stomas and Reservoirs

Various ileostomy procedures have been developed for patients with total colectomy. The conventional ileostomy consists of a loop of ileum that is brought to the skin surface and empties into a bag. Kock's continent ileostomy represents a surgically created internal ileal pouch just beneath the abdominal wall. In the Kock's continent ileostomy, a segment of ileum acts as a valve, and the patient empties the pouch by intubating it at regular intervals.

Ileoanal reservoir represents anastomosis of the ileum to the distal rectum following resection of rectal mucosa. After the ileum is folded upon itself in the shape of a J or S, the ileal pouch is created and ileoanal anastomosis is performed.

INTUSSUSCEPTION

Intussusception is the invagination of one bowel loop into another, with the resulting intestinal peristalsis

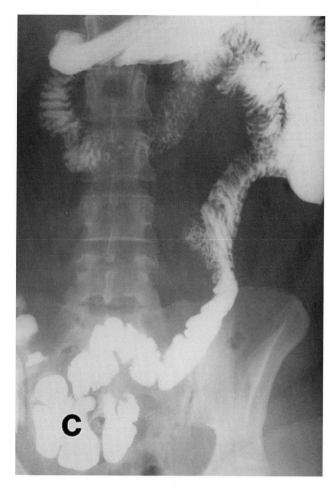

Fig. 3-61   Shortened small bowel secondary to intestinal bypass surgery for obesity. The cecum *(C)* is filled early in the examination.

Box 3-9   Causes of Small Bowel Intussusception

Tumors, primary or metastatic
Idiopathic (typically in children)
Celiac disease (sprue)
Meckel's diverticulum
Intestinal tubes
Cystic fibrosis

---

producing increasing movement of the proximal segment (intussusceptum) into the distal segment (Box 3-9). This can result in obstruction, ischemia, and sometimes even perforation. Typically, an intraluminal lesion such as a polyp serves as a lead point, which gets carried by the peristaltic action into the distal segment. However, a lead point is not necessary for intussusception to occur. Radiographically, an intussusception has a coiled spring appearance as the contrast outlines the intussusceptum (see Fig. 3-10). With cross-sectional imaging techniques,

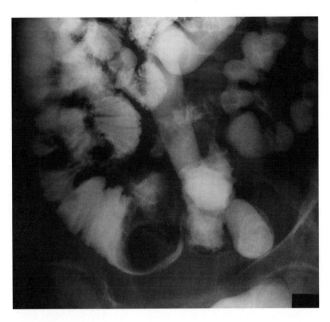

Fig. 3-62   Large intussusception produced by a polyp in Peutz-Jeghers syndrome.

a target appearance is produced by the multiple layers of bowel within each other.

Neoplastic

Neoplasms are the most frequent cause of intussusception in the adult population. Usually, they are benign tumors such as a lipoma or adenoma that serve as lead points for the intussusceptums (Fig. 3-62). These benign tumors often are pedunculated, which aids in the development of intussusception. Malignant tumors such as carcinoma or lymphoma rarely intussuscept because they infiltrate through the bowel wall and not into the lumen. However, malignant sarcomas have the potential for intussuscepting. Also, metastases that develop intraluminal polypoid lesions have often been known to produce intussusception. These include melanoma, breast, and lung.

Nonneoplastic

Approximately a quarter of intussusceptions have no known etiology. This is typically seen in intussusceptions that occur in infants and children. These present with abdominal pain and bleeding. They can sometimes be reduced by a fluoroscopically guided enema, depending upon the duration of the intussusception and the clinical state of the patient.

Sprue is another cause of benign intussusception, although the exact reason why it develops in these patients is uncertain. Intussusception in sprue is usually intermittent or transient in nature and rarely requires any intervention (see Fig. 3-13).

With the increasing use of intestinal tubes, particularly for hyperalimentation, the incidence of intussusception related to tubes is becoming more frequent. Some tubes have a balloon or bag at their end, which serves as a lead point, dragging not only the tube but also a segment of bowel along with it into the distal bowel.

Rarely, diverticula (particularly Meckel's) may invert and be a lead point for an intussusception. Also, ectopic tissue, foreign bodies, and adhesions may serve as a site for intussusception.

POSITIONAL ABNORMALITIES

The intestines develop outside the abdominal cavity and with time return within the abdomen. As they do this, they rotate 270 degrees counterclockwise with the superior mesenteric artery acting as the central axis point. The final location is with the jejunum in the left upper quadrant and the cecum and ileum in the right lower quadrant. Obviously, if this rotation is stopped before completion, any sort of positional variation can occur.

Rotational Abnormalities

Nonrotation is when there is no rotation of the intestines as they return to the abdomen. The ligament of Treitz will not be present, the jejunum and ileum will be on the right side of the abdomen, and the colon will be on the left (Fig. 3-63). Malrotation refers to any degree of rotational abnormality between nonrotation and normal. Often patients are asymptomatic, but there is a predisposition for midgut volvulus as well as aberrant bands producing partial obstruction.

Internal Hernias

Intraabdominal hernias occur as the result of defects, congenital or acquired, in the mesenteries or peritoneal reflections. These defects can incarcerate the small bowel within them, being asymptomatic or producing obstruction and ischemia.

Paraduodenal hernias are the most common, caused by a defect in the parietal peritoneum at the ligament of Treitz. The left paraduodenal hernia is much more common than the right-sided hernia. Radiographically, it can be recognized as a tightly bunched loop of bowel that remains fixed during the study.

Other internal hernias may be due to congenital developmental anomalies or the result of surgically created defects in the mesentery. Again, the diagnosis can be made by identifying several loops of bowel that appear in an unusual location and remain fairly fixed throughout the examination.

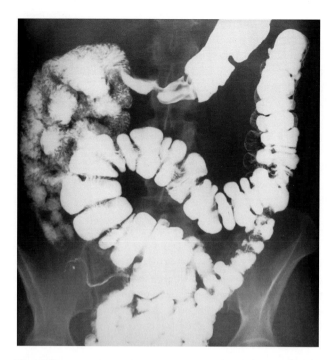

Fig. 3-63 Small bowel loops are in the right upper quadrant in this patient with malrotation.

SUGGESTED READINGS

Balthazar EJ, Gordon R, Hulnick D: Ileocecal tuberculosis: CT and radiologic evaluation, *AJR* 154:499-503, 1990.

Bartnicke BJ, Balfe DM: CT appearance of intestinal ischemia and intramural hemorrhage, *Radiol Clin North Am* 32:845, 1994.

Berk RN, Lee FA: The late manifestations of cystic fibrosis of the pancreas, *Radiology* 106:377-381, 1973.

Berk RN, Wall SD, McArdle CB, et al: Cryptosporidiosis of the stomach and small intestine in patients with AIDS, *AJR* 143:549-554, 1984.

Bhatnagar A, Swaroop K, Behari V, et al: Scintigraphic detection of localized small bowel abnormality, *Clin Nucl Med* 20:367, 1995.

Buck JL, Sobin LH: Carcinoids of the gastrointestinal tract, *Radiographics* 10:1081-1095, 1990.

Carlson HC, Breen JF: Amyloidosis and plasma cell dyscrasias: gastrointestinal involvement, *Semin Roentgenol* 21:128-138, 1986.

Dodds WJ, Geenen JE, Stewart ET: Eosinophilic enteritis, *Am J Gastroenterol* 61:308-312, 1974.

Dudiak KM, Johnson CD, Stephens DH: Primary tumors of the small intestine: CT evaluation, *AJR* 152:995-998, 1989.

Feczko PJ, Collins DD, Mezwa DG: Metastatic disease involving the gastrointestinal tract, *Radiol Clin North Am* 31:1359-1374, 1993.

Feczko PJ, Mezwa DG, Farah MC, et al: Clinical significance of pneumatosis of the bowel wall, *Radiographics* 12:1069-1078, 1992.

Frager D, Mediwd SW, Baer JW, et al: CT of small-bowel obstruction: value in establishing the diagnosis and determining the degree and cause, *AJR* 162:37-41, 1994.

Gardiner R, Smith C: Infective enterocolitides, *Radiol Clin North Am* 25:67-78, 1987.

Gazelle GS, Goldberg MA, Wittenberg J, et al: Efficacy of CT in distinguishing small-bowel obstruction from other causes of small bowel dilatation, *AJR* 162:43-47, 1994.

Glick SN: Crohn's disease of the small intestine, *Radiol Clin North Am* 25:25-45, 1987.

Goldberg HI, Sheft DJ: Abnormalities in small intestine contour and caliber, *Radiol Clin North Am* 14:461-475, 1976.

Gramm HF, Vincent ME, Braver JM: Differential diagnosis of tubular small bowel, *Curr Imaging* 2:62-68, 1990.

Herlinger H: The small bowel enema and the diagnosis of Crohn's disease, *Radiol Clin North Am* 20:721-742, 1982.

Herlinger H, Maglinte DDT: Jejunal fold separation in adult celiac disease: relevance of enteroclysis, *Radiology* 158:605-611, 1986.

Herlinger H, O'Riordan D, Saul S, et al: Nonspecific involvement of bowel adjoining Crohn disease, *Radiology* 159:47-51, 1986.

James S, Balfe DM, Lee JKT, et al: Small-bowel disease: categorization by CT examination, *AJR* 148:863-868, 1987.

Jones B, Kramer SS, Saral R, et al: Gastrointestinal inflammation after bone marrow transplantation: graft-versus-host disease or opportunistic infection? *AJR* 150:277-281, 1988.

Kelvin FM, Gedgaudas RK, Thompson WM, et al: The peroral pneumocolon: its role in evaluating the terminal ileum, *AJR* 139:115-121, 1982.

Laurent F, Drouillard J, Lecesne R, et al: CT of small-bowel neoplasms, *Semin Ultrasound CT MR* 16:102, 1995.

Libshitz HI, Lindell MM, Dodd GD: Metastases to the hollow viscera, *Radiol Clin North Am* 20:487-499, 1982.

Long FR, Kramer SS, Markowitz RI, et al: Radiographic patterns of intestinal malrotation in children, *Radiographics* 16:547, 1996.

Lund EC, Han SY, Holley HC, et al: Intestinal ischemia: comparison of plain radiographic and computed tomographic findings, *Radiographics* 8:1083-1108, 1988.

Maglinte DDT, Chernish SM, DeWeese R, et al: Acquired jejunoileal diverticular disease: subject review, *Radiology* 158:577-580, 1986.

Maglinte DDT, Kelvin FM, O'Connor K, et al: Current status of small bowel radiography, *Abdomin Imag* 21:247, 1996.

Megibow AJ, Balthazar EJ, Hulnick DH: Radiology of nonneoplastic gastrointestinal disorders in acquired immune deficiency syndrome, *Semin Roentgenol* 22:31-41, 1987.

Merine D, Fishman EK, Jones B, et al: Enteroenteric intussusception: CT findings in nine patients, *AJR* 148:1129-1132, 1987.

Merine D, Fishman EK, Jones B: CT of the small bowel and mesentery, *Radiol Clin North Am* 27:707-715, 1989.

Meyers MA: Metastatic seeding along the small bowel mesentery: roentgen features, *AJR* 123:67-73, 1975.

Orel SG, Rubesin SE, Jones B, et al: Computed tomography vs. barium studies in the acutely symptomatic patient with Crohn disease, *J Comput Assist Tomogr* 11:1009-1016, 1987.

Osborne AG, Friedland GW: A radiological approach to the diagnosis of small bowel disease, *Clin Radiol* 24:281-301, 1973.

Ott DJ, Chen YM, Gelfand DW, et al: Detailed per-oral small bowel examination vs enteroclysis, *Radiology* 155:29-34, 1985.

Perez C, Llaugher J, Puig J, et al: Computed tomographic findings in bowel ischemia, *Gastrointest Radiol* 14:241-245, 1989.

Pozniak MA, Scanlan K, Yandow D: Ultrasound in the evaluation of bowel disorders, *Semin Ultrasound CT MR* 8:366-384, 1987.

Rogers LF, Goldstein HM: Roentgen manifestations of radiation injury to the gastrointestinal tract, *Gastrointest Radiol* 2:281-291, 1977.

Rossi P, Gourtsoyiannis N, Bezzi M, et al: Meckel's diverticulum: imaging diagnosis, *AJR* 166:567-573, 1996.

Rubesin SE, Gilchrist AM, Bronner M, et al: Non-Hodgkin lymphoma of the small intestine, *Radiographics* 10:985-998, 1990.

Rubesin SE, Herlinger H, Saul SH, et al: Adult celiac disease and its complications, *Radiographics* 9:1045-1066, 1989.

Scatarige JC, Allen III HA, Fishman EK: Computed tomography of the small bowel, *Semin Ultrasound CT MR* 8:403-423, 1987.

Scholz FJ: Ischemic bowel disease, *Radiol Clin North Am* 31:1197-1218, 1993.

Smith C, Deziel DJ, Kubicka RA: Appearances of the postoperative alimentary tract, *Radiol Clin North Am* 31:1235-1254, 1993.

Szucs RA, Turner MA: Gastrointestinal tract involvement by gynecologic diseases, *Radiographics* 16:1251, 1996.

Teixidor HS, Honig CL, Norsoph E, et al: Cytomegalovirus infection of the alimentary canal: radiologic findings with pathologic correlation, *Radiology* 163:317-323, 1987.

Wall SD, Ominsky S, Altman DF, et al: Multifocal abnormalities of the gastrointestinal tract in AIDS, *AJR* 146:1-5, 1986.

Wiot JF: Intramural small intestinal hemorrhage—a differential diagnosis, *Semin Roentgenol* 1:219-233, 1966.

Yeh H-C, Rabinowitz JG: Ultrasonography of gastrointestinal tract, *Semin Ultrasound CT MR* 3:331-347, 1982.

Pancreas

EXAMINATION TECHNIQUES

The pancreas is a midline retroperitoneal structure located diagonally in the upper abdomen. It consists of the head and uncinate process, body, and tail and lies in close proximity to the stomach, duodenum, left kidney, spleen, aorta, inferior vena cava, portal and splenic veins, and superior mesenteric vessels.

The pancreas performs important exocrine and endocrine functions. Alkaline fluid secreted into the duodenum through the pancreatic duct neutralizes gastric acid, and the enzymes amylase and lipase aid in the digestion of carbohydrates and fats, respectively. Various hormones, most importantly insulin, glucagon, and gastrin, are formed in the pancreatic islets of Langerhans and are secreted directly into the bloodstream to regulate glucose metabolism (insulin and glucagon) and gastric acid secretion (gastrin). Abdominal plain films are useful for demonstrating pancreatic calcifications. An upper gastrointestinal (UGI) series shows deformity of the stomach and duodenum secondary to adjacent pancreatic inflammatory or neoplastic disease. Duodenal and proximal jejunal ulcers may also result from hypersecretion of gastric acid in response to a pancreatic gastrinoma (Zollinger-Ellison syndrome). Various methods of hypotonic duodenography have been developed for improved distention of the duodenum and visualization of ampullary and pancreatic head masses.

Cross-sectional imaging technique revolutionized pancreatic imaging by allowing direct visualization of the pancreas. Percutaneous drainage of pancreatic or peripancreatic fluid collections and aspiration or biopsy of pancreatic masses are also widely performed using ultrasound guidance or computed tomography (CT) guidance.

Ultrasound of the normal pancreas usually shows homogeneous echogenicity that equals or slightly exceeds that of the normal liver. Reported measurements of the normal pancreas vary, but currently accepted values are 2.6 cm for anteroposterior diameter of the head, 2.2 cm for that of the body, and 1.5 cm for that of the tail. Advantages of ultrasound compared with CT include lower cost, absence of ionizing radiation, and multiplanar imaging capabilities. The main disadvantage of ultrasound is poor visualization of the pancreas secondary to obesity or overlying bowel gas. Interference by bowel gas may be overcome by having the patient ingest water, thereby distending the stomach and duodenum and forming an acoustic window. Intravenous injection of glucagon may aid sonographic visualization of the pancreas by decreasing intestinal motility. Supplemental examination in prone, decubitus, upright, or oblique positions may be necessary to evaluate the pancreas completely.

Optimal CT demonstration of the pancreas requires a sufficient amount of oral contrast material to opacify the adjacent stomach, duodenum, and proximal jejunum. Rapid infusion of intravenous contrast material provides opacification of adjacent blood vessels and enhancement of the pancreatic parenchyma (Fig. 4-1). Although 10-mm-thick axial images are routinely used for evaluating the pancreas, dynamic scanning allows rapid acquisition of contiguous 5- or 3-mm-thick axial images during peak vascular enhancement. CT is not limited by obesity or overlying bowel gas, and it provides excellent evaluation of associated peripancreatic and extrapancreatic extension of disease. Magnetic resonance imaging (MRI) of the pancreas offers the advantages of multiplanar imaging capabilities, absence of ionizing radiation, and differentiation between tissue and flowing blood. It is being used more frequently as the relative cost of the examination has decreased. Also, newer imaging sequences have been developed that further enhance the evaluation of

pancreatic ductal structures and parenchyma. Intravenous injection of glucagon decreases motion artifacts caused by intestinal motility, and various negative and positive contrast agents are available for bowel opacification. With increasing advances in MRI, it is slowly becoming an important tool in the evaluation of pancreatic lesions and will in time supplant CT in that regard.

Endoscopic retrograde cholangiopancreatography (ERCP) remains the best method for evaluating the pancreatic duct (Fig. 4-2). Coexistent disease of the biliary tree, such as common bile duct narrowing secondary to pancreatic carcinoma, or choledocholithiasis causing pancreatitis, can also be evaluated by ERCP. ERCP is contraindicated in acute pancreatitis because overinjection of the pancreatic duct may cause parenchymal opacification (acinarization) and worsening of pancreatitis. Other disadvantages of ERCP relate to complications of endoscopy in general and potential trauma to the ampulla of Vater during duct cannulation. Also, the success rate is variable and usually does not exceed 90%. The cost of the procedure and the use of routine sedation prevent it from being a routine procedure.

Because of ERCP's disadvantages, magnetic resonance cholangiopancreatography (MRCP) is being used as a noninvasive method of evaluating the ductal structures. Although its resolution is less than ERCP, it can provide useful information in a variety of circumstances (Fig. 4-3). It is performed using a heavily weighted T2-imaging sequence. Its major advantages are that the ducts can be visualized in multiple planes, both pancreatic and biliary ducts can be imaged simultaneously, success rate is not operator dependent, contrast agents or sedation is not routinely needed, and significant complications are rare. Additionally, the procedure can be performed on almost all patients and the cost is still considerably less than ERCP. Negative aspects include limited resolution, par-

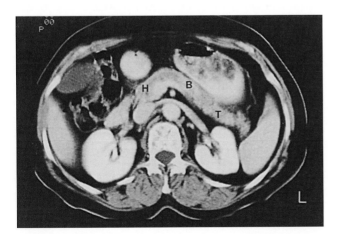

Fig. 4-1 CT demonstrates the normal pancreatic head *(H)*, body *(B)*, and tail *(T)*.

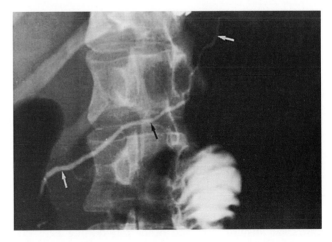

Fig. 4-2 ERCP shows a normal pancreatic duct *(arrows)*.

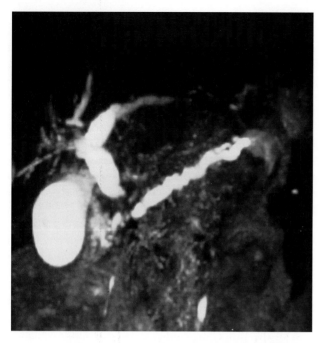

Fig. 4-3   MRCP demonstrates both pancreatic and biliary systems on the same image. Note dilated pancreatic duct secondary to chronic pancreatitis.

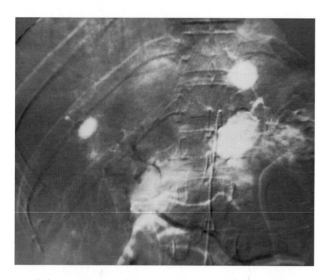

Fig. 4-4   Arteriogram shows multiple hypervascular masses in the pancreas and both lobes of the liver. This is an islet cell tumor of the pancreas with liver metastases.

ticularly of side branches, and inability to perform therapeutic procedures. However, it is likely that MRCP will supplant diagnostic ERCP in the future.

Pancreatic angiography for evaluation of pancreatic carcinoma has been largely supplanted by ultrasound and CT. However, both superselective subtraction arteriography and venous sampling are still used for localizing small insulinomas and other functioning islet cell tumors (Fig. 4-4).

Endoscopic ultrasound is a relatively new method that has shown promising results in the detection of pancre-

---

atic lesions. The instrument consists of an ultrasound transducer attached to the tip of an endoscope. After positioning of the transducer against the gastric or duodenal wall, images of the adjacent pancreas are obtained.

EMBRYOLOGY

Development of the pancreas in utero is a complex mechanism that results in a variety of anomalies and variants. Many of these are asymptomatic, but others can produce symptoms in either children or adults. Understanding the complex nature of this embryological formation aids in the evaluation of the pancreas (Box 4-1).

The pancreas develops from the embryological fusion of dorsal and ventral buds of the foregut, which grow during the fourth week of gestation. The ventral bud begins development to the right of the duodenum, while the dorsal bud develops from the left side of the duodenum (Fig. 4-5). The pancreas comes to occupy a position to the left of the duodenum by rotation of the ventral bud as well as by partial duodenal rotation, which both occur in about the sixth week. The dorsal duct drains the body, tail, and superior portion of the head of the pancreas into the minor papilla, and the ventral duct drains the uncinate process and inferior portion of the pancreatic head (as well as the biliary system) into the major papilla. Under normal circumstances the ventral duct (Wirsung) fuses with the dorsal duct (Santorini), usually around the seventh week. Following fusion of the two ducts, the main duct of Wirsung, consisting of the ventral duct and the proximal segment of the dorsal duct, continues to drain into the major papilla. The distal segment of the dorsal duct, which drains into the minor papilla, partially regresses to form the accessory duct of Santorini.

CONGENITAL ANOMALIES

Annular Pancreas

Annular pancreas is a rare congenital abnormality in which a ring of pancreatic tissue encircles the duodenum at or above the papilla of Vater. Normally, the ventral bud

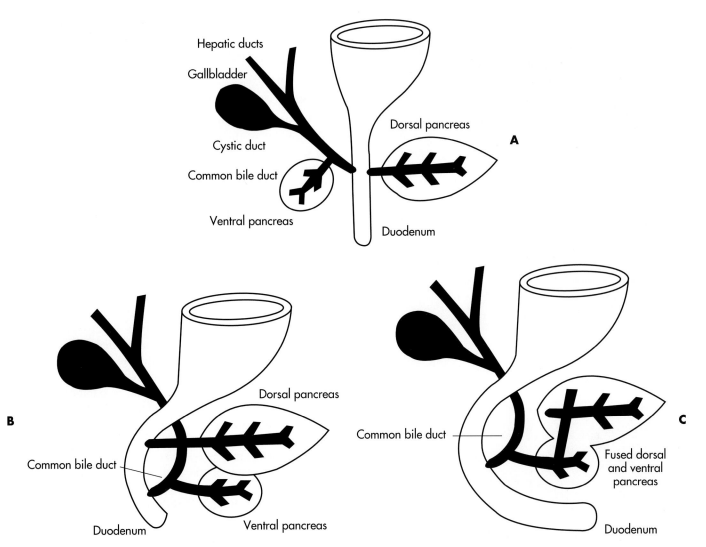

Fig. 4-5   **A,** By the end of the fifth week, ventral and dorsal pancreatic buds are forming along with their ducts and the biliary system. **B,** By the end of the sixth week, the midgut has rotated. Also, the ventral pancreas and distal common duct have rotated to the left of the duodenum. **C,** By the eighth week, the ventral and dorsal pancreatic buds have fused. Their ductal systems have also fused, and the pancreas is now draining through the ventral duct (Wirsung). (Diagrams courtesy of David McVinnie, M.D.)

and the duodenum undergo rotation that places the ventral portion of the pancreas to the left of the duodenum. However, in annular pancreas the ventral pancreas does not completely rotate and there may also be limited rotation of the duodenum. This results in the ventral pancreas forming either a partial or a complete ring around the duodenum. Depending on the degree of obstruction, this may lead to an acute surgical condition in the newborn or be asymptomatic throughout life. Annular pancreas may also first become symptomatic in adulthood, producing epigastric pain, early satiety, and vomiting secondary to duodenal obstruction. Gastric and duodenal peptic ulcer disease and pancreatitis also occur with increased incidence in long-standing annular pancreas. A typical finding of annular pancreas on

UGI series is eccentric or concentric narrowing of the descending duodenum with associated mucosal effacement but without ulceration or mucosal destruction (Fig. 4-6). The proximal duodenum may become dilated, and reversed peristalsis and dilatation of the duodenum distal to the annular narrowing have also been described. CT scan may demonstrate the annulus surrounding and constricting the descending duodenum (Fig. 4-7). On ERCP, opacification of the ventral duct encircling the descending duodenum is diagnostic of annular pancreas. Recommended treatment of annular pancreas presenting in adulthood is surgical bypass of the narrowed segment of duodenum. Simple division of the pancreatic annulus is often insufficient for relief of symptoms because of the frequent association of duodenal stenosis and fibrosis at

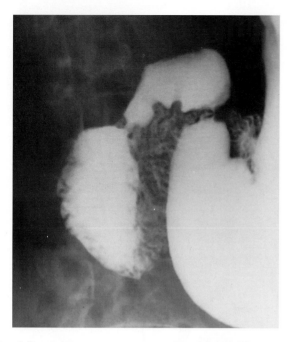

Fig. 4-6   Bandlike narrowing of the duodenal sweep is due to an annular pancreas.

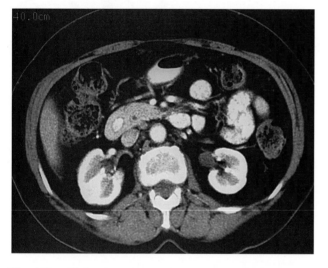

Fig. 4-7   CT demonstrates pancreatic tissue entirely surrounding the duodenum in a patient with annular pancreas.

the site of long-standing narrowing. Division of the annulus with transection of the annular duct may also lead to pancreatitis and pancreatic fistula.

Pancreas Divisum

Pancreas divisum represents a common congenital abnormality of the pancreas, with an incidence of up to 11% recorded in an autopsy series. This anomaly results from failure of fusion of the embryological dorsal and ventral buds. Consequently, the dorsal and ventral ducts remain separate, with the dorsal duct draining the body, tail, and superior portion of the head of the pancreas into the minor papilla, and the ventral duct draining the uncinate process and inferior portion of the pancreatic head into the major papilla (Fig. 4-8).

On ERCP of pancreas divisum, injection of contrast material into the major papilla opacifies the short, tapering ventral duct (Fig. 4-9). Visualization and cannulation of the minor papilla are often difficult because of its small size but when accomplished demonstrate opacification of the long dorsal duct extending along the pancreatic body and tail. Thin-section CT may reveal lobulation of the pancreatic head, separation of the ventral and dorsal portions of the pancreas by a fat cleft, or failure of fusion of the ventral and dorsal ducts. Pancreatitis may occur with increased incidence in patients with pancreas divisum, possibly caused by impeded drainage of the bulk of the pancreatic parenchyma through the small minor papilla. However, the association of pancreatitis and pancreas divisum remains controversial.

Ductal Duplications

There are numerous variants of pancreatic divisum, in which the two ducts join but retain separate drainages to the duodenum (Fig. 4-10). Because of the complex nature of the joining of these ductal structures, there is no typical eventual appearance of the pancreatic ducts. Duplications of the ventral or dorsal pancreatic ducts represent rare embryological abnormalities that have

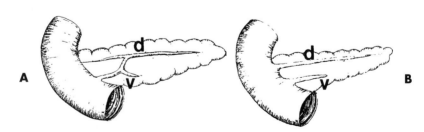

Fig. 4-8   Diagrams illustrate the relationship of the ventral *(v)* and dorsal *(d)* pancreatic ducts, **A,** following fusion and, **B,** in pancreas divisum.

been documented on ERCP (Fig. 4-11). There is no increased association of these anomalies with pancreatitis or other abnormalities.

Ectopic Pancreas

Ectopic or aberrant pancreas (pancreatic rest) represents pancreatic tissue occurring in extrapancreatic sites, most commonly along the greater curvature of

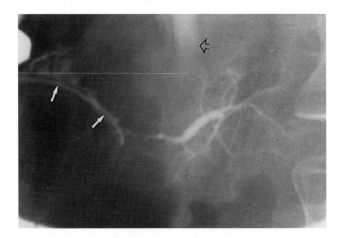

Fig. 4-9   ERCP shows a short, tapering ventral pancreatic duct, indicating pancreas divisum. The cannula of the endoscope extends into the major papilla *(arrows)*. Contrast material partially opacifies the common bile duct *(open arrow)*.

the distal gastric antrum or in the periampullary portion of the descending duodenum. The ectopic tissue is typically small and submucosal in location. A tiny central umbilication that may represent a primitive pancreatic duct is sometimes noted. Ectopic pancreas, although usually asymptomatic, may cause GI hemorrhage or obstruction, biliary obstruction, or small bowel intussusception. Rarely, inflammatory or neoplastic pancreatic lesions arise within ectopic pancreatic tissue.

Short Pancreas

Short pancreas is characterized by congenital absence of the pancreatic body and tail and a rounded appearance of the pancreatic head. This most likely results from agenesis of the dorsal pancreas and may occur as an isolated finding or in association with the polysplenia syndrome (Fig. 4-12).

Long Common Segment of Pancreatic and Common Bile Ducts

The pancreatic duct and the common bile duct normally enter the major papilla either separately or through a short common channel less than 1 cm in length. Abnormally high fusion of the ducts forms a long common channel, usually regarded as greater than 1 cm in length (Fig. 4-13). There is an increase in abnormali-

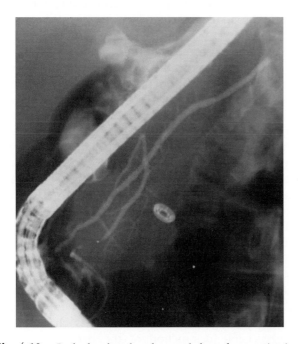

Fig. 4-10   Both the dorsal and ventral ducts have maintained their normal size and have separate drainages into the duodenum. A small connecting channel is still present, however. This is a common variant of pancreas divisum.

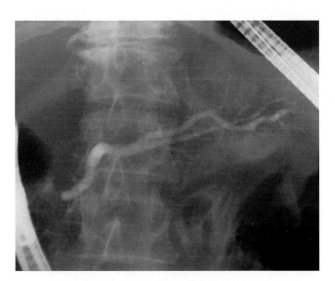

Fig. 4-11   Two distinct ductal systems are seen in the body and tail because of a duplication of the pancreas.

ties of the bile ducts or pancreas when this occurs. One theory is that reflux of pancreatic secretions into the common bile duct may lead to the development of a choledochal cyst, and this anomaly has been reported to be more common in patients with choledochal cysts. There is also an increased incidence of pancreatitis with this anomaly.

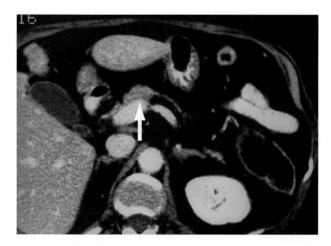

Fig. 4-12   Only the head of the pancreas is present *(arrow)*, and the tail is represented by a thin line of tissue. This is in a patient with congenital absence of the body and tail, probably from failure of development of the dorsal bud.

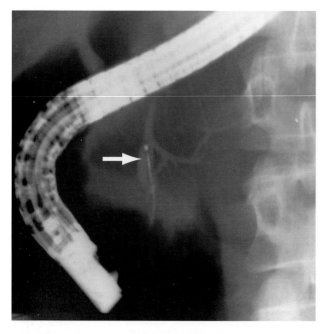

Fig. 4-13   The ventral duct of the pancreas drains the head of the pancreas into the side of the common bile duct, resulting in a long common channel *(arrow)*. This patient also had pancreas divisum and a small choledochal cyst.

PANCREATIC SIZE

Enlarged

Pancreatitis

Acute.   Acute pancreatitis often causes diffuse or focal enlargement of the pancreas secondary to inflammation and edema. Acute pancreatitis is characterized by abdominal pain radiating to the back. Serum amylase and lipase levels are elevated, and the serum calcium level is often reduced. Acute pancreatitis, although most often occurring secondary to alcohol ingestion or gallstone disease, may also result from various infections, medications, surgical or nonsurgical trauma, and metabolic or systemic disorders.

Abdominal plain films may demonstrate generalized or focal ileus (sentinel loop and colon cut-off sign) or abdominal fat necrosis in which hydrolyzed fat produces a mottled appearance. Chest film findings include basilar subsegmental atelectasis, pleural fluid, and elevation of the left hemidiaphragm. On UGI series, acute pancreatitis may cause widening of the duodenal sweep, thickening of duodenal folds, effacement of folds or a reverse figure 3 configuration along the inner aspect of the duodenal sweep, enlargement of the major papilla, or anterior displacement of the stomach. These findings are not specific to acute pancreatitis and may also be seen in chronic pancreatitis and in pancreatic carcinoma.

Ultrasound of acute pancreatitis typically demonstrates diffuse or focal pancreatic enlargement, hypoechoic parenchyma, and poorly defined contour. However, ultrasound in these patients is frequently limited by overlying bowel gas caused by intestinal ileus. CT of acute pancreatitis, in addition to showing enlargement and poorly defined contour of the pancreas, may reveal inflammatory infiltration of peripancreatic and extrapancreatic fat and fascial planes. The pancreatic parenchyma usually shows decreased attenuation secondary to edema or necrosis but on contrast-enhanced scans may appear diffusely hyperdense because of hyperemia. In acute hemorrhagic pancreatitis, a severe form of pancreatitis characterized by parenchymal hemorrhage, inflammation, and destruction, focal areas of increased attenuation are often seen on CT (Fig. 4-14). Both ultrasound and CT are useful for detecting various pancreatic and extrapancreatic fluid collections associated with acute pancreatitis.

Chronic.   ERCP is usually contraindicated in the evaluation of acute pancreatitis because overinjection and manipulation of the pancreatic duct may worsen the pancreatitis. Chronic pancreatitis is characterized by irreversible destruction of the pancreatic parenchyma. Like acute pancreatitis, chronic pancreatitis may cause focal or diffuse pancreatic enlargement. Common clinical manifestations include abdominal pain radiating to the back and severe diabetes mellitus. Amylase and lipase levels may be elevated, normal, or decreased. Chronic pancreatitis most often results from long-term alcohol ingestion but also occurs secondary to hereditary pancreatitis, trauma, hyperparathyroidism, and malnutrition.

Abdominal films commonly show focal or diffuse pancreatic ductal calculi. Most of the plain film and UGI findings seen in acute pancreatitis may also occur in chronic pancreatitis.

Ultrasound and CT may demonstrate focal or diffuse pancreatic enlargement during acute relapses of chronic pancreatitis. With progression of the disease, diffuse parenchymal atrophy and ductal dilatation result. Ultrasound may demonstrate irregular echogenicity with hyperechoic and hypoechoic areas secondary to fibrosis and edema, respectively. These alterations in parenchymal echo texture are a sensitive but nonspecific sign of chronic pancreatitis. Other findings of chronic pancreatitis seen on ultrasound and CT include ductal calculi, pseudocysts and other fluid collections, and biliary ductal dilatation.

ERCP is useful in assessing severity and complications of chronic pancreatitis. Typical findings involving the pancreatic duct include dilatation, irregularity, or beading of the main duct; dilatation of side branches; periampullary ductal stenosis; and filling defects or obstruction caused by ductal calculi. Opacification of the biliary tree during ERCP or percutaneous transhepatic cholangiography (PTC) may reveal smooth stenosis or extrinsic displacement of the common bile duct.

Phlegmon/abscess

In more severe forms of acute pancreatitis, the gland may undergo complete necrosis because of autodigestion. What may be left is a diffuse, necrotic area of tissue occupying the pancreatic bed region (Fig. 4-15). Typically, this has low density and strands of inflammatory changes can be seen extending into the peripancreatic areas. If this becomes infected, abscess formation can result. This type of pancreatitis is often encountered posttraumatically and sometimes as the result of instrumentation or surgery.

Hemorrhage

Hemorrhage into the pancreas is characterized by enlargement of the gland with either focal or diffuse areas of high attenuation (greater than 60 HU). This increased density is distinctive and separates hemorrhage from other inflammatory conditions, which are typically low density.

Malignancy

Pancreatic carcinoma, islet cell tumors, and various other neoplasms may cause focal enlargement of the pancreas (Fig. 4-16). Involvement of peripancreatic nodes secondary to lymphoma or metastatic disease may mimic focal or diffuse enlargement of the pancreas itself. Sometimes there is development of pancreatitis proximal to a tumor of the pancreas, which results in diffuse enlargement of the gland. In these circumstances it may be difficult to separate the neoplastic tissue from the inflammatory changes. However, a distinguishing feature may be focal ductal dilatation proximal to the tumor.

Fatty infiltration

Pancreatic lipomatosis is a disorder in which the parenchyma of the exocrine pancreas is partially or completely replaced by fat. Rarely, massive pancreatic enlargement results from lipomatosis in the form of either diffuse fatty infiltration or multiple nodular fatty masses. This condition, known as lipomatous pseudohy-

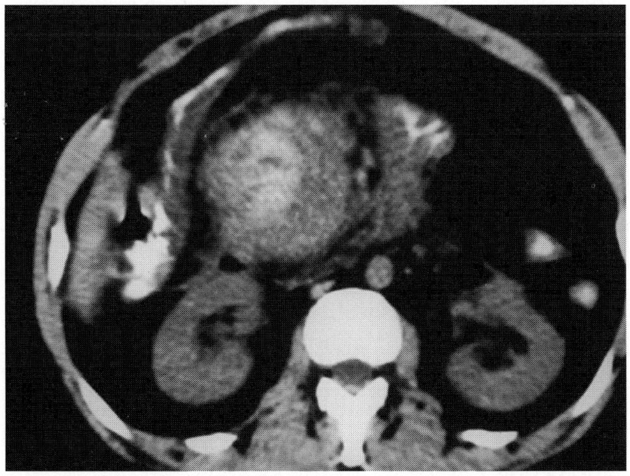

Fig. 4-14 Enlarged pancreatic head in acute pancreatitis. Note the high-density areas representing areas of hemorrhage.

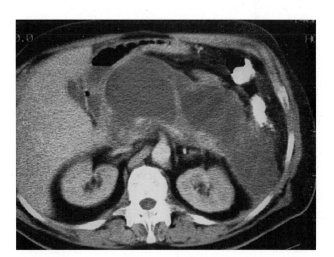

Fig. 4-15 Diffusely enlarged pancreas with multiple low-density areas is due to pancreatic necrosis or phlegmon.

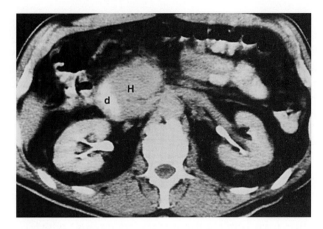

Fig. 4-16 Enlargement of the pancreatic head *(H)* represents pancreatic adenocarcinoma. The adjacent duodenum *(d)* is opacified.

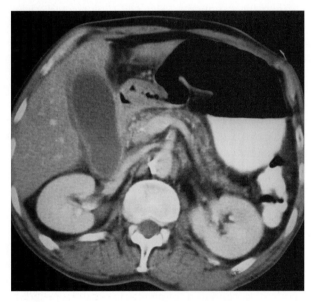

Fig. 4-17 A diffusely thin pancreas is seen above the splenic vein. Atrophy is probably due to chronic pancreatitis.

pertrophy of the pancreas, is of uncertain etiology but may result from various factors, including obesity, cystic fibrosis, diabetes mellitus, alcoholic cirrhosis, and chronic pancreatitis.

Atrophic

Normal aging

The pancreas normally decreases in size with aging and may appear atrophic in elderly patients (without a history of pancreatic disease). Associated findings include pancreatic ductal dilatation and fatty infiltration of the parenchyma. The amount of glandular tissue evident does not reflect the degree of function of the pancreas, and normal pancreatic function may persist despite apparent atrophy on imaging (Fig. 4-17).

Chronic pancreatitis

Chronic pancreatitis often leads to diffuse atrophy of the pancreatic parenchyma. This is associated with parenchymal fibrosis, ductal dilatation, and ductal calculi.

Pancreatic duct obstruction

Long-standing obstruction of the pancreatic duct may result in parenchymal atrophy proximal to the obstructing process, involving the parenchyma surrounding the dilated segment of the duct. The obstruction may be the result of an impacted calculus or a benign or malignant tumor and may be located at the ampulla of Vater or anywhere along the course of the pancreatic duct.

Cystic fibrosis

Cystic fibrosis (mucoviscidosis) is a common genetic (autosomal recessive) disorder in which abnormally thick mucous secretions lead to pulmonary, pancreatic, and GI dysfunction. The disease may first become evident in the neonate as meconium ileus or in childhood or early adulthood as recurrent pneumonia and progressive pulmonary or pancreatic insufficiency.

In the pancreas, mucus precipitates in the ducts and obstructs the secretion of pancreatic enzymes into the duodenum. This leads to intestinal malabsorption and steatorrhea, as well as eventual fibrotic or fatty replacement of the exocrine pancreatic parenchyma. The pancreas may become diffusely atrophic with or without fatty replacement.

Other abnormalities

Congenital pancreatic hypoplasia (Shwachman syndrome) is a rare genetic disorder characterized by abnormalities of the exocrine pancreas similar to those seen in cystic fibrosis. In pancreatic hypoplasia, atrophy and fatty replacement of the pancreas are associated with various skeletal and hematological abnormalities.

Viral infection, hemochromatosis, and malnutrition may also cause atrophy and fatty replacement of the pancreas.

PANCREATIC MASSES

Solid

Focal acute pancreatitis

Acute pancreatitis, although usually a diffuse process, may cause focal enlargement of any portion of the pancreas. The localized inflammatory mass may appear solid, cystic, or inhomogeneous on CT and hyperechoic, normal, or hypoechoic on ultrasound. Focal pancreatic enlargement may also be seen in chronic pancreatitis.

Table 4-1   Epithelial neoplasms

Tumor type	Texture	Histology
Ductal adenocarcinoma	Solid	Malignant
Acinar cell carcinoma	Solid (partially necrotic)	Malignant
Microcystic adenoma	Cystic (numerous small cysts)	Benign
Mucinous cystic neoplasm	Cystic (fewer and larger cysts)	Premalignant or malignant
Solid and papillary epithelial neoplasm	Solid and cystic	Malignant (low-grade)

Phlegmon

Pancreatic phlegmon represents diffuse pancreatic enlargement and peripancreatic inflammation secondary to acute pancreatitis. It appears inhomogeneous on CT and ultrasound and may resolve completely or worsen, leading to fluid collections, necrosis, or abscess formation.

Ductal adenocarcinoma

Pancreatic ductal adenocarcinoma (pancreatic carcinoma) is the most common neoplasm of the pancreas (Table 4-1). It represents 80% of all tumors originating from the ductal epithelium of the exocrine pancreas. Approximately two thirds of pancreatic carcinomas arise in the head of the pancreas, and only 10% to 15% of the tumors are surgically resectable when first diagnosed. Even when surgical resection is performed, median postoperative survival is less than 20 months.

Clinical signs and symptoms of pancreatic carcinoma are nonspecific and may include abdominal pain, weight loss, jaundice, UGI bleeding, thrombophlebitis (Trousseau's syndrome), and new onset of diabetes mellitus or pancreatitis. Barium studies may demonstrate extrinsic compression or mural invasion of the adjacent stomach, duodenum, or transverse colon. However, ultrasound and CT have proved more useful for evaluating the pancreas, pancreatic and biliary ducts, liver parenchyma, and peripancreatic nodes, thereby improving detection of pancreatic carcinoma and allowing determination of resectability. They also provide accurate guidance for percutaneous aspiration and biopsy of primary or metastatic pancreatic carcinoma.

Pancreatic carcinoma typically appears as a focal hypoechoic mass on ultrasound and a hypodense mass on CT (Fig. 4-18). Obstruction of the pancreatic duct by the mass often causes ductal dilatation and atrophy of the adjacent pancreatic parenchyma (Box 4-2). Coexistent obstruction of the intrapancreatic segment of the biliary duct may also be seen in cases of carcinoma involving the head of the pancreas. Dilatation of both the pancreatic and biliary ducts is known as the double-duct sign. Although this may also result from intrapancreatic extension of cholangiocarcinoma, it is most commonly caused by carcinoma of the pancreatic head (Fig. 4-19).

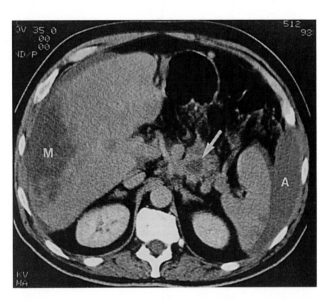

Fig. 4-18   Irregular hypodense mass in the pancreatic tail *(arrow)* represents pancreatic adenocarcinoma. Hepatic metastasis *(M)* and ascites *(A)* indicate disseminated disease.

Box 4-2   CT Signs of Pancreatic Adenocarcinoma

Focal mass (low density)
Diffuse enlargement
Ductal dilatation
Proximal atrophy
Perivascular encasement
Local extension
Metastases

Various CT criteria have been established for determining unresectability of pancreatic carcinoma (Box 4-3). These include local extrapancreatic extension of tumor, invasion of contiguous organs, hepatic or regional nodal metastases, malignant ascites, and encasement or obstruction of major peripancreatic vessels. Obliteration of fat surrounding the celiac and superior mesenteric arteries, although usually secondary to vas-

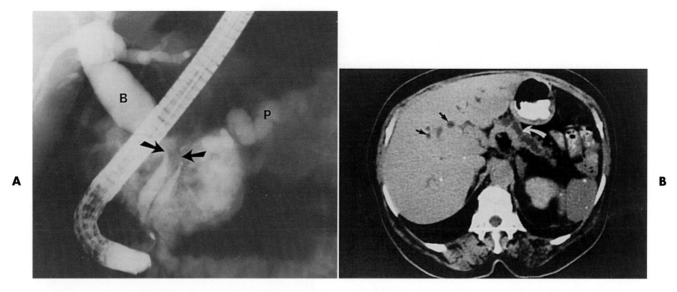

Fig. 4-19   **A,** ERCP shows adjacent narrowing *(arrows)* and proximal dilatation of the biliary *(B)* and pancreatic *(P)* ducts in a patient with pancreatic adenocarcinoma. **B,** CT demonstrates dilatation of the biliary ducts *(arrows)* and pancreatic duct *(curved arrow).*

Box 4-3   Important Signs in Evaluating Resectability of Pancreatic Carcinoma

Liver metastases
Vascular encasement
Peritoneal implants
Peripancreatic extension
Size >3 cm
Adenopathy

---

cular encasement by pancreatic carcinoma, has been reported in chronic pancreatitis and various nonpancreatic tumors including metastatic disease and lymphoma.

An ERCP finding in pancreatic carcinoma is obstruction or encasement of the pancreatic duct (Fig. 4-20). Although involvement is usually irregular and abrupt, it occasionally appears smooth and tapering, mimicking inflammatory disease. Obstruction or encasement of the biliary duct typically affects the intrapancreatic portion of the duct. Less commonly, the proximal common duct or intrahepatic ducts appear narrowed secondary to metastatic disease involving portal nodes or liver parenchyma, respectively. Opacification of an irregular cavity within the pancreas may result from tumor necrosis and subsequent communication between the tumor and the pancreatic duct. In cases of biliary duct obstruction, an internal biliary stent can be placed endoscopically during ERCP in order to achieve decompression.

Similarly, PTC may be performed to detect the level and degree of biliary duct obstruction secondary to pancreatic carcinoma. Pancreatic carcinoma may cause irregular or smooth narrowing of the biliary duct. Internal or external biliary drainage can be achieved by percutaneous stent placement immediately following PTC. The most common angiographic finding in pancreatic carcinoma is encasement of peripancreatic arteries or veins (Box 4-4). Less common findings include vascular occlusion, angulation, and displacement. Neovascularity is not a typical feature of pancreatic carcinoma.

Acinar cell carcinoma and other epithelial tumors

Acinar cell carcinoma is a rare tumor arising from acinar cells of the exocrine pancreas (Table 4-1). This tumor may be associated with elevated serum lipase levels and disseminated intraosseous and subcutaneous fat necrosis. Acinar cell carcinomas usually appear large, lobulated, and partially necrotic when first detected, and liver metastases are often present. Angiography shows moderate vascularity as well as vascular encasement and neovascularity.

Other rare pancreatic tumors of epithelial cell origin include pleomorphic carcinoma, adenosquamous carcinoma, and pancreatoblastoma. Radiographic findings are similar to those of pancreatic ductal adenocarcinoma.

Islet cell tumors

Tumors arising from the islet cells of the pancreas produce a variety of clinical and radiographic findings. Islet cells, classified as APUD cells because of their

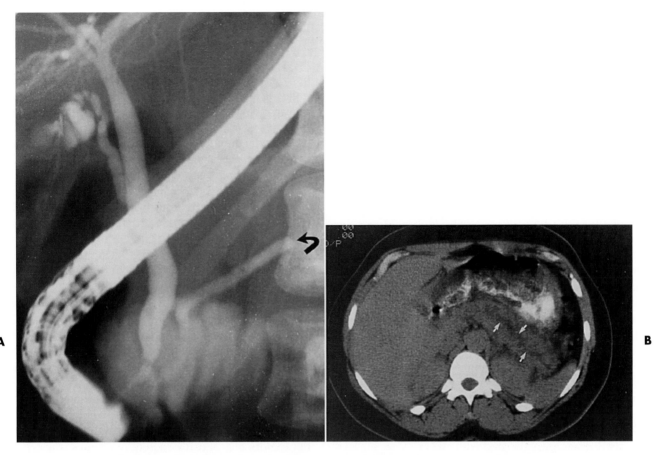

Fig. 4-20   A, ERCP shows abrupt occlusion of the midportion of the pancreatic duct *(arrow)* caused by pancreatic adenocarcinoma. **B,** CT reveals the dilated, obstructed duct in the pancreatic body and tail *(arrows)*.

Box 4-4   Vascularity of Pancreatic Masses

HYPOVASCULAR

Adenocarcinoma
Lymphoma
Mucinous cystic neoplasms
Most metastases
Focal pancreatitis

HYPERVASCULAR

Islet cell tumors
Microcystic adenoma
Rare metastases (melanoma, hypernephroma)

---

chemical properties of **a**mine **p**recursor **u**ptake and **d**ecarboxylation, elaborate various hormones, including insulin, glucagon, gastrin, and somatostatin (Table 4-2). APUD cells migrate from neural crest tissue during embryological development and are found not only in the pancreas but also throughout the GI tract and in endocrine organs, including the thyroid, parathyroid, and adrenal medulla.

Pancreatic islet cell tumors are divided into functioning and nonfunctioning types. The functioning types are hormonally active and are further divided according to the hormone that they produce and the subset of islet cells from which they arise (Table 4-2). Functioning islet cell tumors may be associated with multiple endocrine neoplasia type I (MEN I or Wermer's syndrome), an autosomal dominant disease characterized by hyperplasia or neoplasia of the pituitary and parathyroid glands. Islet cell tumors occur in 45% to 80% of cases of MEN I. These tumors are usually multiple and may involve any subset of islet cells. Islet cell tumors are also found in approximately 20% of patients with von Hippel-Lindau disease, an autosomal dominant syndrome that includes central nervous system hemangioblastomas, retinal angiomas, renal cell carcinoma, and pheochromocytoma.

Insulinoma, the most common type of functioning islet cell tumor, originates from the beta islet cell and produces insulin. Approximately 90% of these tumors are benign, solitary, and less than 2 cm in diameter at the time of diagnosis. They produce a symptom complex known as Whipple's triad, which consists of hypoglycemia, central nervous system abnormalities related to hypoglycemia (including confusion, loss of consciousness, and seizures), and rapid response to oral or intravenous administration of glucose.

Clinical symptoms and laboratory evaluation usually lead to early diagnosis of insulinoma, and radiologic studies are indicated primarily for localizing the tumor before surgical resection. Angiography using superselective injections can detect 80% to 90% of insulinomas and typically demonstrates a well-defined hypervascular mass. CT typically shows a small enhancing mass that may deform the pancreatic contour. Ultrasound reveals a hypoechoic, solid mass. Because of the small size of most insulinomas, careful technique is essential for radiographic detection (CT with dynamic bolus and thin axial slices, real-time or high-frequency intraoperative ultrasound). Gastrinoma, the second most common type of functioning islet cell tumor, arises from the alpha-1 islet cell and produces gastrin. Approximately 60% of these tumors are malignant, and 50% to 66% have metastasized when diagnosed. Elevated serum gastrin levels produce the Zollinger-Ellison syndrome, in which increased output of gastric acid in the stomach leads to an ulcer diathesis in the duodenum and proximal jejunum. In 10% to 40% of patients with Zollinger-Ellison syndrome, pancreatic gastrinomas are associated with MEN I.

As a result of the small size and sometimes ectopic location of primary gastrinomas, imaging studies have not proved reliable in their detection. However, because gastrinomas frequently metastasize, CT and ultrasound are useful for demonstrating extrapancreatic disease and determining an appropriate course of treatment. In the absence of metastases, surgical resection of the primary tumor is curative. If metastases are present, however, gastric acid hypersecretion can be controlled by either total gastrectomy or medical treatment with histamine H_2 receptor antagonists or omeprazole.

Glucagonoma arises from the alpha-2 islet cell and produces glucagon. This slow-growing tumor is malignant in approximately 80% of cases and is often large and metastatic when first diagnosed. It usually occurs in the body or tail of the pancreas and metastasizes to the regional lymph nodes or liver (Fig. 4-21). Pancreatic glucagonomas and their liver metastases are typically hypervascular (see Fig. 4-4). Clinical findings include diabetes mellitus, anemia, weight loss, hypoaminoacidemia, and necrolytic migratory erythema (a recurrent skin rash that may blister and crust).

Vipoma (VIPoma) originates in the delta-1 islet cell and secretes vasoactive intestinal polypeptide (VIP). This tumor is malignant in 50% of cases and occurs most often in the pancreatic body and tail. Originally described by Verner and Morrison in 1958, vipoma produces a syndrome characterized by watery diarrhea, hypokalemia, achlorhydria, and hypovolemia (WDHA or WDHH syndrome). The primary tumor typically appears large and hypervascular on angiography.

Somatostatinoma, a rare tumor arising in the delta islet cell, produces somatostatin. Of the few reported cases of somatostatinoma, most were hypervascular, malignant, and associated with diarrhea and weight loss.

Nonfunctioning (or nonhyperfunctioning) islet cell tumors do not produce the clinical symptoms typical of their functioning counterparts. Although nonfunctioning tumors may actually secrete hormones, the type or amount of hormone produced cannot be detected or measured.

Nonfunctioning islet cell tumors are usually large and metastatic at the time of diagnosis. They cause nonspecific clinical symptoms related to focal mass effect, including abdominal pain, jaundice, and GI bleeding or obstruction. Although typically hypervascular, nonfunctioning tumors may undergo focal necrosis because of their large size. Imaging studies are useful for demonstrating both the large primary tumor and local or distant metastases.

Table 4-2 Functioning islet cell tumors

Tumor type	Cell of origin	Hormone produced	Malignancy (% cases)	Clinical findings
Insulinoma	Beta	Insulin	10	Hypoglycemia
Gastrinoma	Alpha-1	Gastrin	60	Zollinger-Ellison syndrome
Glucagonoma	Alpha-2	Glucagon	80	Diabetes mellitus, necrolytic migratory erythema
Vipoma	Delta-1	VIP	50	WDHA syndrome
Somatostatinoma	Delta	Somatostatin	67 (4/6 reported cases)	Diarrhea, weight loss

VIP, Vasoactive intestinal polypeptide; *WDHA*, watery diarrhea, hypokalemia, and achlorhydria.

Lymphoma and other nonepithelial tumors

Lymphoma rarely occurs as a primary tumor of the pancreas. More commonly, pancreatic involvement results from secondary spread of non-Hodgkin's lymphoma. Lymphoma may affect the pancreas, peripancreatic lymph nodes, or both (Fig. 4-22). Although typically large with solid, uniform texture, pancreatic lymphoma may appear cystic or inhomogeneous on cross-sectional imaging studies. Other radiographic findings of lymphoma include displacement of the pancreatic duct and vessels by the mass and displacement of the pancreas itself by adjacent peripancreatic adenopathy. Lymphoma may mimic pancreatic carcinoma but is less likely to cause vascular or ductal encasement. Other rare pancreatic tumors of nonepithelial cell origin include hemangiomas, lymphangiomas, and sarcomas.

Metastases

Metastasis to the pancreas usually occurs through contiguous spread from adjacent organs, including the colon and stomach. Hematogenous metastases that may involve the pancreas include renal cell carcinoma, hepatoma, melanoma, leiomyosarcoma, and carcinoma of the breast, lung, ovary, or prostate. Pancreatic metastases are usually asymptomatic but may cause recurrent acute pancreatitis (Fig. 4-23). Radiographically, pancreatic metastases may appear solid or cystic and demonstrate variable degrees of vascularity. Metastatic disease involving peripancreatic lymph nodes surrounding the head of the pancreas may mimic a primary pancreatic tumor.

Cystic

Inflammatory pancreatic cystic lesions include focal acute pancreatitis, acute fluid collections, pseudocysts, retention cysts, necrosis, and abscesses. A variety of neoplastic processes may also appear cystic on CT (Box 4-5).

Focal acute pancreatitis and acute fluid collection

Focal acute pancreatitis may produce a cystic-appearing pancreatic mass resulting from localized edema. This appears hypoechoic on ultrasound and shows low attenuation on CT. Acute fluid collections (phlegmon) occur secondary to release of pancreatic secretions from ruptured pancreatic ductules in acute pancreatitis. These collections may be confined to the pancreas or extend into the surrounding tissues. Acute fluid collections lack a fibrous capsule but can be either well defined or poorly marginated. Most resolve spontaneously over several weeks.

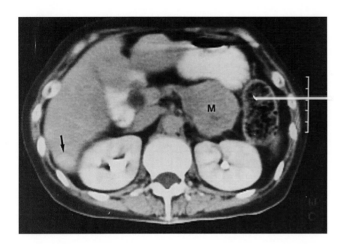

Fig. 4-21 Contrast-enhanced CT shows a large soft tissue mass *(M)* in the pancreatic tail and an enhancing mass in the right lobe of the liver *(arrow)* in a patient with metastatic pancreatic glucagonoma. (From Goodman P, Kumar R: Diagnostic radiology case number 11, *Intern Med* 12:46, 1991.)

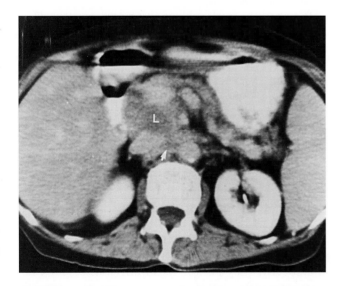

Fig. 4-22 Hypodense masses occupying the peripancreatic *(L)* and interaortocaval regions *(arrow)* represent non-Hodgkin's lymphoma.

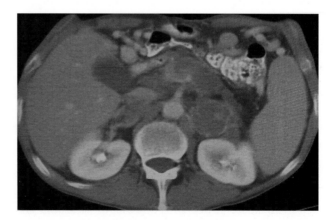

Fig. 4-23 Multiple low-density solid lesions in the pancreas are from metastatic small-cell carcinoma of the lung.

Box 4-5   Cystic Masses of the Pancreas

INFLAMMATORY

Pseudocysts and phlegmons
Abscess
Echinococcal cyst

TRUE CYSTS

Solitary
Cystic fibrosis
Multiple
    Adult polycystic kidney disease
    von Hippel-Lindau disease

NEOPLASTIC

Benign
    Microcystic adenoma
    Cystic teratoma
Malignant
    Mucinous cystic adenocarcinoma
    Papillary epithelial neoplasm
    Cystic islet cell tumors (rare)

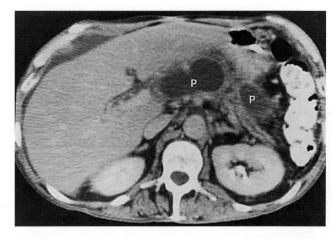

Fig. 4-24   Cystic masses *(P)* represent pancreatic pseudocysts.

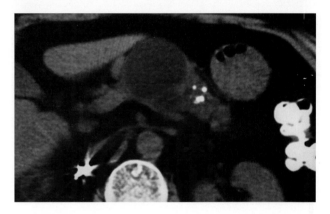

Fig. 4-25   Large pancreatic pseudocyst is seen in the body. Note the pancreatic calcifications proximally, caused by chronic pancreatitis.

Pseudocysts

Pseudocysts are well-encapsulated collections of fluid that develop after pancreatitis. They begin as collections of necrotic tissue, secretions, and blood from one or more episodes of pancreatitis. Unlike acute fluid collections, pseudocysts are surrounded by a fibrous capsule. However, they lack an epithelial lining and therefore are not considered true cysts. Pseudocysts occur in approximately 10% of patients with acute pancreatitis but are more commonly associated with chronic pancreatitis (Figs. 4-24 and 4-25). Although usually located in the pancreas or peripancreatic region, pseudocysts may occur in areas distant from the pancreas (Fig. 4-26). Other causes of pseudocysts include trauma and surgery. Although uncomplicated pseudocysts appear cystic on CT and ultrasound, superimposed hemorrhage or infection may cause the fluid contents to appear complex or inhomogeneous.

Retention cysts

Retention cysts result from focal obstruction of pancreatic ductules. The cysts are usually small and lined with epithelium. Although most often seen in chronic pancreatitis, retention cysts may also occur in pancreatic carcinoma, gallbladder disease, ampullary stenosis, acute pancreatitis, and various parasitic diseases associated with acute pancreatitis, including ascariasis and clonorchiasis. Hydatid disease of the pancreas may demonstrate multiseptated cysts that represent the echinococcal daughter cysts.

Necrosis and abscess

Pancreatic necrosis (phlegmon) represents devitalized pancreatic tissue secondary to acute pancreatitis and resultant ischemia (Fig. 4-27). This produces diffuse or localized decrease in density of the pancreatic parenchyma on CT. Pancreatic abscess formation or fistulization to an adjacent hollow viscus may complicate pancreatic necrosis, forming gas collections within the pancreatic parenchyma in 25% of cases (Box 4-6). Pancreatic abscess develops in approximately 4% of patients with pancreatitis and may require prompt surgical debridement and drainage (Fig. 4-28).

Congenital pancreatic cysts

Congenital pancreatic cysts have an epithelial lining and are therefore classified as true cysts. Solitary congenital cysts vary in size and may appear unilocular or multilocular. They are seen mostly in neonates and result from abnormal segmentation of rudimentary pancreatic ducts. CT and ultrasound demonstrate their fluid content and thin wall.

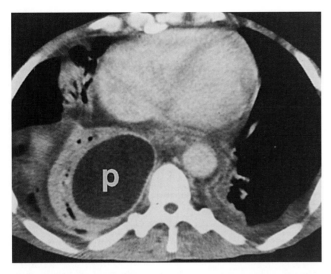

Fig. 4-26 Fluid collection *(p)* in the posterior right hemithorax represents a pseudocyst surrounded by pulmonary consolidation.

Box 4-6 CT Differentiation of Inflammatory Cystic Lesions of the Pancreas

PSEUDOCYST
Low density
Well-defined wall
Possible calcification

PHLEGMON
Variable density
Poorly defined wall
Inflammatory changes present

ABSCESS
Variable density
Wall variable
Gas (≈ 30%)

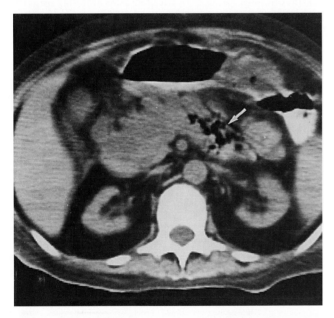

Fig. 4-27 Numerous air bubbles *(arrow)* in the pancreatic tail of a patient with pancreatitis and pancreatic necrosis.

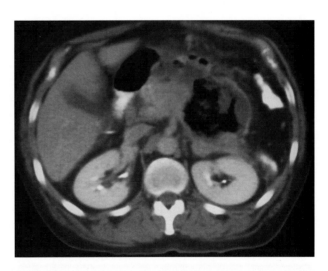

Fig. 4-28 Large cavity with irregular walls is seen in the tail. This represents a pancreatic abscess.

Multiple congenital cysts are usually associated with adult polycystic kidney disease, von Hippel-Lindau disease, or cystic fibrosis. Multiple pancreatic cysts occur in 10% of patients with adult polycystic kidney disease and in 25% to 72% of patients with von Hippel-Lindau disease. The pancreatic cysts occurring in cystic fibrosis represent the sequelae of chronically dilated pancreatic ductal structures.

Intrapancreatic choledochal cysts and duodenal duplication cysts are other congenital lesions that can mimic true pancreatic cysts. Duplication or enterogenous cysts of the pancreas itself are extremely rare.

Microcystic adenoma

Cystic tumors of the pancreas represent 5% to 15% of pancreatic cystic masses (see Table 4-1). Approximately half of these tumors are classified as microcystic adenoma (serous cystadenoma or glycogen-rich cystadenoma) and the other half as macrocystic or mucinous cystic neoplasms (mucinous cystadenoma and cystadenocarcinoma). These tumors arise from ductal epithelium of the exocrine pancreas and together account for approximately 6% of nonfunctioning pancreatic neoplasms.

Microcystic adenomas can occur in any portion of the pancreas and are composed of numerous small cysts, each 0.1 to 2 cm in diameter. The cysts are lined by low cuboidal epithelium containing glycogen. These slow-growing tumors, although often discovered incidentally, may become large and produce symptoms of bowel or biliary duct obstruction. About 80% of cases are first detected after age 60, and the female to male ratio is 1.5:1. Microcystic adenoma occurs with increased incidence in patients with von Hippel-Lindau disease. Although microcystic adenoma is generally considered a benign lesion, a single case of malignancy was recently reported.

CT of microcystic adenoma typically demonstrates a low-attenuation mass on noncontrast scans and a honey-combed or spongy appearance on contrast-enhanced scans as a result of hypervascularity of the septa (Fig. 4-29). Overall attenuation of the mass on contrast-enhanced scans varies from solid to cystic. A central scar with or without calcification is often present.

On ultrasound, microcystic adenoma appears primarily hyperechoic or hypoechoic, depending on the size of cysts and the number of fibrous septa. Angiography typically reveals hypervascularity and neovascularity, but hypovascular lesions have also been described.

Mucinous cystic neoplasms

Mucinous cystic neoplasms occur most often in the tail of the pancreas and are rarely seen in the pancreatic head. They are typically composed of no more than six cysts with each cyst measuring more than 2 cm in diameter. The cysts are lined by tall columnar epithelium that produces mucin. The tumors are usually large and bulky when first detected. The mean age of patients with mucinous cystic neoplasms is 50 years old, and females are affected 6 to 8 times more often than males. Mucinous cystadenoma, the benign form of mucinous cystic neoplasm, is generally considered premalignant.

CT and ultrasound of mucinous cystic neoplasms show a multilocular or, less often, unilocular cystic lesion that may contain septations, papillary projections, or mural nodules (Figs. 4-30 and 4-31). Although contrast-enhanced CT may show enhancement of the septa and cyst wall, these areas are better visualized using ultrasound. Angiography reveals a hypovascular mass, and peripheral curvilinear calcifications are found in approximately 15% of cases. In the absence of metastatic disease, benign and malignant lesions are difficult to distinguish radiographically.

Mucinous pancreatic duct ectasia

Mucinous pancreatic duct ectasia (ductectatic mucinous cystadenoma and cystadenocarcinoma) is a rare tumor of the pancreatic duct that demonstrates histological features similar to those of mucinous cystic neoplasms. This tumor consists of clusters of small, thin-walled cysts that cause dilatation of the side branches of the main pancreatic duct. This tumor occurs most often in the uncinate process of the pancreas and may undergo malignant transformation.

Solid and papillary epithelial neoplasms

Solid and papillary epithelial neoplasms of the pancreas (papillary cystic tumors) are rare tumors arising from acinar cells (see Table 4-1). They most often affect young women and can arise in any portion of the pancreas. These large, well-circumscribed masses usually contain both solid and cystic areas resulting from focal necrosis and hemorrhage (Fig. 4-32). Calcifications and septations rarely occur. These tumors are considered low-grade malignancies with good prognosis following resection.

Other pancreatic cystic tumors

Cystic islet cell tumors of the pancreas result from central necrosis of nonfunctioning or functioning islet

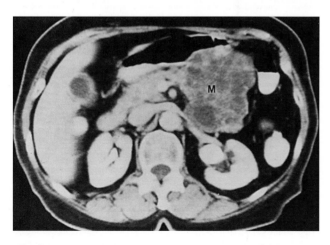

Fig. 4-29   Large mass *(M)* composed of numerous small cysts represents a microcystic adenoma of the pancreatic tail.

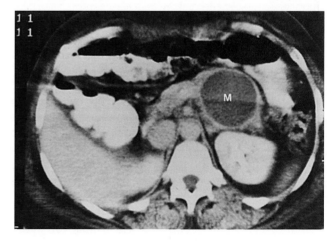

Fig. 4-30   Large unilocular cystic mass *(M)* in the pancreatic tail represents a mucinous cystic neoplasm.

cell tumors. These lesions are locally invasive and potentially or frankly malignant. A similar cystic appearance may be seen in necrotic pancreatic ductal adenocarcinoma and in metastatic lesions involving the pancreas (Fig. 4-33). Other rare pancreatic tumors that may appear cystic on radiographic studies include acinar cell carcinoma, cystic teratoma (Fig. 4-34), lymphoma, hemangioma, lymphangioma, sarcoma, and various types of anaplastic carcinoma.

PANCREATIC DUCT

The normal pancreatic duct size is variable, but there are some guidelines by which to evaluate the duct. Typically, the duct is largest in the head, usually not exceeding 5 mm in diameter. It gradually tapers towards the tail, and the distal duct is typically less than 3 mm in diameter. Along its course, however, there are mild

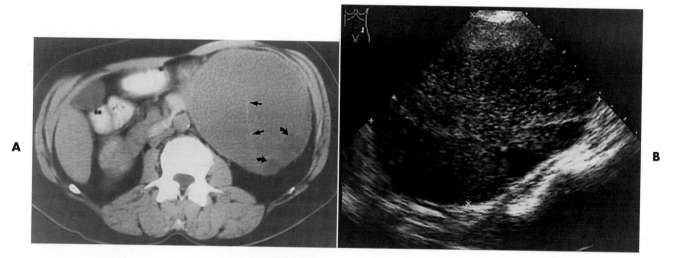

Fig. 4-31   **A,** CT shows a large cystic mass containing septations *(arrows)* and mural nodules *(curved arrows)* in a patient with mucinous cystic neoplasm of the pancreas. **B,** Ultrasound demonstrates numerous internal echoes throughout the mass.

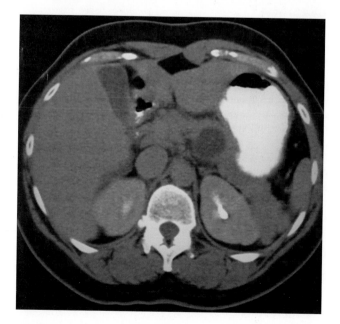

Fig. 4-32   Small low-density cystic lesion in the body is a cystic adenoma.

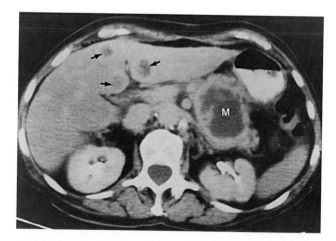

Fig. 4-33   Irregular cystic mass *(M)* represents necrotic adenocarcinoma of the pancreatic tail. Hypodense hepatic lesions *(arrows)* indicate metastases.

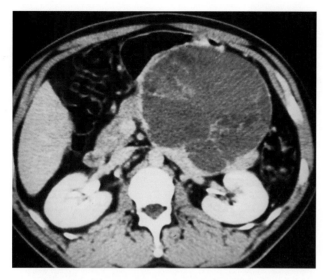

Fig. 4-34 Large cystic mass with septations was found to be a cystic teratoma at surgery.

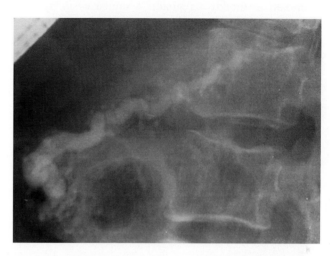

Fig. 4-35 Dilated, tortuous main pancreatic duct and dilated side branches in a patient with chronic pancreatitis.

undulations in diameter in normal individuals. Typically, these have smooth margins and are not abrupt changes in caliber.

Dilated

Normal aging

As people age, the pancreatic duct becomes slightly larger. This is probably the result of mild atrophy of the gland rather than any type of obstructive condition. It is not unusual with the newer CT scanners to identify the pancreatic duct in normal older individuals and even younger persons. This does not indicate disease, however. A distinguishing feature, particularly on ERCP, is that the duct shows diffuse enlargement and the changes are not focal.

Pancreatitis

Chronic pancreatitis (but not acute) will also result in enlargement of the duct. This enlargement is the result of both parenchymal loss and strictures that may develop as the result of repeated inflammation (Fig. 4-35). The changes of chronic pancreatitis include multifocal to diffuse areas of dilatation with scattered bandlike areas of narrowing. The side branches of the pancreatic duct are also dilated or blunted and may show some clubbing. The degree of pancreatic duct change usually mirrors the severity of repeated inflammation, as well as the degree of pancreatic dysfunction.

Neoplasms

Neoplasms also produce pancreatic ductal dilatation. This is the result of dilatation proximal to the strictured area (Fig. 4-36). As the degree of neoplastic stricturing increases, the proximal dilatation worsens

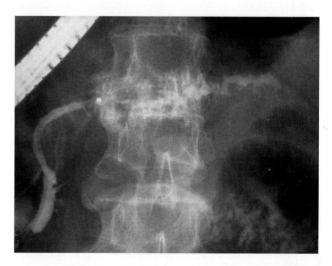

Fig. 4-36 Dilated pancreatic duct is seen in the body and tail, with a normal duct in the head. This is due to a pancreatic carcinoma partially obstructing the duct and producing changes of pancreatitis proximally.

and begins to resemble chronic pancreatitis. There is also associated glandular atrophy in the areas proximal to the tumor. This dilatation is identifiable because it can be seen only proximal to the stricture. Typically, neoplastic strictures are much longer than those seen with chronic pancreatitis.

Narrowed

Pancreatitis

The most common cause of narrowing of the pancreatic duct is prior inflammation, as from pancreatitis. Strictures secondary to pancreatitis can have a variety of appearances. Some features that are more typical of

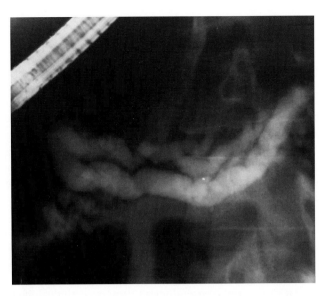

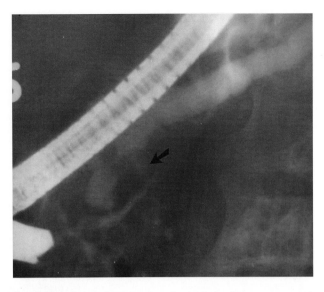

Fig. 4-37 Bandlike areas across the ducts are a sequela of chronic pancreatitis. Note the duplication of the pancreatic ducts as well.

Fig. 4-38 Area of narrowing *(arrow)* is due to pancreatic carcinoma.

pancreatitis are multifocal, short, and bandlike (Fig. 4-37). Occasionally the strictures of pancreatitis are solitary or focal, which makes it much more difficult to distinguish from malignant strictures. If a pseudocyst is present, it may produce a focal compression of the pancreatic duct, and also may be difficult to distinguish from malignancy.

Neoplasms

Typical strictures produced by pancreatic malignancy are focal and have tapered margins. This is because pancreatic cancer infiltrates around the duct and produces circumferential narrowing. Because the process begins outside the lumen of the duct, the margins are tapered or smooth, not abrupt like other gastrointestinal malignancies (Fig. 4-38).

Developmental variation

In certain circumstances there may be focal areas of narrowing of the pancreatic ducts in normal individuals. As mentioned previously, the pancreatic duct normally has mild undulations along its course. Where the ventral duct of Wirsung fuses with the dorsal duct of Santorini, there may be a naturally occurring bend or narrowing. To distinguish these physiological narrowings from pathological strictures, one must look for proximal dilatation and delayed emptying on the postdrainage film.

CALCIFICATIONS

Pancreatitis

Radiographically visible pancreatic calcifications occur in approximately 50% of patients with chronic

Box 4-7 Differentiation of Pancreatic Calcifications

SMALL, PUNCTATE

Pancreatitis
Hyperparathyroidism
Cystic fibrosis

ROUND, LARGER

Hereditary pancreatitis
Ductal calculi

CURVILINEAR

Pseudocyst
Hematoma

STELLATE (STARBURST)

Mucinous cystadenocarcinoma
Microcystic adenoma

pancreatitis secondary to alcohol ingestion. The calcifications lie within the pancreatic ducts and vary in size, shape (Box 4-7), and distribution (Fig. 4-39).

Hereditary pancreatitis is an unusual form of chronic pancreatitis that demonstrates autosomal dominant genetic transmission. The disease begins in childhood and recurs throughout adult life. It is characterized by a high incidence of pancreatic calculi, which typically appear larger than those occurring in other forms of chronic pancreatitis. These calculi reside within the ducts and are much larger calculi than are seen in conventional chronic pancreatitis (Fig. 4-40). Patients with hereditary

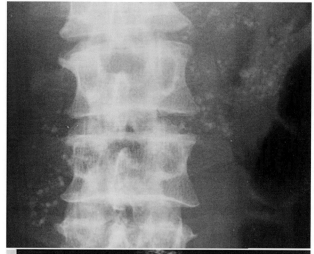

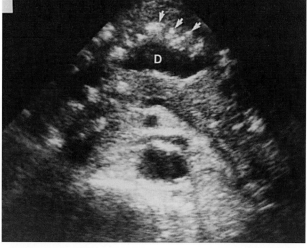

Fig. 4-39   **A,** Speckled calcifications in the midabdomen represent pancreatic calculi secondary to chronic pancreatitis. **B,** Ultrasound demonstrates a markedly dilated pancreatic duct *(D)* and multiple pancreatic calcifications *(arrows)*.

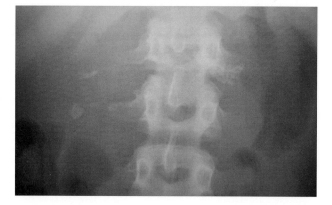

Fig. 4-40   Large calculi reside in the head of the pancreas (actually in the main pancreatic duct) in this patient with congenital pancreatitis.

pancreatitis have a 20% chance of developing pancreatic carcinoma.

Pseudocysts

Pancreatic pseudocysts sometimes demonstrate curvilinear calcification in the cyst wall (Fig. 4-41). These calcifications can be thick and diffuse and may involve the entire periphery of the pseudocyst. When they involve only a portion of the cyst, they are curvilinear and indistinguishable from calcifications seen in cystic neoplasms.

Neoplasms

Mucinous cystic neoplasms contain peripheral curvilinear calcifications in approximately 15% of cases (Fig. 4-42). Compared to pseudocysts, however, the calcification involves only a portion of the wall or septation and is curvilinear in appearance. Microcystic adenomas occasionally demonstrate stellate calcification within a central fibrous scar on plain films or CT.

Dystrophic calcification may occur in solid and papillary epithelial neoplasms. Calcifications have also been reported in nonfunctioning islet cell tumors and rarely in gastrinomas associated with MEN I syndrome. Cavernous lymphangiomas of the pancreas are rare tumors that may contain calcifications in dilated lymphatic channels.

Hyperparathyroidism

Hyperparathyroidism may cause pancreatitis and pancreatic calcifications, most likely as a result of hypercalcemia.

Cystic Fibrosis

Pancreatic calcifications in cystic fibrosis typically appear granular and may be either focal or diffuse. Calcium precipitates within dilated pancreatic ductules secondary to obstruction by mucous plugs or within the pancreatic parenchyma secondary to extravasation of pancreatic enzymes from ruptured ductules and acini. Pancreatic calcifications in cystic fibrosis are often associated with marked pancreatic fibrosis and diabetes mellitus.

Malnutrition and Other Causes

In tropical countries an idiopathic form of pancreatitis associated with pancreatic ductal calculi may result from malnutrition caused by a diet low in protein and high in carbohydrates.

Peripheral calcifications have been reported in con-

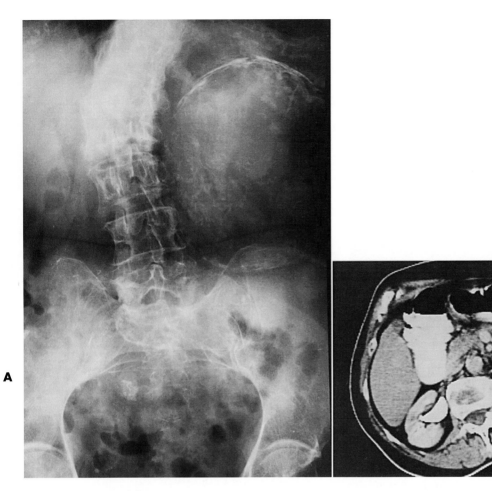

Fig. 4-41   **A,** Large, peripherally calcified mass in the left upper quadrant represents a pancreatic pseudocyst. **B,** CT demonstrates homogeneous cystic contents *(P)*.

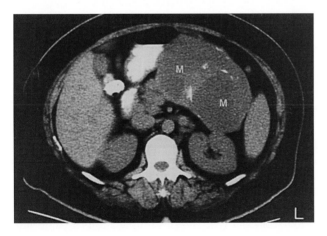

Fig. 4-42   Large cystic mass *(M)* containing partially calcified septations represents mucinous cystic neoplasm of the pancreas.

genital pancreatic cysts associated with von Hippel-Lindau disease. Hydatid cysts, although rarely occurring in the pancreas, may also calcify peripherally.

Other unusual causes of intraparenchymal pancreatic calcifications include previous trauma, hematoma, ab-scess, and infarction. A calcified aneurysm of the adjacent celiac or splenic artery may simulate an intra-pancreatic mass.

TRAUMA

Pancreatic injury occurs in 3% to 12% of patients with blunt abdominal trauma. Clinical symptoms suggesting pancreatic injury are nonspecific. However, elevated se-rum amylase levels are found in 90% of patients with blunt trauma to the pancreas. Pancreatic injuries include contusion, laceration, and transection (fracture) and most often result from compression of the pancreatic body against the spine. Thin-section contrast-enhanced CT scan of the pancreas may demonstrate focal or diffuse pancreatic enlargement and extension of blood into the peripancreatic and retroperitoneal tissues. An area of decreased density perpendicular to the long axis of the pancreas may be seen immediately following trauma, suggesting a contusion or hematoma (Fig. 4-43). Within hours to days a clear zone of disruption through the

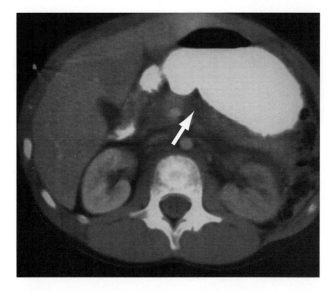

Fig. 4-43   Low-density area *(arrow)* between the body and head of the pancreas is actually an area of laceration following an automobile accident.

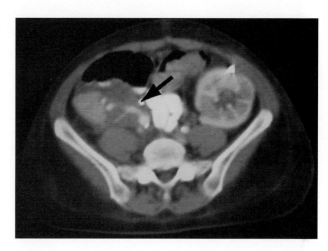

Fig. 4-44   Note transplanted pancreas *(arrow)* on the right side of the pelvis and transplanted kidney on the left side in the patient with diabetes mellitus.

pancreatic parenchyma may become evident, indicating a laceration or transection. Ultrasound is sometimes able to demonstrate these findings but frequently is limited by overlying bandages or by bowel gas secondary to intestinal ileus. Laceration of the pancreatic duct resulting from pancreatic transection is best evaluated by ERCP.

Pancreatic injury is accompanied by trauma to other visceral structures in 75% of cases and is fatal in 10% to 20% of cases. Surgical treatment of pancreatic transection usually consists of partial resection (when the body or tail is injured) or repair (when the head is injured). Complications of pancreatic trauma occur frequently and include chronic pancreatitis, pseudocysts, pancreatoenteric fistulas, and abscesses.

POSTOPERATIVE PANCREAS

Resection

Surgical resection of the pancreas may be partial or complete. After resection of the tail or of the body and tail, the residual pancreas appears shortened.

The standard Whipple's procedure consists of resection of the pancreatic head and neck, subtotal gastrectomy, duodenectomy, gastrojejunostomy, pancreaticojejunostomy, and choledochojejunostomy. A total rather than a partial pancreatectomy is sometimes performed, leading to severe diabetes mellitus.

Cystogastrostomy

Cystogastrostomy or marsupialization represents a surgical anastomosis of a pancreatic pseudocyst to the

adjacent gastric wall. This procedure allows the pseudocyst to drain internally and eventually resolve. A UGI series or CT scan using oral contrast material typically demonstrates opacification of the pseudocyst through the patent anastomosis.

Puestow's Procedure

Puestow's procedure represents an end-to-end pancreaticojejunostomy. It is performed to allow drainage of the dilated but nonobstructed pancreatic duct in chronic pancreatitis. It may also involve resecting portions of the pancreas. It may be performed in instances of tumors in the head of the pancreas or ampullary region of the duodenum.

Pancreatic Transplantation

Pancreatic transplantation is an increasingly performed procedure for managing patients with severe diabetes mellitus. A cadaver donor pancreas and adjacent periampullary segment of duodenum are placed in the recipient's pelvis with vascular anastomoses to iliac vessels and duodenal anastomosis to the dome of the urinary bladder (Fig. 4-44). Complications include acute and chronic transplant rejection, intraperitoneal or extraperitoneal leakage, fluid collections (hematomas, abscesses, and pseudocysts), fistulas, and various vascular abnormalities (Box 4-8).

Cystography has proved useful for detecting anastomotic leaks and fistulas by allowing opacification of the adjacent duodenal segment (Fig. 4-45). CT is useful for evaluating intraabdominal fluid collections and providing

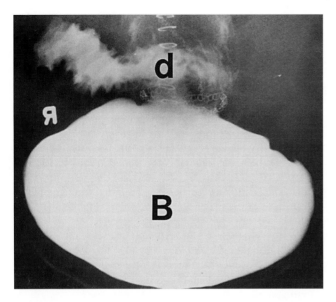

Fig. 4-45 Cystogram following pancreatic and renal transplantation shows opacification of the urinary bladder *(B)* and transplanted duodenum *(d)*.

Box 4-8   Complications of Pancreatic Transplantation

Rejection
Peripancreatic effusions (common after surgery)
Ascites (usually indicates leakage)
Leakage
Ischemia/thrombosis
Pancreatitis and pseudocysts
Infection/abscess

---

guidance for percutaneous drainage procedures and pancreatic biopsies. MRI has shown some promising results in detecting pancreatic transplant rejection.

SUGGESTED READINGS

Axon ATR: Endoscopic retrograde cholangiopancreatography in chronic pancreatitis: Cambridge classification, *Radiol Clin North Am* 27:39-50, 1989.

Balthazar E: CT diagnosis and staging of acute pancreatitis, *Radiol Clin North Am* 27:19-37, 1989.

Balthazar EJ, Robinson DL, Megibow AJ, et al: Acute pancreatitis: value of CT in establishing prognosis, *Radiology* 174:331-336, 1990.

Bolondi L, LiBassi S, Gaiani S, et al: Sonography of chronic pancreatitis, *Radiol Clin North Am* 27:815-833, 1989.

Bret PM, Reinhold C, Taourel P, et al: Pancreas divisum: evaluation with MR cholangiopancreatography, *Radiology* 199:99, 1996.

Buck JL, Hayes WS: Microcystic adenoma of the pancreas, *Radiographics* 10:313-322, 1990.

Buetow PC, Miller DL, Parrino TV, et al: Islet cell tumors of the pancreas: clinical, radiologic, and pathologic correlation in diagnosis and localization, *Radiographics* 17:453-472, 1997.

Burdeny DA, Kroeker MA: CT appearance of the ventral pancreas, *J Can Assoc Radiol* 39:190-194, 1988.

Clark LR, Jaffe MH, Choyke PL, et al: Pancreatic imaging, *Radiol Clin North Am* 23:489-501, 1985.

Dodds WJ, Wilson SD, Thorsen MK, et al: MEN I syndrome and islet cell tumors of the pancreas, *Semin Roentgenol* 20:17-63, 1985.

Donovan PJ, Sanders RC, Siegelman SS: Collections of fluid after pancreatitis: evaluation by computed tomography and ultrasonography, *Radiol Clin North Am* 20:653-665, 1982.

Freeny PC: Radiology of the pancreas: two decades of progress in imaging and intervention, *AJR* 150:975-981, 1988.

Freeny PC: Radiologic diagnosis and staging of pancreatic ductal adenocarcinoma, *Radiol Clin North Am* 27:121-128, 1989.

Freeny PC, Marks WM, Ryan JA, et al: Pancreatic ductal adenocarcinoma: diagnosis and staging with dynamic CT, *Radiology* 166:125-133, 1988.

Friedman AC, Edmonds PR: Rare pancreatic malignancies, *Radiol Clin North Am* 27:177-190, 1989.

Fugazzola C, Procacci C, Bergamo Andreis IA, et al: Cystic tumors of the pancreas: evaluation by ultrasonography and computed tomography, *Gastrointest Radiol* 16:53-61, 1991.

Glazer GM, Margulis AR: Annular pancreas: etiology and diagnosis using endoscopic retrograde cholangiopancreatography, *Radiology* 133:303-306, 1979.

Gunther RW: Ultrasound and CT in the assessment of suspected islet cell tumors of the pancreas, *Semin Ultrasound CT MR* 6:261-275, 1985.

Hill MC, Barkin J, Isikoff MB, et al: Acute pancreatitis: clinical vs. CT findings, *AJR* 139:263-269, 1982.

Jeffrey RB Jr: Sonography in acute pancreatitis, *Radiol Clin North Am* 27:5-17, 1989.

Jeffrey RB, Federle MP, Crass RA: Computed tomography of pancreatic trauma, *Radiology* 147:491-494, 1983.

Kettritz U, Semelka RC: Contrast-enhanced MR imaging of the pancreas, *MRI Clin North Am* 4:87, 1996.

Kloppel G, Maillet B: Classification and staging of pancreatic nonendocrine tumors, *Radiol Clin North Am* 27:105-119, 1989.

Lane MJ, Mindelzun RE, Jeffrey RB: Diagnosis of pancreatic injury after blunt abdominal trauma, *Semin Ultrasound CT MR* 17:177, 1996.

Low RA, Kuni CC, Letourneau JG: Pancreas transplant imaging: an overview, *AJR* 155:13-21, 1990.

Luetmer PH, Stephens DH, Ward EM: Chronic pancreatitis: reassessment with current CT, *Radiology* 171:353-357, 1989.

Mathiu D, Guigui B, Valette PJ, et al: Pancreatic cystic neoplasms, *Radiol Clin North Am* 27:163-176, 1989.

Megibow AJ, Zhou XH, Rotterdam H, et al: Pancreatic adenocarcinoma: CT versus MR imaging in the evaluation of resectability, *Radiology* 195:327, 1995.

Mergo PJ, Helmberger TK, Buetow PC, et al: Pancreatic neoplasms: MR imaging and pathologic correlation, *Radiographics* 17:281-301, 1997.

Mitchell DG: MR imaging of the pancreas, *MR Clin North Am* 3:51, 1995.

Moulton JS, Munda R, Weiss MA, et al: Pancreatic transplants: CT with clinical and pathologic correlation, *Radiology* 172:21-26, 1989.

Op den Orth JO: Sonography of the pancreatic head aided by water and glucagon, *Radiographics* 7:85-100, 1987.

Reinhold C, Bret PM, Guibaud L, et al: MR cholangiopancreatography: potential clinical applications, *Radiographics* 16:309-320, 1996.

Rizzo RJ, Szucs RA, Turner MA: Congenital abnormalities of the pancreas and biliary tree in adults, *Radiographics* 15:49-68, 1995.

Ros P, Hamrick-Turner JE, Chiechi MV, et al: Cystic masses of the pancreas, *Radiographics* 12:673-686, 1992.

Rosch T, Lorenz R, Braig C, et al: Endoscopic ultrasound in pancreatic tumor diagnosis, *Gastrointest Endosc* 37:347-352, 1991.

Rossi P, Allison DJ, Bezzi M, et al: Endocrine tumors of the pancreas, *Radiol Clin North Am* 27:129-161, 1989.

Simeone JF, Edelman RR, Stark DD, et al: Surface coil MR imaging of abdominal viscera: the pancreas, *Radiology* 157:437-441, 1985.

Taylor AJ, Carmondy TJ, Schmalz MJ, et al: Filling defects in the pancreatic duct on endoscopic retrograde pancreatography, *AJR* 159:1203-1208, 1992.

Thoeni RF, Gedgaudas RK: Ectopic pancreas: usual and unusual features, *Gastrointest Radiol* 5:37-42, 1980.

Tscholakoff D, Hricak H, Thoeni R, et al: MR imaging in the diagnosis of pancreatic disease, *AJR* 148:703-709, 1987.

Weinstein BJ, Weinstein DP: Sonographic anatomy of the pancreas, *Semin Ultrasound* 1:156-165, 1980.

Weinstein DP, Wolfman NT, Weinstein BJ: Ultrasonic characteristics of pancreatic tumors, *Gastrointest Radiol* 4:245-251, 1979.

Weyman PJ, Stanley RJ, Levitt RG: Computed tomography in evaluation of the pancreas, *Semin Roentgenol* 16:301-311, 1981.

White EM, Wittenberg J, Mueller PR, et al: Pancreatic necrosis: CT manifestations, *Radiology* 158:343-346, 1986.

Woolsey EJ, Tauscher JR, Dafoe DC: Pancreas transplantation with pancreato-duodeno-cystostomy for exocrine drainage: cystographic findings, *AJR* 149:507-509, 1987.

Yuh WTC, Hunsicker LG, Nghiem DD, et al: Pancreatic transplants: evaluation with MR imaging, *Radiology* 170:171-177, 1989.

Zeman RK, McVay LV, Silverman PM, et al: Pancreas divisum: thin-section CT, *Radiology* 169:395-398, 1988.

Liver and Spleen

LIVER

The liver is the largest organ in the abdomen. Classically, the liver is divided into right and left lobes by the falciform ligament. However, anatomical division with respect to vascular supply and biliary drainage differs in that the division of the right and left lobes is actually to the right of the falciform ligament, along a plane of intralobar division that is determined by a line drawn from the inferior vena cava to the superior recess of the gallbladder fossa. Medial to this is the medial segment of the left lobe, which, in turn, is separated from the lateral segment by the vertical cleft in the surface of the left lobe, in which runs the ligamentum teres.

Segmental liver anatomy based on the internal vascular supply has a much more practical application with respect to hepatic surgical resection. With aggressive hepatic resection for limited metastatic disease becom-

ing more common, segmental vascular anatomy has become more important. A numbering system developed by Couinaud divides the liver into eight segments, each of which has a major portal vein division and bile duct, drained by a distinct hepatic vein (Fig. 5-1).

Examination Techniques

The standard of practice for liver imaging has undergone a significant change over the last two decades. The primary radiological evaluation of the liver using nuclear scintigraphy and angiography has given way to computed tomography (CT), ultrasound, and magnetic resonance imaging (MRI).

The primary radiological technique for evaluating the liver is CT. CT techniques for hepatic evaluation have evolved at a rapid pace over the last decade. Helical CT scanning has markedly reduced scanning times, and resolution continues to improve with each generation of scanners introduced. Indeed, the continuous technical developments of CT being made available as diagnostic tools (e.g., subsecond scanning and CT fluoroscopy) will continue to make CT the modality of choice well into the future. Ultrasound occupies a position just behind CT in liver evaluation.

MRI shows great promise for the detection of selected disease entities. However, some difficulties remain in bringing this mode of imaging to the forefront of liver disease detection.

The usefulness of radionuclide imaging in evaluating hepatic disease has become more focused over the last few decades and tends now to be limited to evaluation of bile duct or cystic duct obstruction.

Computed tomography

CT is the acknowledged standard for liver tumor imaging. However, it should be understood that meticulous attention to the technical aspects of the examination is required to fulfill its promise. In some instances (especially when evaluating for certain metastatic lesions, breast and colorectal being the most common), both unenhanced and enhanced evaluations of the liver are required (Fig. 5-2). In addition to considerations of vascular enhancements, attention to good opacification of the stomach and duodenum is one of the hallmarks of high-quality CT liver imaging. The contrast examination is almost uniformly performed using dynamic bolus technique and a power injector. Helical scanning has replaced the older individual slice acquisition tech-

niques, and as a result, scanning times are greatly reduced and resolution is increased. With newer software, image reconstruction times have markedly lessened. A case is made in the literature for using CT arterial portography (CTAP) in tumor evaluation, in both primary and metastatic disease, in patients who may be candidates for hepatic resection. This technique, particularly using splenic artery injections, appears to be more sensitive than the routine examination.

For the purposes of organizing this chapter on the liver, radiological problems related to the CT evaluation of liver abnormalities are the basis for discussion. The role of other imaging modalities is appropriately included wherever possible.

Ultrasound

Ultrasound is a relatively inexpensive and noninvasive method of evaluating the upper abdomen. It is especially useful in evaluating for the presence of bile duct obstruction and the presence or absence of gallstones. Because of the high incidence of gallstones throughout our population, some argument can be made for the primary use of ultrasound in the evaluation of upper abdominal pain when gallstones are suspected. In addition, ultrasound is especially useful in distinguishing between cystic and solid lesions. However, there are limitations. Although tumor masses can be detected, the false negative rate for liver metastatic disease is thought to be higher than with CT, and both findings and lack of findings necessitate additional evaluation, most likely by CT. For this reason ultrasound is generally not the primary screening technique in patients whose clinical presentation suggests something other than gallstone disease.

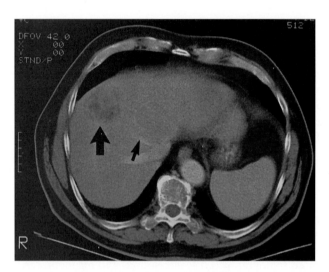

Fig. 5-1   A 72-year-old patient with breast carcinoma and a solitary hepatic metastatic lesion. The lesion *(large arrow)* is located on the boundary between segment 4a *(left lobe)* and segment 8 *(right lobe)*. The boundary between the segments is defined by the middle hepatic vein *(small arrow)*.

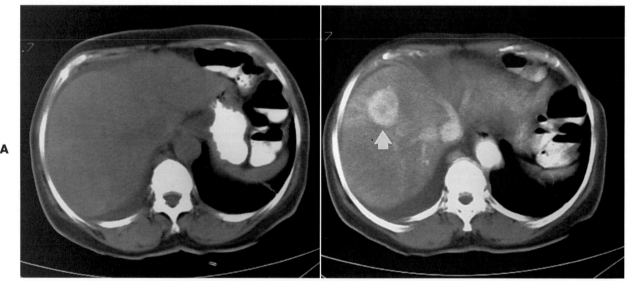

Fig. 5-2   Patient with metastatic carcinoid. Unenhanced CT image **(A)** of liver shows no defects. Postenhancement image **(B)** reveals a hypervascular liver metastatic lesion *(arrow)*.

Magnetic resonance imaging

Although there continues to be considerable discussion in the literature of the comparative value of CT and MRI, helical CT remains the standard. This is not only for technical reasons but also for practical ones because CT imaging facilities are ubiquitous, whereas MRI facilities, although on the increase, are still centered largely in major medical centers. Even so, the great bulk of the work being done in MRI imaging is in the neuroradiological and musculoskeletal area. However, some progress is being made in MRI abdominal technique, and with its capability of multiplanar imaging it may very well become an even more important imaging tool for the abdomen, particularly for liver disease, in the coming decade (Fig. 5-3).

Before MRI can assume a prominent role, several problems must be resolved. These include problems arising from cardiac, vascular, respiratory, and peristaltic motion within the abdomen. In addition, no generally acceptable intraluminal contrast material that is specific for MRI of the gastrointestinal (GI) tract has proved effective at this time. Moreover, the examination is still lengthy compared with CT evaluation of the abdomen. But the promise and potential of MRI of the liver are great. The basis of MRI image formation is much more complex than CT and involves a number of different factors, such as hydrogen ion tissue density, T1 and T2 relaxation times, vascular flow characteristics, and chemical shift. Various operator-dependent factors can be manipulated that also contribute to the image formation and contrast.

The physics of MRI is beyond the scope of this text. But some elemental knowledge is necessary to interpret the images appropriately, and readers are encouraged to avail themselves of the many excellent books and courses that are currently being offered in this area.

Enlarged Liver without Focal Disease

Fatty liver

Diffuse fatty infiltration almost invariably results in an enlarged liver on cross-sectional imaging of the abdomen. The liver normally appears slightly denser than the spleen on CT scanning. Where the liver is fatty, this normal density relationship is reversed. The diffuse form of fatty infiltration can result in a relative increase in the contrast of the vascular structures of the liver, making them more prominent (Fig. 5-4).

Ultrasound examination of the fatty liver demonstrates degrees of diffuse increased echotexture.

Conventional MRI techniques have not been shown to be highly sensitive for the diagnosis of fatty infiltration of the liver (Fig. 5-5). However, alternative techniques using the spectroscopic capabilities of MRI, as in proton spectroscopic imaging, have been found to be an alternative method for detecting fatty infiltration.

Fatty infiltration of the liver, although most commonly diffuse, can occur in focal form as either isolated or multiple focal lesions. Normally less than 5% of the liver is composed of fat. In diffuse fatty infiltration this can rise to as high as 40% to 50%. These patients may be asymptomatic, but occasionally patients report vague abdominal pain. Jaundice is unusual but has been reported in a small number of patients. A large liver can be detected clinically and radiologically, although splenomegaly is unusual.

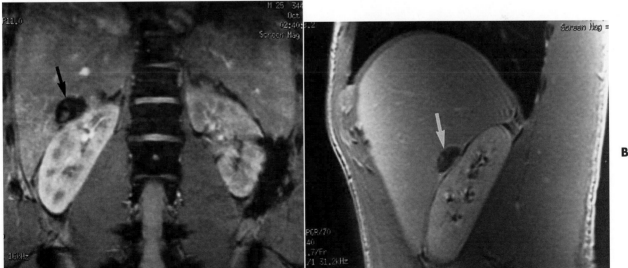

Fig. 5-3   Patient with subcapsular hematoma. MR imaging in two planes shows hematoma to advantage. Hematoma seen on (**A**) coronal image *(black arrow)* and sagittal oblique (**B**) image *(white arrow)*.

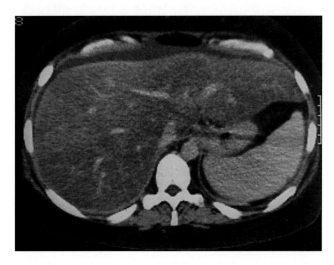

Fig. 5-4   CT section through the liver and spleen demonstrates hepatic enlargement and decreased density throughout the hepatic substance as a result of fatty infiltration.

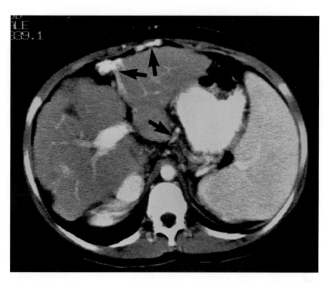

Fig. 5-6   Patient with alpha$_1$-antitrypsin deficiency with fatty and cirrhotic liver. CT images reveal marked collaterals with varices seen in the anterior abdominal wall, over the surface of the liver, and around the gastroesophageal junction *(arrows)*.

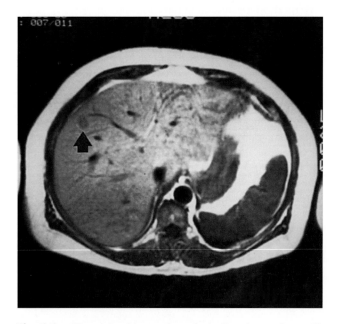

Fig. 5-5   T1-weighted image through the liver in a patient with known fatty infiltration of the liver. Note the small, rounded metastatic lesion seen in the periphery of the right lobe of the liver *(arrow)*.

Box 5-1 Some Common Causes of Fatty Changes in the Liver
Alcoholic hepatotoxicity Toxicity from chemotherapy Hepatitis Hyperalimentation Alpha$_1$-antitrypsin disease

The causes of fatty liver are numerous (Box 5-1) and can generally be divided into two categories, alcoholic and nonalcoholic. The histological, radiological, and clinical differences between these two are not discernible.

It is probably appropriate to say that most fatty livers result from chronic alcohol intake. It has been demonstrated that relatively small amounts of alcohol can increase hepatic fat content over a short period. This probably represents the earliest of the toxic changes induced in the liver by alcohol. Ordinarily these short-term changes in liver fat content are of no consequence, although they can precede more significant hepatotoxic changes of alcohol, progressing from fatty liver through alcoholic hepatitis and cirrhosis in a group of patients who either are genetically susceptible or indulge in regular high alcohol intake.

Numerous conditions can cause nonalcoholic fatty liver. Viral hepatitis may produce mild fatty changes in the liver. Also included are nutritional causes, such as starvation and prolonged hyperalimentation. Fatty liver has been described in Reye's syndrome in children. It is a common finding in patients undergoing chemotherapy. Fatty liver has also been demonstrated in patients who have undergone intestinal bypass surgery or hyperalimentation. Some cases have been associated with inflammatory bowel disease. Fatty liver has been described in patients with diabetes mellitus and metabolic abnormalities, such as Cushing's disease, alpha$_1$-antitrypsin disease (Fig. 5-6), and certain types of porphyria. Administration of exogenous steroids is associated with fat deposition at several sites within the body, including the liver. The acute fatty liver of pregnancy is a relatively rare disorder in which diffuse fatty infiltration of the liver occurs during the latter part of pregnancy. This condition is distinct from the well-known preeclampsia or toxemia of pregnancy. It has serious prognostic implications and often results in hepatic failure and GI bleeding.

Viral hepatitis

Inflammation of the liver as a result of viral infection can be divided into hepatitis A and hepatitis B. When neither the A nor B viral etiology can be identified, the hepatitis is usually referred to as non-A/non-B type (hepatitis C). There are no specific clinical or radiological distinctions in the course of either hepatitis A or hepatitis B. The route of transmission for hepatitis A is known to be the fecal-oral route, and the disease tends to be milder. The disease is of worldwide distribution and is related to contaminated water supplies and undercooked foods, among other factors. About 85% of patients with hepatitis A have some degree of hepatomegaly, and about 15% have some splenomegaly. The incubation phase is about two weeks. The prodromal phase is characterized by fatigue, weakness, and possibly vague abdominal pain. Most infections are anicteric, especially in children. Most patients completely recover within 2 to 3 months, and the illness is generally a benign and self-limiting illness.

Hepatitis B is usually transmitted parenterally, sexually, or by perinatal exposure. About 5% of the world population are said to be carriers. The incubation period is 60 to 120 days, and jaundice is more common than with the A type. Complications include the risk of chronicity (5%) or an acute, fulminant, often fatal, overwhelming infection (less than 1%). Patients with chronic disease are at increased risk for cirrhosis, portal hypertension, varices, and hepatocellular carcinoma.

Hepatitis C type is transmitted via blood route (transfusion, needle stick) or sexually. The prevalence of hepatitis C in intravenous (IV) drug abusers is 40% to 80%. Transfusion risk has declined with more sensitive screening of donors and is expected to decline further as yet more sensitive screening tests are introduced. The overwhelming clinical presentation of chronic disease is marked fatigue, while acute disease is often asymptomatic. The incubation period for hepatitis C is probably between those of A and B.

Hepatitis C has become an important factor in liver transplantation, partly because it is one of the primary indications of transplant (about 25% of liver transplants). Since these patients are universally viremic at transplantation, recurrence is almost entirely predictable. The risk is also increased by transmission via the donor organ or blood product transfusions.

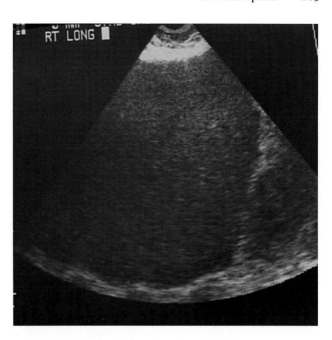

Fig. 5-7   Ultrasound of the liver in patient with acute hepatitis demonstrating hepatomegaly and generalized decreased echogenicity of the liver.

In the last two decades both viral hepatitis D and E have been described.

Certain ultrasonographic patterns have been described with acute hepatitis, and these generally are described as accentuated brightness and prominence in the demonstration of the portal vein radicle walls, with generalized decrease in echogenicity of the liver (Fig. 5-7). The role of imaging in the diagnosis of viral hepatitis is limited but can be one method used to differentiate obstructive from nonobstructive jaundice. CT of the abdomen in such patients reveals nonspecific liver enlargement, possibly some mild fatty infiltration in the acute phase but little else.

Liver and spleen imaging using technetium sulfur colloid may be normal or demonstrate hepatic enlargement. If the hepatocellular disease is sufficiently severe, there may be patchy, inhomogeneous uptake and reversal of the normal pattern of greater liver activity than splenic activity. Shift of the radionuclide to adjacent bone marrow or even lungs may also be seen in severe cases.

Diffuse metastatic disease

Diffuse involvement of the liver by metastatic disease can result in an enlarged liver (Fig. 5-8). This type of metastatic involvement of the liver is most commonly encountered with breast and lung primary lesions and colorectal carcinomas.

Budd-Chiari syndrome

The Budd-Chiari syndrome (hepatic venous occlusive disease) can result in hepatomegaly. There are many possible causes for hepatic vein occlusion. These range from local disease, such as hepatocellular carcinoma, and adjacent disease (carcinoma of the pancreas and kidney) to more generalized causes, such as thrombosis secondary to polycythemia vera, and blood dyscrasias, such as leukemia and sickle cell disease. There is an increasing suspicion that estrogen-containing birth control medication may be responsible for some cases. The imaging findings depend on the acuteness or chronicity of the condition. Acute hepatic vein occlusion often results in a dramatic presentation of symptoms with some cases presenting with severe abdominal pain and shock. In most chronic cases the patients present with ascites and hepatomegaly. This is accompanied by abdominal pain in about half of the cases. Jaundice is much less common. Clinical findings center on intraperitoneal fluid and a large, tender liver.

The CT appearance of hepatic venous occlusion is that of hepatomegaly and accompanying ascites. During dynamic imaging of the liver, an inhomogeneous, patchy appearance of may be observed, and the hepatic veins may not be clearly seen as a result of thrombosis and obliteration. In patients for whom the condition has been present for several weeks, the caudate lobe is enlarged. This enlarged caudate lobe of the liver is readily detectable on both CT and ultrasound examination of the liver. MRI features of Budd-Chiari syndrome also include reduction of the size and number of hepatic veins. On both CT and MRI, collateral circulation may be observed, particularly involving the azygos and hemiazygos veins in the retrocrural area.

Other uncommon causes

Hepatomegaly can be seen when performing imaging on patients with a number of other, relatively uncommon conditions. Patients with congestive heart failure can experience hepatic enlargement and even right upper quadrant tenderness as a result of capsular distention on the basis of chronic passive congestion (Fig. 5-9).

A number of hepatotoxic drugs can sometimes result in hepatomegaly. These include methotrexate, methyldopa, isoniazid, acetaminophen, nitrofurantoin, tetracycline, and halothane.

In Weil's disease (leptospirosis) an enlarged liver and spleen are a common clinical presentation. This is a spirochete infection that is spread to humans via animals. In addition to the enlarged liver and spleen, these patients demonstrate constitutional symptoms of fever and generalized myalgias, as well as varying degrees of central nervous system (CNS) involvement.

Hepatic enlargement may also be seen as part of the clinical picture of abnormal iron deposition within the liver (hemochromatosis) and Wilson's disease (hepatolenticular degeneration), which is a hereditary disorder of copper metabolism and resultant copper deposition within the liver and brain. The striking CT finding in these diseases, particularly hemochromatosis, is not so much the enlarged liver but the increased density of the liver seen on noncontrast studies. This can be missed if the liver is studied only during contrast enhancement.

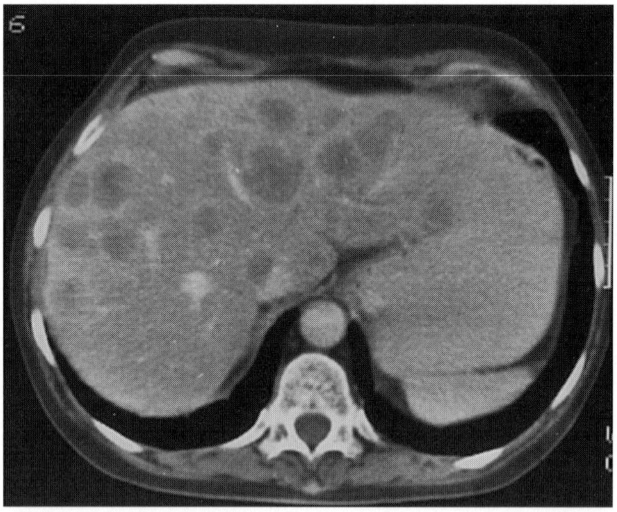

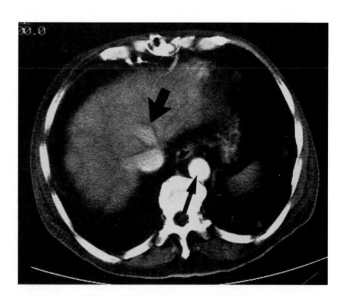

Fig. 5-8 Patient with carcinoma of the lung. Patient has hepatic enlargement. CT image obtained through the liver shows multiple intrahepatic metastatic lesions.

Fig. 5-9 Patient with congestive heart failure. Note patchy appearance of liver and distention of the hepatic veins *(large arrow)*. The sluggishness of the circulation causes the aorta to remain quite bright *(smaller arrow)*.

Small or Shrunken Liver

Cirrhosis

Liver cirrhosis involves a chronic increase in fibrotic tissue throughout the liver, resulting in distortion of the normal liver architecture, fibrotic deposition around the portal vein tributaries, degrees of portal vein occlusion, portal vein hypertension, and redistribution of blood within the upper abdomen through collateral circulations. The ongoing fibrotic process results in decreasing liver size, although individual segments of the liver may maintain their size or even increase slightly. These latter changes are often seen in the lateral segment of the left lobe and the caudate lobe. The liver margins become nodular and irregular. There is often evidence of fatty infiltration in the less severe cases. Other associated imaging findings include splenomegaly secondary to portal hypertension, as well as ascites and varices.

Generally, cirrhosis can be divided into Laënnec's and postnecrotic types. From an imaging perspective, there is little to distinguish between these two. A third type of cirrhosis associated with hemochromatosis and Wilson's disease is rare.

In the United States, cirrhosis constitutes a relatively common cause of death in the adult age group with the greater bulk of the cases secondary to alcoholic hepatitis (Laënnec's cirrhosis). A small number of cases may be attributed to the postnecrotic condition.

Primary biliary cirrhosis, which is a chronic progressive form of bile duct inflammation and fibrosis, may also be included in the discussion. The diagnostic designation is somewhat misleading, since most of these patients present with an enlarged liver and spleen. However, in severe progressive disease, the typical appearance of cirrhosis may develop. This condition is seen mostly in women and usually has an insidious onset with patients often presenting with jaundice, pruritus, and constitutional symptoms, including vague abdominal pain.

CT evaluation of the upper abdomen of patients with advanced cirrhosis demonstrates a small, shrunken liver (Fig. 5-10). Some relative increase in the size of the caudate lobe and lateral segment of the left lobe can be easily identified along with the accompanying findings of ascites, splenomegaly, and varices. CT may also demonstrate diffuse or focal fatty changes throughout the liver.

Superimposed disease is always a possibility, particularly hepatocellular carcinoma; the cirrhotic liver presents a potential imaging dilemma because the superimposed lesion may be masked by the cirrhotic changes, which can include areas of focal fatty changes, regenerating nodules, and fibrosis (Fig. 5-11).

Ultrasound has been helpful in detecting the hepatic changes seen in cirrhosis along with the accompanying findings of ascites. The increased echogenicity of the liver is similar to the findings described for fatty liver, and differentiation cannot be made on the basis of echotexture alone. The cirrhotic liver may appear smaller and there may be accompanying ascites. Regenerating nodules may be detected as areas of decreased echogenicity within the cirrhotic liver. Although ultrasound evaluation of the liver is sensitive in detecting the diffuse changes, it may not be able to differentiate between fatty infiltration and cirrhosis or other diffuse hepatocellular diseases.

The radionuclide liver/spleen scan shows the changes typical of hepatocellular disease with inhomogeneous take-up and shift of colloid to bone marrow and lungs. The spleen appears enlarged. MRI evaluation of patients with cirrhotic liver demonstrates morphological findings similar to those seen on CT. MRI can often nicely demonstrate the portal venous system and its patency in addition to the presence of collateral circulation around the spleen and stomach.

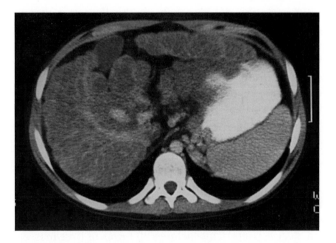

Fig. 5-10   Patient with marked cirrhotic changes. The liver is shrunken and fatty infiltrated and has lobular contours.

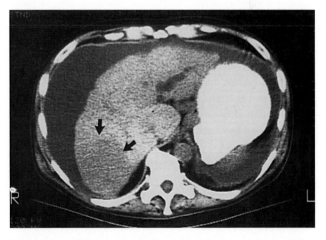

Fig. 5-11   Patient with a small cirrhotic liver. A poorly defined, low-attenuation lesion (*arrows*) is seen on the posterior right lobe of the liver, representing hepatocellular carcinoma.

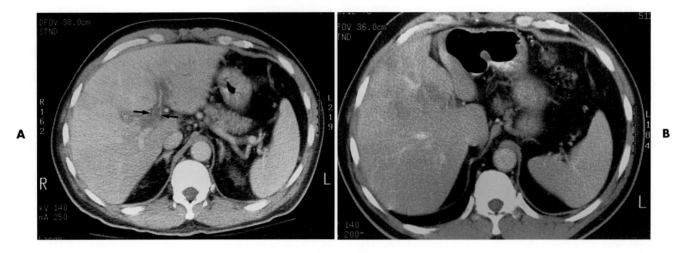

Fig. 5-12   **A,** Patient with thrombus of the left portal vein *(arrows).* **B,** Four months later CT images show atrophy of the left lobe of the liver with the lateral segment almost completely absent.

Lobar atrophy

Because the blood supply to the liver is rich and derived from both the hepatic arterial and portal venous systems, hepatic infarction is highly unusual. However, since the perfusion of normal hepatocytes is about 80% supplied from the portal venous system, prolonged obstruction of the portal vein may result in atrophy of the involved lobe (Fig. 5-12).

Other causes of contour abnormalities

Most of the conditions that result in contour abnormalities of the liver are also covered in the consideration of other radiological problems of the liver, in particular, those parenchymal focal lesions that involve the edge of the liver, resulting in some focal bulging or deformity of the liver capsule. This includes all forms of liver masses, particularly adenomas and hepatic cysts. Hepatic trauma can also result in deformity of the hepatic margins as a result of blood either within or outside the hepatic capsule. The same may be said of subdiaphragmatic abscesses indenting the capsular surface of the dome of the liver (Fig. 5-13).

Dissemination of peritoneal metastatic disease can result in metastatic deposits along the peritoneal surface adjacent to the liver, as well as along the capsular surface. The most common of these lesions is ovarian cancer, although cancer of the pancreas, stomach, and colon can present with a similar pattern and appearance. Early diffuse peritoneal metastatic spread can be subtle and is often undetected by CT. Small peritoneal metastatic implants visualized along the peritoneal or visceral surface of liver or spleen may be the earliest sign. These may occur before the development of ascites and the more obvious mesenteric conglomerate masses known as *omental cakes.*

To some extent, hepatic venous occlusive disease

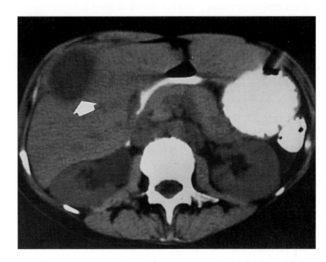

Fig. 5-13   CT section showing a low-density extrahepatic lesion *(arrow)* impressing the anterior lateral surface of the liver. This lesion proved to be actinomycosis.

(Budd-Chiari syndrome) can result in hepatic contour abnormalities. The CT evaluation in such cases generally demonstrates ascites and an enlarged liver. Hepatic veins may be poorly delineated. Because of the separate and direct drainage of the caudate lobe into the vena cava, the caudate lobe is spared and appears enlarged in chronic cases. However, apart from the enlarged and apparently bulging caudate lobe, the hepatic contours should otherwise be smooth.

Solitary Defects

Hemangiomas

Although hepatic hemangiomas had been considered rare by clinicians, the experience of cross-sectional CT and ultrasound imaging over the last two decades has

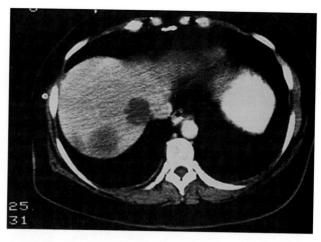

Fig. 5-14   CT section through the dome of the liver demonstrates multiple low-attenuation lesions in the right lobe, representing multiple hemangiomas.

confirmed what pathologists have always maintained: this lesion is much more common than is clinically suspected (Box 5-2). It is thought to be the most common neoplastic lesion of the liver, with an incidence range between 2% and 5%. It is more common in females, and some lesions may enlarge with age. This lesion demonstrates a predilection for the posterior right lobe of the liver, and almost 70% of hepatic hemangiomas are subcapsular. They are mostly solitary, although multiple lesions sometimes occur.

Hemangiomas can be of the capillary or the cavernous variety, with the former being considerably more common. The capillary hemangioma is, as its name implies, a lesion made up of tiny capillary-like vessels. A cavernous hemangioma, on the other hand, is made up of large cystic, blood-filled spaces lined with epithelium. The larger the lesion, the more likely that it is a cavernous hemangioma.

Virtually all hemangiomas are asymptomatic. Only when the lesion becomes quite large (greater than 4 to 5 cm) do any symptoms appear. Symptoms are often nonspecific, usually vague right upper quadrant discomfort.

Although hepatic hemangiomas are rarely a clinical dilemma, they commonly result in a diagnostic dilemma for the radiologist. Unfortunately, the appearance of hepatic hemangiomas can simulate other serious diseases, such as primary hepatic cancer or metastasis to the liver (Box 5-3).

This diagnostic problem can often be resolved by obtaining CT images of the liver using dynamic-enhanced technique. A low-attenuation lesion with varying configuration and a zone of increased density along its margin is the initial finding (Fig. 5-14). Delayed images at the level of the lesion over the next 5 to 15 minutes demonstrate centripetal opacification of the lesion. A dynamic series of images at a predetermined level within the lesion, following a rapid bolus injection, demonstrates similar findings with the initial enhancement at the margin and delayed enhancement centrally (Fig. 5-15).

Unfortunately, a sizeable percentage of cavernous hemangiomas do not demonstrate the classic findings during CT. This usually occurs when the lesions are quite small (less than 2 cm) or quite large (greater than 5 to 6 cm). The extremely small lesions may fill in quickly, while the extremely large lesions may fill in incompletely or not at all. In the case of larger lesions this is thought to result from the presence of thrombus and fibrosis within the lesion (Fig. 5-16). This can cause considerable diagnostic confusion in attempting to correctly differentiate between a cavernous hemangioma and more serious disease, such as primary and secondary malignancies.

Characteristic acoustic patterns in the ultrasonic evaluation of hemangiomas have been described. These have been shown to be well-defined, echogenic focal areas within the liver (Fig. 5-17). However, in very small lesions, less than 1 cm, or extremely large lesions in which there are fibrotic, cystic changes or even thrombotic elements within the lesion, ultrasonic examination of the liver is not definitive.

MRI of the liver can be useful in the diagnosis of hemangioma. On T2-weighted images, a high signal intensity is characteristically encountered (Fig. 5-18). Unfortunately, other lesions can occasionally give similar

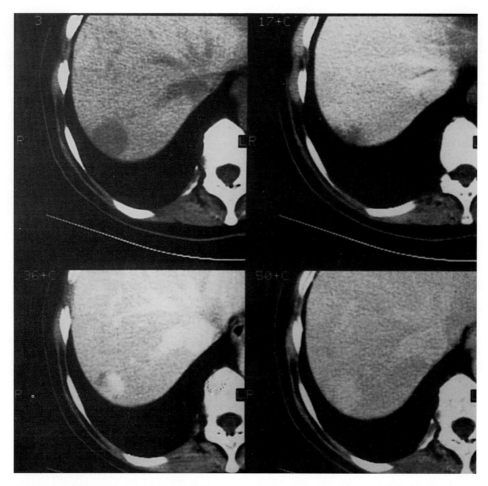

Fig. 5-15 Patient with a rounded, low-attenuation lesion in the posterior right lobe of the liver *(upper left image)* undergoing dynamic scans during bolus injection at the level of the lesion. Progressive enhancement and fill-in of the lesion are seen on the subsequent three images, consistent with hemangioma.

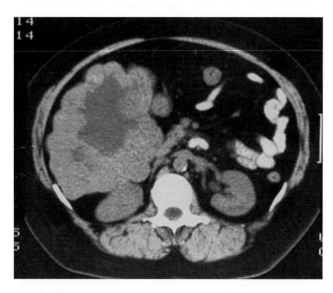

Fig. 5-16 CT section through the inferior aspect of the liver shows a large lobulated mass that is arising from the inferior margin of the right lobe with central area of low density representing thrombus and fibrosis within this large cavernous hemangioma.

appearances, such as simple cysts or even some metastatic lesions. Although cysts usually have a long T1 value, this is not always the case in small lesions (Fig. 5-19). Gradient echo technique using in-phase and out-phase imaging is extremely helpful. Larger cavernous hemangiomas with fibrosis and thrombus formation may also give an atypical appearance on MRI and can be confused with other liver lesions. However, newer MRI protocols continue to show more promise in the specificity of hemangioma diagnosis.

Radionuclide imaging using tagged red blood cells has been used occasionally in an attempt to clarify a questionable hepatic lesion that may be a hemangioma (Fig. 5-20). In similar fashion, uptake is seen at the edge of the lesion and delayed imaging shows gradual fill-in. The nuclear scan suffers from exactly the same weaknesses as that described for CT.

Although there has been a general hesitancy about doing direct aspiration biopsy of these questionable lesions, there is a slowly developing consensus that a thin-needle aspiration biopsy is the method of definitive clarification and diagnosis. Relative contraindications in this diagnostic approach are patients with coagulopathies and patients in whom the lesion is immediately subcapsular.

Metastatic disease

Secondary metastatic lesions to the liver are common. Generally, the detection of such lesions is a grave prognostic indicator. In the past, it has been observed

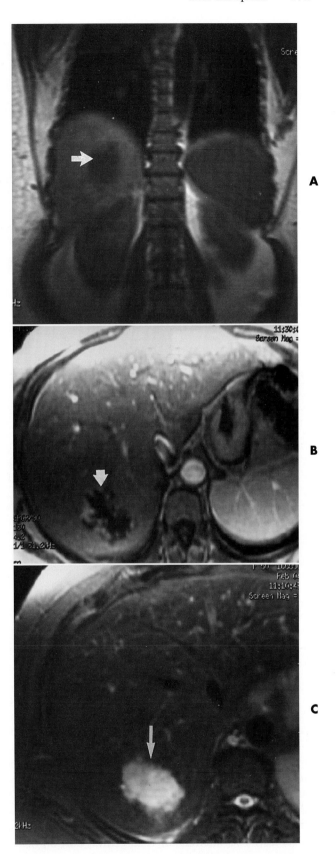

A

B

C

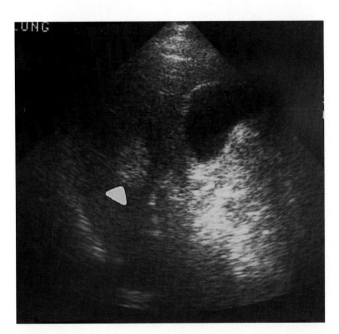

Fig. 5-17 Ultrasound of the liver shows a well-defined echogenic lesion within the liver *(arrowhead)*, representing the most common ultrasonic finding in small- to moderate-sized hemangiomas.

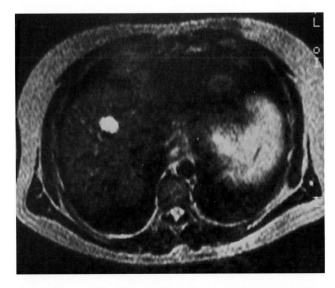

Fig. 5-18 Image obtained through the liver on T2-weighted MRI scan demonstrates a high signal intensity in a rounded hepatic hemangioma.

Fig. 5-19 **A,** T1-weighted MR image shows high signal of hemangioma in posterior right lobe of liver *(arrow).* **B,** Axial T2 fast spin echo image shows hemangioma as bright signal *(arrow).* **C,** Coronal T2-weighted image demonstrates lesion *(arrow).*

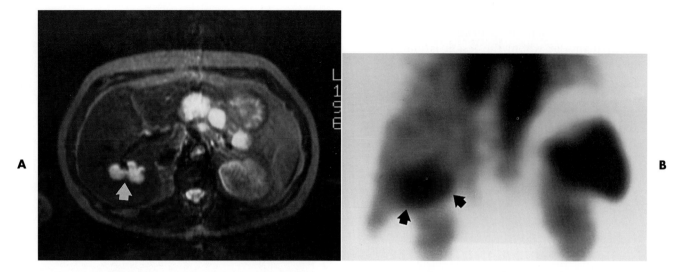

Fig. 5-20   Patient with suspected hepatic hemangioma. **A,** MR shows high-signal lobulated lesion in right lobe *(arrow)*. **B,** Red blood–tagged radionuclide scan confirms diagnosis of hemangioma *(arrows)*.

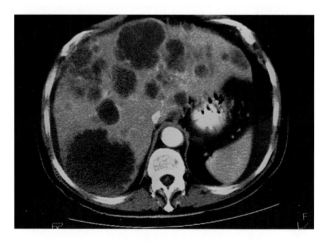

Fig. 5-21   Patient with widespread metastatic lesions of the liver with markedly varying sizes and resultant hepatomegaly.

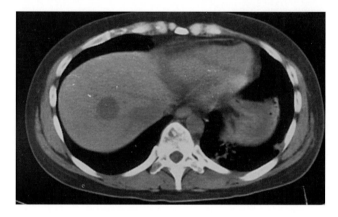

Fig. 5-22   CT through the dome of the liver demonstrates an isolated metastatic lesion.

that only about 5% of patients with untreated liver metastatic disease survive one year beyond detection.

CT imaging of liver metastatic lesions has demonstrated that they come in all sizes, shapes, and numbers. The lesions can be focal or diffuse (Fig. 5-21). By far the most common appearance of hepatic metastatic disease on CT is a low-attenuation lesion with respect to the surrounding liver, although isodense and hyperdense lesions are encountered (Figs. 5-22 and 5-23). There may be degrees of peripheral ring enhancement similar to that observed in hemangioma, although the centripetal opacification is uncommon. The central portion of the lesion may be near fluid density in lesions large enough to undergo central necrosis. Calcifications are uncommon and tend to be seen in younger patients with

aggressive primary lesions, such as mucinous adenocarcinomas of the colon, stomach, or ovary.

In general, focal metastatic disease is not difficult to detect if the lesion is greater than 1 cm. However, metastatic disease superimposed on a fatty liver can present a diagnostic dilemma.

The diffuse form of metastatic involvement of the liver does occasionally occur and can be especially difficult if IV contrast enhancement is not used. Moreover, certain types of diffuse metastatic disease that are hypervascular in nature, such as islet cell tumors and carcinoids, may become isodense during the contrast enhancement of the liver. To further confuse the issue, occasionally a lesion is isodense on the enhanced images and well defined on only the postenhanced images (see Fig. 5-2).

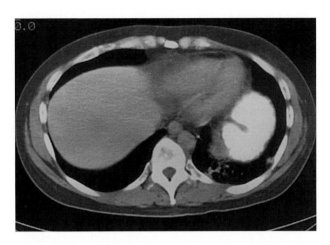

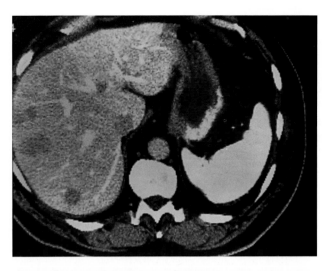

Fig. 5-23   In the same patient as in Fig. 5-22 after IV administration of contrast material, the well-defined lesion seen on the preenhancement scan has become isodense.

Fig. 5-24   Demonstration of CTAP with injection of the splenic artery. Note the hyperdense appearance of the spleen and a portion of the gastric wall. Several defects are now clearly demonstrated predominantly in the right lobe of the liver.

For this reason both preenhancement and postenhancement images of the liver are recommended routinely for the evaluation of the liver for possible metastatic disease.

In the late 1970s, interest in the possible resection of solitary liver metastatic lesions was revived. Indeed, this approach has resulted in increased survival times in a select subgroup of patients.

Of course, imaging techniques are not sufficiently sensitive to ensure that the liver is truly free from disease. At best, we can attest to the fact that no metastatic disease is seen or that there is disease apparently limited to one lobe. The presence of extrahepatic nodal disease, of course, negates the possibility of hepatic resection regardless of the state of the liver.

The increasing interest in the possibility of selective hepatic resection for metastatic disease has resulted in several attempts to refine the CT evaluation of the liver and thus its sensitivity for metastatic disease detection.

At the moment the best approach appears to be CTAP. Most lesions are believed to be supplied largely by blood drawn from the hepatic arterial system, whereas normal liver tissue derives most of its blood supply from the portal venous system. In CTAP the portal system is flooded with contrast material while the liver is dynamically scanned. This results in increased contrast at the lesion/parenchymal interface and makes subtle, smaller, or otherwise invisible lesions more discernible. Indeed, CTAP has resulted in improved sensitivity in the detection of liver metastatic disease.

CTAP requires arterial puncture and the advancement of a catheter tip to the celiac axis and subsequent selective catheterization of the splenic artery or superior mesenteric artery. The splenic artery may be preferred because of dilution factors and streaming artifacts associated with superior mesenteric artery injection portography. After placement of the catheter tip in the splenic artery, an injection bolus of 60 to 80 ml is given, followed by dynamic imaging of the liver (Fig. 5-24).

Sonography has not proved to be the diagnostic imaging method of choice for hepatic metastatic disease when CT or MRI capabilities are available. The false negative rate is generally higher than with CT, and apart from distinguishing fluid from solid tissue, lesion characterization is often limited and nonspecific.

At the moment, CT continues to be the primary imaging modality for the detection of hepatic metastatic disease. Recent studies comparing CTAP and MRI sensitivity in the detection of hepatic metastatic lesions have been conflicting. MRI sensitivities have been reported ranging between 57% to 95% (Fig. 5-25). The sensitivity using CTAP has been reported to be around 85%.

Cysts

The simple congenital hepatic cyst is extremely common. These lesions probably arise from developmental defects in bile duct development in utero. They are rarely symptomatic, and liver function is usually unaffected. They tend to be more common in females and more commonly localized to the right lobe of the liver. They range in size from 5 mm to 10 to 12 cm. Most of these congenital cysts have an epithelial lining and are filled with clear or cloudy fluid.

Cysts can occur as an isolated hepatic lesion or as multiple lesions involving both lobes of the liver. When the cysts are multiple, concomitant cystic disease of the kidneys, pancreas, and ovaries may be present. In 20% to 50% of patients with polycystic disease of the kidneys, hepatic cysts can be identified.

CT imaging of hepatic cysts discloses a sharp, well-circumscribed, low-attenuation lesion with extremely thin or no discernible walls (Fig. 5-26). Cysts are usually round. The internal content is homogeneous and low density, with Hounsfield numbers approaching those of water. Generally, no change occurs in the internal density of the cysts with IV enhancement, although the cyst itself gives the appearance of being more lucent because of the increased density in the surrounding liver tissue. Very small cysts are difficult to evaluate and difficult to get a cursor on to obtain accurate density numbers (Fig. 5-27).

Ultrasound is often helpful in distinguishing a simple cyst from a low-density solid lesion, such as an abscess, necrotic tumor, echinococcal cyst, or cystic neoplasm. The ultrasound characteristics are a focal, well-defined anechoic defect within the liver, through-transmission, and acoustic enhancement of the far wall.

MRI characteristics of hepatic cysts are also characteristic with a low signal on T1-weighted images and a very high signal on T2-weighted images. The relatively long T1 and T2 values are helpful in differentiating simple cysts from most hepatic neoplasms. However, a hemangioma can give a similar signal pattern. In addition, difficulties may be encountered when imaging infected or bloody cysts.

Trauma

Blunt trauma to the abdomen resulting in hepatic laceration is most commonly seen as a solitary laceration within the substance of the liver (Fig. 5-28). A fractured liver with multiple lacerations is uncommonly seen because these patients usually die before CT imaging. In the uncommon event that they do survive, their condition is usually unstable and they are candidates for emergency exploratory surgery. Trauma can be contained within the liver capsule or result in capsular tear and intraperitoneal bleeding (Fig. 5-29).

Hepatocellular carcinoma

Hepatocellular carcinoma or hepatoma is a slow-growing but, nevertheless, malignant lesion originating in liver parenchymal cells (Box 5-4). It is the seventh most common tumor in men and the ninth in women. Distant metastatic involvement is unusual but has been reported. However, 75% of patients have contiguous or

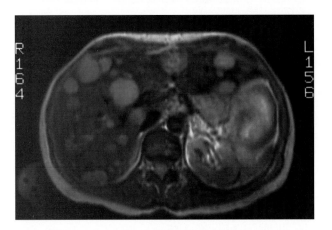

Fig. 5-25 Proton density MR images of patient with suspected liver metastatic disease. Liver images reveal widespread lesions in both lobes.

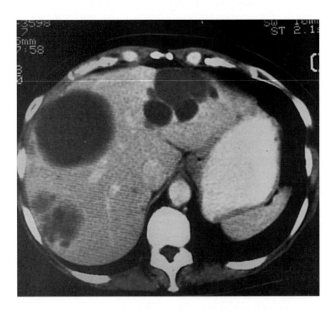

Fig. 5-26 CT scan through the liver of female patient demonstrates multiple, benign hepatic cysts of varying size.

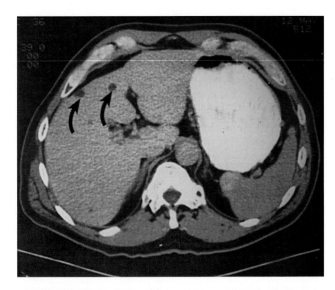

Fig. 5-27 Two small cysts *(curved arrows)* seen near the margin of the liver and measuring approximately 1 cm, confirmed by ultrasound.

lymphatic extrahepatic spread of tumor at the time of diagnosis and are unresectable. In addition, portal vein thrombosis is seen in up to 50% of patients. Invasion of the hepatic venous system can result in a Budd-Chiari–type picture. An elevated serum alpha-fetoprotein (AFP) level is a good (but not absolute) serum indicator of the presence of hepatocellular carcinoma (or hepatoblastoma in children).

The tumor appears to be more common in females and is relatively common in the Far East, where it is attributable to the presence of various parasites (especially liver flukes), diet, and a high incidence of hepatitis B or hepatitis C.

In the West the tumor is much less common. However, a definite relationship between hepatic cirrhosis and hepatocellular carcinoma does exist. Almost 75% of patients with hepatocellular carcinoma have either cirrhosis or a history of cirrhosis. The risk of hepatocellular carcinoma may be higher in patients with hemochromatosis of the liver.

Certain other risk factors have been described. The use of oral contraception is thought to relate to an increased incidence over the last three decades. Moreover, in recent years the use of anabolic steroids has been thought to place individuals at an increased risk for this disease.

Patients often present with cachexia, weakness, right upper quadrant pain, and weight loss. Clinically, an enlarged liver is commonly detected.

CT may demonstrate a solitary mass or multiple masses with a dominant lesion and multiple satellite lesions. The mass is usually of low attenuation (Fig. 5-30). A small number of patients (fewer than 10%) have

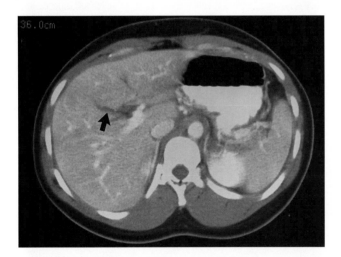

Fig. 5-28 Patient with blunt trauma to abdomen. CT images of liver reveal an irregular linear defect *(arrow)*. No blood is seen around liver.

Box 5-4   The Facts about Hepatoma

Risk factors: hepatitis B infection, cirrhosis, exposure to hepatocarcinogens
Associated with elevated alpha-fetoprotein (AFP)
Relatively uncommon in the United States but common in parts of Asia
Imaging assessment by CT, CT-portography, MR, angiography
Poor prognosis

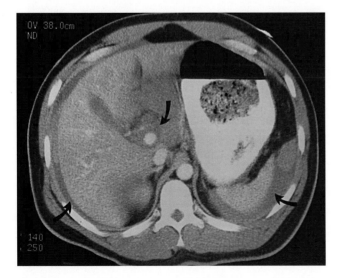

Fig. 5-29 Patient in motor vehicle accident with blunt trauma to the abdomen and lacerated liver. Blood is seen around the liver, around the spleen, and in the porta hepatis region *(curved arrows)*. Laceration is not shown on this image.

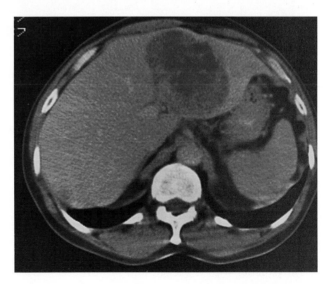

Fig. 5-30 Large inhomogeneous lesion occupying and expanding most of the left lobe of the liver, representing a hepatocellular carcinoma.

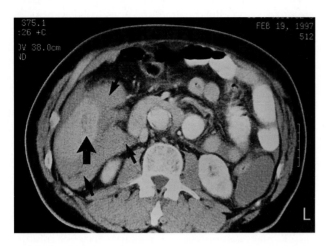

Fig. 5-31 An 83-year-old male with hepatocellular carcinoma (hepatoma) presents with orthostatic hypotension. CT images show lesion in tip of liver *(large arrow)* and surrounding blood in lower perihepatic space *(small arrows)*.

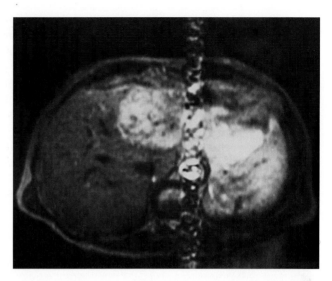

Fig. 5-32 MRI scan in the same patient as in Fig. 5-30 demonstrates high signal within the lesion on T2-weighted image.

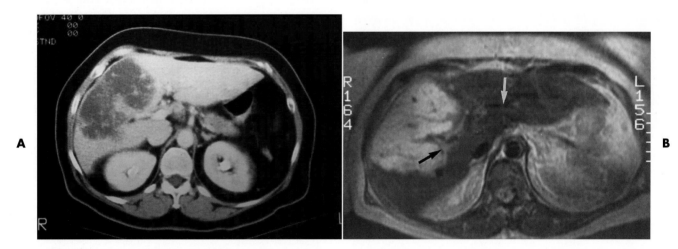

Fig. 5-33 **A,** CT of patient with hepatoma. Lesion is large and lobulated. **B,** Spin echo T2-weighted MR images show lesion with tumor in portal veins *(black arrow)*. Uninvolved veins are seen distal to the lesion *(white arrow)*.

some calcification within the lesion. In addition, the size of the lesion may be exaggerated on CT evaluation by the presence of regional portal vein thrombosis in up to 50% of patients. This may be seen on CT imaging as regional wedgelike shapes of low density projecting peripherally. Extrahepatic bleeding sometimes occurs, and a positive peritoneal tap for blood in suspected cases of hepatoma in the pre-CT era was considered a strong diagnostic sign (Fig. 5-31).

In patients with a background of cirrhosis, involvement of the liver with hepatocellular carcinoma tends to be more diffuse and thus presents a diagnostic difficulty in differentiating among regenerating nodules, metastatic disease, and primary hepatic carcinoma.

Multiple patterns have been described for the ultrasonographic presentations of this lesion. These range from discrete echogenic to relatively echo-free lesions. They can have a mixed echo pattern, or there may be diffuse disease. MRI of hepatocellular carcinoma approaches CT in its accuracy. In large lesions, findings can be nonspecific and to some extent depend on the amount of fibrosis and necrosis within the lesion (Fig. 5-32). Generally, this lesion displays low-signal intensity on T1-weighted images with an increase in signal intensity on T2-weighted images. However, MRI has proved to be quite superior in demonstrating vascular involvement by this tumor (Fig. 5-33).

Fibrolamellar hepatocellular carcinoma is a rare vari-

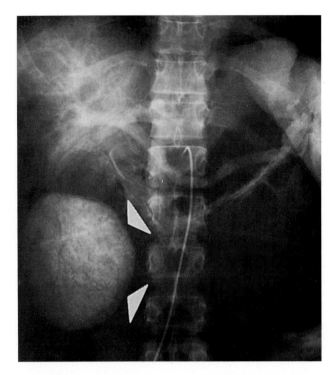

Fig. 5-34   Vascular study during venous phase on patient with pedunculated hepatic adenoma demonstrates well-defined hypervascular lesion *(arrowheads)*.

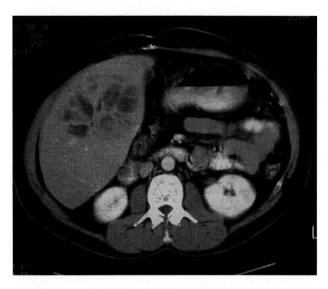

Fig. 5-35   Large heterogeneous lesion involving the lower portion of the right lobe of the liver that proved to be a hepatic adenoma in a 30-year-old female.

ety of hepatocellular carcinoma more commonly seen in younger patients. There is a tendency for intralesional calcification, and a better prognosis.

Adenomas

Hepatic adenomas are focal, well-differentiated benign lesions of the liver. They are usually solitary. Ninety percent or more of these lesions are found in females. The lesions are generally well encapsulated. The incidence of hepatic adenomas has increased over the last three decades, possibly relating to the increased use of oral contraception. The incidence of hepatic adenomas in some glycogen storage diseases has also increased.

Generally, the malignant potential of hepatic adenomas is considered low. Yet the suspected increased incidence of hepatocellular carcinoma in the female population taking birth control pills does raise the question of some degree of malignant potential.

Adenomas tend to be hypervascular, and internal hemorrhage can lead to blood-filled cysts within the adenoma (Fig. 5-34). They are usually asymptomatic. Serum AFP levels are normal. When symptoms do occur, they are usually acute and in 50% of the cases result from bleeding. The adenomas can be subcapsular or pedunculated on the edge of the liver, and bleeding can occur into the peritoneal cavity, resulting in a surgical emergency. The incidence of bleeding in hepatic ad-

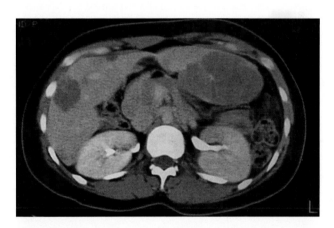

Fig. 5-36   CT scan of the abdomen obtained on a young female after abdominal trauma demonstrates multiple inhomogeneous low-density lesions of the liver that proved to be multiple adenomas.

enomas is increased among women taking birth control pills.

Hepatic adenomas present as discrete masses, usually solitary on dynamic CT scanning. They are commonly hyperdense. If hemorrhage or internal necrosis has occurred, the tumor can be heterogeneous in its appearance with focal areas of low attenuation (Figs. 5-35 and 5-36). Ultrasound demonstrates variable patterns, depending on the presence of intralesional bleeding. This results in a decreased echogenicity within the lesion. Otherwise, the adenoma is seen as a hyperechoic solid lesion (Fig. 5-37).

Like hepatocellular carcinomas, hepatic adenomas are best demonstrated on T2-weighted MRI images.

Focal nodular hyperplasia

Focal nodular hyperplasia is a relatively uncommon lesion best described as a well-defined hepatic lesion, commonly solitary, composed of bundles of benign hyperplastic hepatocytes arranged around a stellate fibrous central scar. The etiological origins are unclear, although there is evidence to suggest that some degree of hormonal dependency is involved in either its origin or its growth. Unlike hepatic adenomas (Table 5-1), differences in incidence between men and women are less striking and there is much less of a tendency

for the lesion to bleed or rupture. Generally, focal nodular hyperplasia (FNH) is asymptomatic. A small proportion of the patients has vague right upper quadrant pain.

Most patients are female (70% to 80%), in the 30 to 40 years of age range. Again a relationship between FNH and the use of birth control pills has been postulated but not proven.

The lesions can be single or less commonly multiple. The mass is composed of hyperplastic liver parenchymal elements often partitioned into bundles by fibrous bands radiating from a large central scar. This configuration is seen in approximately 60% of patients with FNH. The size of the lesions can vary from 1 to 20 cm. They are most commonly seen in the right lobe of the liver.

CT imaging may demonstrate an isodense or hypodense lesion on the unenhanced scans (Fig. 5-38).

Table 5-1 Distinctions between hepatic adenoma and focal nodular hyperplasia		
	Hepatic adenoma	**Focal nodular hyperplasia**
Sex distribution	Predominantly women	Predominantly women
Relationship to oral contraceptives	Related to long-term use of oral contraceptives	Relationship not well understood; may be no etiological relationship, but oral contraceptives may contribute to growth of lesion
Clinical presentation	50% will bleed	Often asymptomatic; may complain of abdominal pain or mass
Pathology	Usually solitary adenomatous lesion	Proliferation of hepatocytes divided by fibrous septa
Radiology	Can be difficult to distinguish from FNH	Tc-99 sulfur colloid liver scan can be helpful in 60% to 70% of cases

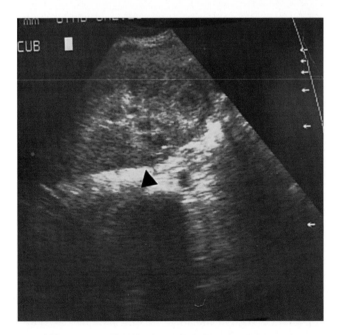

Fig. 5-37   Ultrasound in young female with hepatic adenoma demonstrates a large hyperechoic lesion *(arrowhead)*.

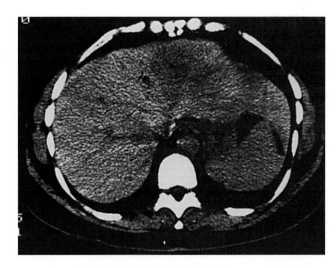

Fig. 5-38   FNH of the liver seen in a female as ill-defined area of low attenuation in the left lobe of the liver.

Like hepatic adenomas, the lesion shows an increase in homogeneous enhancement following IV contrast enhancement (Fig. 5-39). There may be an area of low attenuation in the center of the lesion if a central stellate area of scarring is present. It is difficult to differentiate between hepatic adenoma and FNH on CT scanning.

The ultrasound appearance is of a mass that may appear somewhat less echogenic than the surrounding normal liver. Unfortunately, it can also appear isoechoic with the surrounding liver. Identification of the central scar may be helpful and is manifested by dense internal echoes.

MRI may be helpful. There is a tendency for the lesion to be isodense on all pulse sequences. If the central scarring complex is present, this tends to have a low signal on T1-weighted images and a somewhat higher signal on T2-weighted images (Fig. 5-40). On technetium

sulfur colloid scans, FNH, because of the presence of Kupffer's cells, can show normal or near normal uptake and may be indistinguishable from surrounding liver (60% to 70%) tissue, whereas a hepatic adenoma is almost always a cold defect.

Abscesses

Hepatic abscesses can be bacterial, parasitic, or mycotic. The bacterial or pyogenic abscesses are focal collections of pus within the liver. They are relatively uncommon today. Most pyogenic abscesses occur as an extension of infection ascending through the biliary tree (ascending cholangitis). Hematogenous spread through the portal vein or the hepatic artery or direct contiguous spread from an adjacent site of infection can also be a cause for hepatic abscess formation. It can be also seen in posttraumatic events involving the liver.

Most commonly a gram-negative organism is involved. The clinical course without therapeutic intervention is almost uniformly a rapid downhill decline and death.

The early symptoms vary and include fever, chills, sweating, right upper quadrant pain, pleuritic pain, nausea, and vomiting. Many patients have abnormal liver function tests, and up to one third of the patients have some degree of jaundice. The size of the lesions is quite variable, from 1 cm to 18 to 20 cm. The smaller the abscess, the higher the probability of multiple sites within the liver. In fact, approximately two thirds of patients have multiple lesions. Eighty percent of the lesions occur in the right lobe of the liver. The CT evaluation of the liver generally discloses a low-attenuation lesion with a peripheral rim that usually enhances following IV contrast. Internally the liver may have septations or papillary projections (Fig. 5-41). In

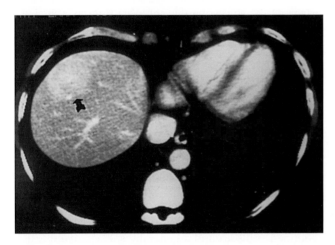

Fig. 5-39   Postenhancement CT image through the dome of the liver demonstrates increased enhancement *(arrow)* within solitary FNH lesion in a female patient.

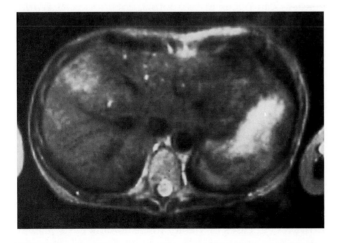

Fig. 5-40   In the same patient as in Fig. 5-39, an MRI scan through the same region shows relative increase in signal intensity at the lesion site.

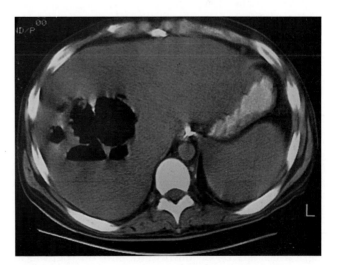

Fig. 5-41   Large hepatic abscess occupying most of the right lobe of the liver. Note the internal septations, air-fluid levels, and wall irregularity of the lesion.

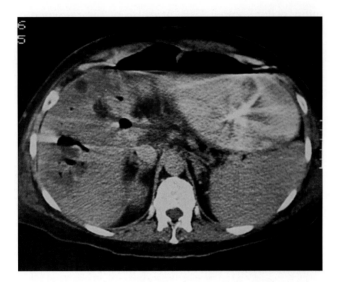

Fig. 5-42 CT images obtained through liver of patient with multiple, small hepatic abscesses in the right lobe of the liver.

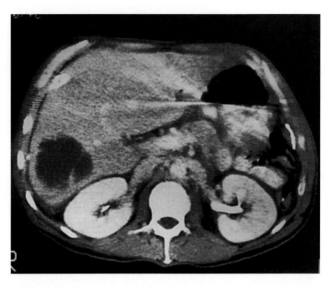

Fig. 5-43 CT scan through the liver of a patient with known amebic abscess of the posterior right lobe. Note the well-defined margins of the abscess on this enhanced scan, as well as the internal septation.

about one fifth of the cases gas bubbles can be detected. Air-fluid levels are identified on occasion. Lesions may be solitary or multiple, or there may be a grouping of lesions, generally in the right lobe with one large and several small adjacent lesions (Fig. 5-42). The CT appearance can be simulated by metastatic disease, although the clinical presentations are different. Needle aspiration is the most helpful method of differentiation. MRI of hepatic abscesses provides no additional specificity above CT imaging. Ultrasound generally demonstrates a focal area of decreased echogenicity. If there is gas within the abscess, or internal septations, internal echoes are generated.

Hepatic amebic abscesses, although common in many parts of the world, are rarely seen in the United States and Canada. It is thought that they are secondary to colonic amoebiasis. It is estimated that approximately 5% of these patients will have hepatic abscesses. Amebic abscesses can also be seen within the lungs and brain. The organism, *Entamoeba histolytica,* is thought to enter the liver through the portal venous system. For that reason the lesions tend to be peripheral in location. The classic "anchovy sauce" appearance of the contents of hepatic amebic abscess results from a combination of internal liquefaction, hepatonecrosis, and bleeding. The cysts are mostly solitary with thick, shaggy walls. Complications of these amebic abscesses include rupture upward through the diaphragm into the pleural or pericardial spaces or downward into the peritoneal cavity.

Patients almost always present with abdominal pain. Fever, weight loss, and symptoms relative to colonic

involvement may also be present. Diagnosis is usually based on history, clinical presentation, and positive hemagglutination titers. Although considerable reluctance to perform needle aspiration of these lesions existed in the past, this procedure is being done today, with little or no occurrence of the catastrophic complications once anticipated. The CT appearance of amebic abscesses in the liver is similar to that of pyogenic abscesses. However, amebic abscesses tend to be unilocular (Fig. 5-43). Ultrasound often demonstrates ill-defined walls around a generally solitary ovoid lesion located near the liver capsule. Echogenicity within the lesion is decreased.

Echinococcal infection of the liver (hydatid cyst disease) can occur in two forms, *Echinococcus granulosus* or *Echinococcus multilocularis.* The former is more likely to involve the liver with large encapsulated cysts.

Although the parasite primarily involves the colon, at least half of the cases with extracolonic disease have hepatic involvement. Animals, particularly dogs, are the chief mediators of hydatid disease. The ingested eggs hatch in the patient's stomach and upper small bowel and reach the liver through the portal system. In the liver the larvae encyst, and for a long time the patient may be asymptomatic. Symptoms develop as the cyst grows. Occasionally, the parasite will die, the fluid is absorbed, and an encapsulated, calcified lesion is all that remains. However, in cases of viable, long-standing cysts, calcification may also occur in the wall. The major clinical problems arise as a result of complications associated with the cysts. These can result from the pressure on the biliary system, raising the possibility of obstructive jaundice. The most significant complication is rupture into the peritoneal cavity, alimentary canal, or biliary tree. Indeed, cephalad development of the cysts could result in rupture into the pleural cavity. Rupture, especially into the peritoneum, is accompanied by profound shock, peritonitis, and possibly anaphylaxis. Prognosis following intraperitoneal rupture is poor.

As would be expected, the disease is relatively common in sheep-raising and to a lesser extent cattle-raising areas in the world. However, with increased mobility and worldwide travel common today, the dissemination of this along with other diseases that were relatively confined to endemic regions of the world is now seen with more frequency in North America.

Hydatid cyst involvement of the liver is manifested by low-attenuation lesions on CT. Focal areas of additional attenuation within the cysts are usually indicative of daughter cysts. Calcification may be identified in the rims. Infection or bleeding can alter the CT appearance. Occasionally the detached cyst membrane is seen on CT. This is analogous to the well-known water lily sign seen in the lungs of patients with pulmonary involvement. This finding has been described after cyst aspiration and is highly specific for hydatid disease. The sonographic findings can be variable. Cyst wall calcification may be present. Otherwise, a well-defined mass with good through-transmission may be identified. Daughter cysts within the lesion are particularly helpful in making the diagnosis.

Mycotic abscesses of the liver are almost always multiple and small. These are commonly seen in immunocompromised patients and frequently are accompanied by multiple small abscesses within the spleen. The most common organism is *Candida albicans* (Fig. 5-44).

Angiosarcoma Angiosarcoma is a rare tumor of particular interest because of its association with Thorotrast and the industrial carcinogen vinyl chloride. During the 1940s and 1950s a radioactive colloid suspension of thorium dioxide, called Thorotrast, was injected intravenously for hepatosplenic imaging. Unfortunately, the radioactivity put the individual at high risk for malignant induction. Patients chronically exposed to arsenic or to vinyl chloride in the manufacture of plastics are also at significant risk for this tumor. Generally, CT evaluation of these patients discloses a large, irregular low-attenuation lesion within the liver that may manifest peripheral enhancement during the dynamic phase (Fig. 5-45).

Other causes of solitary low-attenuation lesions of the liver include lipomas. These are unusual but do occur in about 10% of patients with renal angiomyolipomatosis. The CT appearance of this lesion is characteristic.

Biliary cystadenoma and cystadenocarcinoma Biliary cystadenoma and cystadenocarcinoma are rare tumors arising from the bile ducts but most commonly

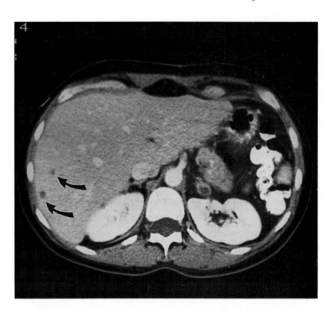

Fig. 5-44   CT scan through the liver of patient who has recently undergone bone marrow transplant. At least two small abscesses are seen in the periphery of the right lobe of the liver *(curved arrows),* representing hepatic candidiasis.

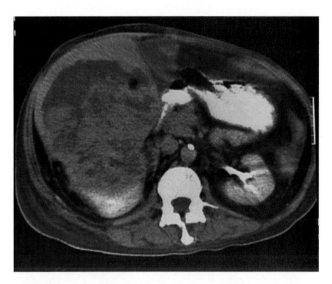

Fig. 5-45   CT scan through the lower portions of the right lobe of the liver demonstrates a huge inhomogeneous mass occupying and expanding most of the inferior portion of right lobe of the liver, representing an angiosarcoma of the liver.

appearing as a liver lesion on CT. Eighty percent are seen in middle-aged women. They are usually large, solitary lesions with low-attenuation characteristics on CT. They often demonstrate multiple loculations, which are lined with biliary epithelium.

The patients present with abdominal pain, upper abdominal mass, and occasionally jaundice, as well as constitutional symptoms. The tumor tends to be slow growing. CT evaluation demonstrates enhancement along the margin and the septum of the lesion. This unusual septal enhancement occurs as a result of papillary growth along the septum, which is seen in the cystadenocarcinoma. Lesser degrees of papillary growth can be seen in the cystadenoma. The cystadenoma, however, usually demonstrates a thin septum and little or no enhancement. Absolute differentiation between the cystadenoma and the cystadenocarcinoma ultimately requires surgical removal and pathological evaluation of the lesion. Surgical resection of these lesions often yields excellent results.

Intrahepatic cholangiocarcinoma Intrahepatic cholangiocarcinoma arises from the epithelium of the bile ducts and is covered in more detail elsewhere. It is usually a sclerosing tumor with little or no mass effect. However, it is occasionally seen as a solitary intrahepatic lesion. The lesion is usually central (Fig. 5-46).

Multiple Defects

Many of the lesions that have been previously discussed and can present as a solitary lesion within the liver may also present as multiple lesions. To avoid redundancy, they are only briefly discussed here.

Metastatic disease

Multiple bilobar metastatic involvement is a common presentation and results in the typical low-attenuation lesions previously described. Hypervascular metastatic lesions are much less common but include such malignancies as carcinoid, islet cell carcinomas, renal cell carcinomas, and some pancreatic cancers.

Lymphoma involves the liver in 20% to 50% of the cases of Hodgkin's disease. The hepatic involvement may be higher in non-Hodgkin's lymphomas. It can be multiple and nodular, giving multiple, low-attenuation lesions on CT examination. Alternatively, the involvement may be diffuse, resulting in an inhomogeneous enlarged liver (Fig. 5-47). Primary hepatic lymphoma has been described in the literature, although the existence of such a lesion is disputed. Other lesions that can rarely involve the liver with focal nodular lesions include Burkitt's lymphoma and leukemia.

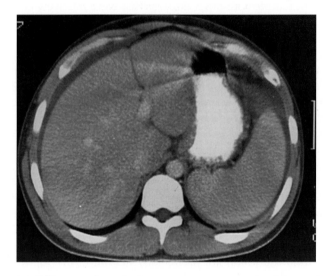

Fig. 5-47 CT through the liver in a 27-year-old patient with lymphoma. The liver is diffusely and homogeneously infiltrated with lymphoma. Note the perihepatic fluid.

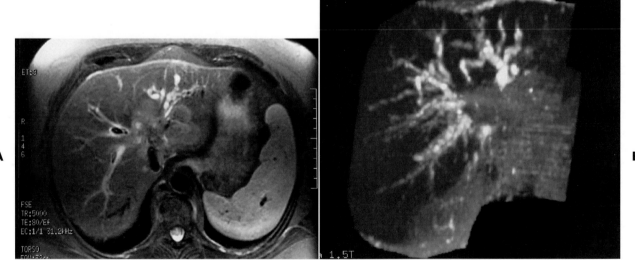

Fig. 5-46 **A,** T2-weighted axial MR images of the liver show large central lesion. **B,** MR cholangiography (heavily weighted T2 imaging making bile appear white) shows central nature of the lesion and suggests the origins of the lesion that proved to be cholangiocarcinoma.

Focal nodular hyperplasia

Although usually solitary, FNH can present as multiple hepatic lesions.

Cysts

Hepatic cysts are commonly multiple. Along with hemangiomas, they represent the most common lesions incidentally encountered in CT and ultrasound of the liver.

Abscesses

In about 50% of the cases abscesses are multiple in the liver. Most abscesses that result from bacteremia and the entrance of microorganisms through the hepatic artery are multiple and bilobar. In adults, as previously mentioned, most pyogenic hepatic abscesses are associated with bile duct infections (Fig. 5-48).

Hemangiomas

In about 10% of patients, hemangiomas are multiple.

Caroli's disease

Cavernous ectasia of the biliary tract (Caroli's disease) is actually an autosomal recessive disease of bile ducts in which cystic dilatation of the ducts occurs. In its severe form it can look like multiple cystic lesions of the liver on CT. Recently a central dot sign within the apparent cystic lesions in the liver on CT, following IV contrast administration, has been described. This central dot is thought to represent portal vein surrounded by the dilated biliary ducts. This finding when present may result in an increased degree of specificity for the diagnosis on CT examination. The liver is usually enlarged, and the disease has an association with polycystic disease of the kidney, despite differences in genetic expression. The incidence of biliary stasis,

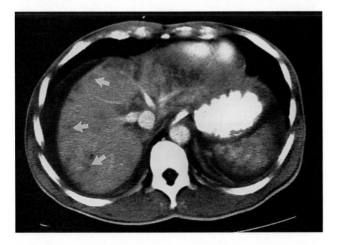

Fig. 5-48   Immunosupressed patient with multiple small hepatic abscesses *(arrows)*.

sepsis, stone formation, and ultimately cholangiocarcinoma is increased.

Epithelioid hemangioendothelioma

Epithelioid hemangioendothelioma is a rare vascular tumor most commonly seen in adults. It often starts as a multinodular lesion of the liver and may progress to a more diffuse pattern. The usual CT finding is multiple low-attenuation lesions with a low-attenuation halo around all the lesions. These are slow-growing, indolent, but progressive lesions.

Regenerating nodules

Regenerating nodules, seen in cirrhotic livers, are also referred to as adenomatous hyperplasia or nodular hyperplasia of the liver. There is no definite capsule or fibrous scarring in or around the lesion. They are generally considered precancerous lesions in cirrhotic livers. Often these nodules contain malignant foci. A small, well-differentiated hepatocellular carcinoma is extremely difficult to distinguish from a regenerating nodule. CT portography probably provides the best imaging method to differentiate the two at this time. Because regenerating nodules tend to have an abundance of portal blood supply as opposed to diminished portal blood supply for hepatocellular carcinomas, portography provides a helpful method in distinguishing them. MRI of regenerating nodules tends to show a low signal on T2-weighted images, as opposed to hepatocellular carcinoma, which tends to have a high signal on T2-weighted images.

Peliosis hepatis

Peliosis hepatis is considered a rare lesion but has been seen with increasing frequency over the last decade. This is thought to relate to the increasing use of androgenic anabolic steroids. The condition is manifested as multiple, blood-filled cysts throughout the liver. The earliest cases were thought to be a result of advanced tuberculosis or cancer. Recently, however, peliosis hepatis in human immunodeficiency virus (HIV)-infected patients with associated cutaneous bacillary angiomatosis, a pseudoneoplastic vascular proliferation containing bacteria, has been reported. Peliosis involving the spleen has also been reported. Multiple small intrahepatic cystic lesions may be seen on CT and ultrasound of the liver.

Biliary dilatation

Dilated bile ducts sometimes give the appearance of multiple hepatic defects (Fig. 5-49). This is usually the case if the obstruction is at the level of the major bifurcation of the common hepatic duct in the porta hepatis. Enhanced views and a branching pattern usually suggest the nature of the defects. Otherwise the identification of a dilated common bile duct or dilated gallbladder (Courvoisier's sign) confirms the biliary obstruction (Fig. 5-50).

Calcifications

Granulomatous diseases

Granulomatous diseases excite the immune system in a specific manner that results in a characteristic inflammatory response. The particular response results in the

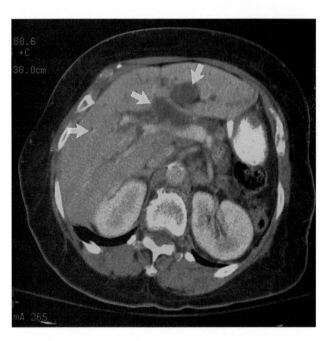

Fig. 5-49   Patient with obstruction of the common bile duct by a pancreatic lesion and multiple defects in the liver *(arrows)* representing dilated bile ducts. Note how the left biliary system tends to dilate before the right *(upper arrows).*

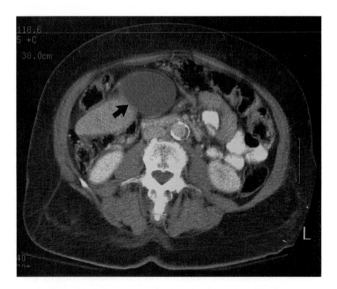

Fig. 5-50   Painless enlargement of the gallbladder *(arrow)* in patient with biliary obstruction (Courvoisier's sign).

formation of a granuloma that commonly calcifies after a time. Granulomatous inflammatory responses, especially without caseation, are nonspecific, and frequently the offending organism cannot be identified unless associated with other systemic or laboratory findings.

The most common granulomatous disease seen in North America is histoplasmosis, which is endemic in certain regions of the United States. In its postinfectious state it is seen as tiny punctate calcifications scattered throughout the liver and possibly the spleen. However, tuberculosis, rickettsial infection, and bacterial, viral, fungal, or even parasitic involvement of the liver can give a similar pattern. In addition, patients with sarcoid may have liver involvement in a similar pattern.

Primary hepatic granulomatous disease tends to have little or no calcification associated with it. Such disease includes primary biliary cirrhosis and so-called granulomatous hepatitis, as well as granulomatous hepatic lesions resulting from drug toxicities.

Metastatic disease

Calcifications within hepatic metastatic lesions are unusual. They have been described in association with mucinous (colloid) lesions of the colon or stomach. These are typically tiny stippling calcifications seen focally within the liver (Fig. 5-51).

Hepatocellular carcinoma

Calcification within hepatocellular carcinoma is unusual, and it is said that fewer than 10% of these lesions calcify. If the calcification is present in the right clinical circumstances, the possibility of a fibrolamellar hepatocellular carcinoma may be considered because these lesions more frequently (30%) demonstrate calcification.

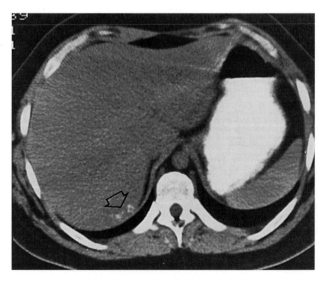

Fig. 5-51   Calcifications seen in a small metastatic lesion in the posterior aspect of the right lobe of the liver *(arrow).* The primary tumor was a mucinous carcinoma of the colon.

Abscesses

Calcification may be seen in the wall of old pyogenic or amebic abscesses. Often this is a result of chronic, organized inflammation, secondary infection, or even bleeding into the wall of the lesion (Fig. 5-52).

Cysts

Simple hepatic cysts do not calcify. On the other hand, echinococcal cysts (hydatid disease) commonly develop wall calcifications over several years. This occurs whether the cyst is viable or nonviable. The calcification tends to be denser in nonviable cysts. A typical ring of calcification of varying thickness is seen within the liver, and lesions range from 2 to 15 cm.

Hemangiomas

Although hemangioma is a common hepatic lesion, it only rarely calcifies. A large cavernous hemangioma on rare occasion calcifies centrally in its fibrotic component, and there may be some calcification along the radiating strands of fibrosis. This is a typical sunburst pattern seen in hemangiomas elsewhere in the body. The typical phlebolith-like calcification seen in hemangiomas elsewhere is exceedingly rare in the liver.

Hematomas

Old subcapsular hematomas may calcify on the liver margin, giving linear or coarse focal areas of calcification.

Tertiary syphilis

Tertiary syphilis lesions are only rarely seen today. However, medical practitioners in the tropics or developing countries have an increasing possibility of encountering a hepatic gumma, known to an older generation of physicians as hepar lobatum. This is a manifestation of late or tertiary syphilis that may calcify.

Parasites

An uncommon cause of hepatic calcification rarely encountered in the West is parasitic infestation. Parasites, such as the tongue worm (*Armillifer armillatus*), can involve the liver and result in numerous tiny, comma-shaped hepatic calcifications.

Increased Density

Hemochromatosis

Hemochromatosis is an uncommon disorder in which the total iron deposition within the liver and other organs progressively increases. It can be regarded as either a primary idiopathic disease or a secondary disorder. The primary condition is autosomal recessive in its genetic manifestation. Secondary forms are seen in patients with a history of multiple blood transfusions, chronic anemia, and erythroid hyperplasia, such as in thalassemia or sideroblastic anemia. Secondary hemochromatosis can also occur as a consequence of high dietary intake of iron.

From whatever cause, excessive iron deposition in the liver over a period of many years results in an enlarged liver with evidence of cirrhosis. Hemosiderin is found both in the hepatic cells and in Kupffer's cells, as well as within the fibrous matrix of the liver.

CT demonstrates varying degrees of diffuse homogeneous high attenuation throughout the liver (Fig. 5-53).

The effects of hemochromatosis are systemic and involve other organs, including the pancreas and the

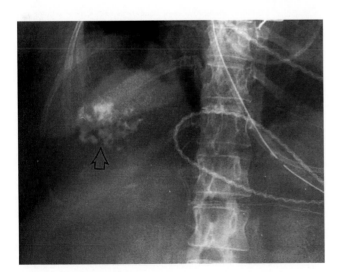

Fig. 5-52   Plain film of the abdomen demonstrates flocculent calcification *(arrow)* in an old intrahepatic abscess.

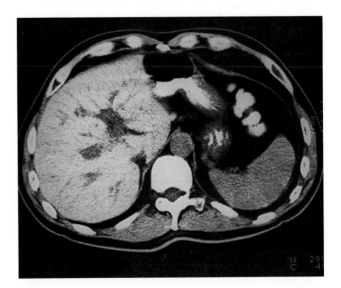

Fig. 5-53   CT of the liver of a patient with hemochromatosis during the preenhancement phase. Note the marked density of the liver parenchyma.

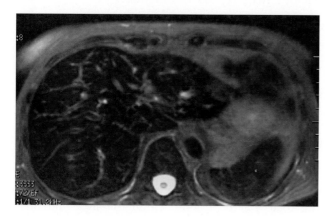

Fig. 5-54   Patient with hemochromatosis secondary to hemosiderosis. MR image (T2 fast spin echo) with low signal in liver, marrow, and spleen typical of hemosiderosis. Low signal would be confined to the liver in hemochromatosis of other causes.

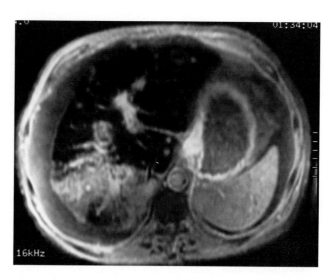

Fig. 5-55   Patient with hemochromatosis and cirrhosis complicated by hepatoma. T1-weighted spin echo MR image shows low signal in the anterior liver and brighter signal at the site of hepatocellular cancer (hepatoma) in the posterior liver.

heart (Fig. 5-54). As a result, in addition to impairment of hepatic function, cirrhosis, and possible portal hypertension, patients also manifest symptoms secondary to disease in other organ systems. These patients also are at increased risk for hepatocellular carcinoma (Fig. 5-55). Cardiac failure or arrhythmias, in addition to diabetes, are not unusual.

Chronic cirrhotic liver disease

In severe chronic cirrhosis the liver may appear small and contracted and demonstrate density above the normal expectations on unenhanced CT images. Conversely, because of the distortion and redistribution of the intrahepatic vascular system in these patients, enhanced CT images may show little increase in density when compared with the unenhanced images (Fig. 5-56).

The relative increase in density on unenhanced images may be explained on the basis of increased diffuse fibrosis throughout the liver and decreased fat content.

Thorotrast

The radioactive colloid suspension of thorium dioxide, injected intravenously and used during the 1940s to 1950s, was taken up primarily in the reticuloendothelial cells of the liver, spleen, and lymph nodes. This was done for imaging of the liver and spleen. Unfortunately, the radionuclide is a long-term, alpha-emitting agent, resulting in many patients' developing bone marrow dyscrasias, neoplasms, or local malignancy in the liver. This agent has not been used in many years, and patients with high-density liver and spleen secondary to Thorotrast injection are becoming rare.

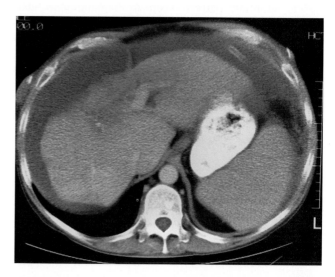

Fig. 5-56   Patient with cirrhosis and ascites. Note the small liver with nodular margins and the free fluid in the perihepatic spaces.

Drug-induced causes

Certain drugs increase hepatic density. The use of parenteral gold injections for the treatment of rheumatoid arthritis over a prolonged period may lead to hepatic deposition and an increase in liver density.

Many drugs can result in hepatic toxicity or cholestasis. However, it is extremely unusual for a drug or its metabolites to accumulate in the liver and result in increased liver density. One such drug is amiodarone (Fig. 5-57). This is an effective antidysrhythmic drug containing 40% iodine by weight. Because of its prolonged half-life, the significance of serum therapeutic levels is difficult to interpret. In response to this, it has

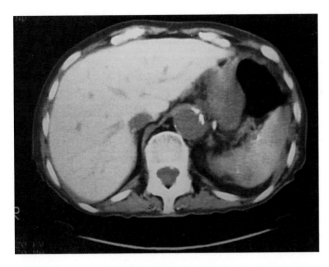

Fig. 5-57   CT scan of the liver of a patient being treated for cardiac dysrhythmia with the drug amiodarone, resulting in increased density throughout the liver.

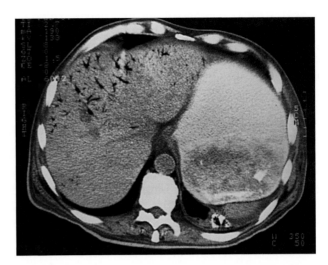

Fig. 5-58   CT scan demonstrates air in the portal venous system of the liver in a postoperative patient. This was not related to bowel necrosis, and the patient had an uneventful recovery.

been suggested that the density of the liver be evaluated in patients who are receiving this medication and still experiencing cardiac dysrhythmias in an attempt to determine whether insufficient medication or a toxic side effect of the medication is the basis of the dysrhythmia. It is postulated that normal liver densities during the administration of the drug and continuing dysrhythmias may indicate insufficient therapeutic levels of the medication, whereas increased liver density suggests adequate to toxic levels of the drug.

Portal Venous Air

Air in the portal venous system is an occasional dramatic finding on plain films or CT of the abdomen (Fig. 5-58). It can be benign in a distinct minority of patients, secondary to recent GI surgery, gastric or duodenal ulcers, instrumentation associated with mucosal tears, or occasionally a patient with severe gastric outlet obstruction who develops mucosal defects as a result of the gross acute distention. It has been reported in some patients who have undergone recent barium enemas. However, many GI radiologists have not seen this phenomenon in their entire careers. Given that the risk of bowel perforation is some 10 times greater in colonoscopy, one would expect the incidence of this side effect to be much higher in that procedure. However, even there it remains relatively uncommon.

When making the diagnosis of portal venous air, the radiologist should expect the worst and hope for the best. A proper clinical history is invaluable in deciding how much concern and activity the finding will generate. Unfortunately, the finding in the great majority of cases carries grave prognostic implications, most commonly associated with bowel infarction, breakdown of the mucosal barrier, and leakage of air and toxins into the portal venous system. There it eventually percolates into the liver. These patients are usually toxic and obviously ill, although in older patients the symptoms may not be quite so pronounced. The findings must be correlated to the clinical situation. In a patient with minimal or no abdominal findings, this radiological finding may be benign and close observation and monitoring are the appropriate actions.

This particular radiological problem, with its emphasis on clinical correlation, as in so many other conditions, is yet another example of how the historical and expected role of the radiologist as a physician, practicing the specialty of radiology, must be defended. No physician would attempt a physical examination without a clinical history, and it seems equally foolish for a radiologist to undertake an examination or interpretation without an appropriate medical history. Radiologists who do otherwise are doing both themselves and the patient an injustice. Clinicians who expect radiologists to practice in such a manner have misguided and foolish perceptions of the role of the radiologist.

The most important initial task for the radiologist when linear branching collections of air are seen in the liver is to distinguish between portal venous air and air in the hepatic biliary system, which is almost always benign. The difference is based on the physiological flow characteristics of the two systems. Bile flows in a centripetal pattern from the liver periphery to the liver hilum, and as a result, air collections in the biliary system tend to be central in the common hepatic and main hepatic ducts. Conversely, portal venous flow is centrifugal from hilum to periphery and hence, air in the portal venous system is found in the periphery along the margins of the liver. However, if sufficient air has leaked into the portal system, it can also be seen in the liver hilum, within the portal vein, or even backed up into the splenic pulp. Air is also occasionally seen within the superior mesenteric vein on CT. Additionally, a careful search of the abdominal plain films or CT images is in order to identify intramural air collections in the bowel.

SPLEEN

The spleen is the largest component of the reticulo-endothelial system, comprising white pulp (lymphoid tissue) and red pulp (vascular sinuses and end arterial vessels) contained within a thin fibrous capsule. It is located in the left upper quadrant and may be found in considerable variations of size and shape in normal people. The normal dimensions given for the spleen in various textbooks are of relatively little use in evaluating for splenomegaly because of the marked variation from person to person in the size and configuration of the spleen. In imaging of the spleen the most accurate method for evaluating the possibility of splenomegaly may well be the observations of an experienced radiologist, or even better, a previous study. In general, the normal spleen occupies approximately 15% to 25% of the volume of a normal liver and weighs between 100 and 250 gm.

Accessory spleens are a common CT finding and most often are seen in the region of the splenic hilum around or near the tail of the pancreas. Approximately 20% of patients undergoing CT of the abdomen demonstrate this finding.

Enlarged Spleen

Common causes of an enlarged spleen are summarized in Box 5-5.

Passive congestion
Although chronic right-sided congestive heart failure occasionally results in some degree of splenomegaly, by

---

Box 5-5   Some Common Causes of Oversized Spleen

Portal hypertension
Trauma
Lymphoma
Leukemia
Infection
Hemolytic anemias
Metabolic storage diseases

---

far the most common cause of splenomegaly is congestion within the portal venous system secondary to cirrhotic changes within the liver. Portal hypertension secondary to hepatic cirrhosis of any cause, most commonly alcoholic, almost always results in some degree of splenic enlargement. Fifty percent of patients with portal hypertension have a palpable spleen. It is an even more common CT finding. The splenic enlargement is secondary to obstructive and congestive changes within the spleen, particularly the red pulp. The term *Banti's syndrome* is occasionally used in describing passive congestion of the spleen secondary to portal hypertension and hepatic cirrhosis. However, the original description of this syndrome postulated a splenomegaly that preceded the cirrhotic changes within the liver and, in fact, is the reverse of the sequence of events seen in portal hypertension. Any condition that can result in intrahepatic vascular congestion can secondarily cause splenomegaly. This includes not only any cause of cirrhosis, but also any cause of hepatic venous occlusive disease, as well as congenital hepatic fibrosis. Splenic vein thrombosis may cause acute congestive splenomegaly, as can Budd-Chiari syndrome. Chronic passive congestion can result in a spleen that is a number of times its original size and can weigh up to 1000 gm.

CT findings in cirrhotic patients with splenomegaly, as a result of portal hypertension, show characteristic changes within the liver, as well as prominence of the vascular structures in the region of the splenic hilum, the gastrohepatic ligament, and around the gastroesophageal junction. Ultrasound scans of such a spleen may demonstrate an isoechoic or hypoechoic pattern. Liver and spleen radionuclide scans show a relative increase in the uptake of the radionuclide in the spleen compared with the liver (colloid shift). Uptake in bone marrow may also be demonstrated.

Trauma
Posttraumatic splenic injury with an intact capsule or tamponaded splenic capsule can also result in transitory splenic enlargement. This is often associated with lower left rib injuries, although this associated finding need not be present.

Hodgkin's lymphoma
Outside of the usual nodal sites, the spleen is the organ most commonly involved with Hodgkin's disease. Splenic involvement is demonstrated in approximately one third of patients undergoing staging laparotomies. Although CT can be extremely helpful in evaluating the possibility of splenic involvement (particularly with focal disease), the definitive assessment for splenic involvement is splenectomy. Splenic enlargement in most cases signifies splenic involvement, while a normal spleen size, in most cases, suggests noninvolvement. However,

the incidence of false positives and false negatives, based on size criteria alone, is significant.

CT evaluation of splenic involvement with Hodgkin's disease can include a number of presentations, from numerous small nodules to a solitary splenic tumor mass to diffuse enlargement without focal defects (Fig. 5-59).

Because involvement of the spleen with Hodgkin's disease has significant therapeutic and prognostic implications, the determination of splenic involvement is crucial, hence the necessity of splenectomy in the staging process.

Non-Hodgkin's lymphomas

Involvement of the spleen with non-Hodgkin's–type lymphomas is more common than Hodgkin's disease and occurs in over 50% of patients. The lymphomatous involvement of the spleen may present as diffuse enlargement without focal disease, as a round tumor mass, or as multiple, small nodules. Unlike in Hodgkin's disease, splenomegaly usually is a more accurate indication of tumor involvement. Discrete lymphomatous lesions often show increased signal on T2-weighted MRI. Focal lesions can also be detected with ultrasound and are demonstrated as hypoechoic foci.

Leukemia

Splenomegaly is a relatively common occurrence in leukemia, but its presence and severity depend on the type and duration of the leukemia. Although a common presenting finding in hairy cell leukemia, it is rare in acute lymphoblastic leukemia. The presence of splenomegaly does give rise to the possibility of splenic rupture as a complication of some of the chronic leukemias.

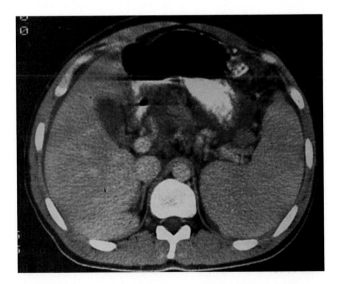

Fig. 5-59   CT image of the hepatosplenic area in a patient with Hodgkin's lymphoma and known splenic involvement shows diffuse homogeneous enlargement of the spleen.

Chronic myeloid leukemia is associated with significant splenomegaly that can often reach massive proportions. In patients with chronic lymphocytic leukemia, splenomegaly may also be a prominent feature, although the size of the spleen is less striking than that seen in chronic myeloid disease.

Generally speaking, splenomegaly is more commonly associated with the chronic forms of leukemia and is probably a poor prognostic sign.

CT evaluation generally demonstrates an enlarged spleen with a homogeneous appearance. Enlargement of the spleen in leukemia is almost always associated with disease involvement. Often the involved spleen demonstrates an isoechoic ultrasound pattern.

Chronic myeloproliferative disorders

The chronic myeloproliferative disorders represent a group of related disease processes that are thought to be clonal disorders of the hematopoietic stem cell. They include such entities as polycythemia vera, myeloid metaplasia, essential thrombocythemia, and chronic myeloid leukemia. Various authors overlap the myeloproliferative disorders and the leukemic disorders, and some include the acute nonlymphocytic leukemias in the myeloproliferative group.

Splenomegaly is common in chronic proliferative conditions, with the degree varying from condition to condition. The most prominent example of splenomegaly in this group tends to occur in myeloid metaplasia. Lesser degrees of splenomegaly are seen in polycythemia vera and essential thrombocythemia. Imaging generally demonstrates an obviously enlarged, homogeneous-appearing spleen.

Protozoan infection

Splenomegaly is characteristically associated with malaria. In the acute presentations the spleen may become grossly enlarged, reaching gigantic proportions. With chronic disease and gradual development of fibrosis and scarring, the degree of splenomegaly is diminished.

Systemic infections

Mild to moderate degrees of splenic enlargement may be seen in patients with mononucleosis, and indeed splenic rupture is a rare but known complication of infectious mononucleosis.

Splenomegaly is a relatively common finding in patients with subacute bacterial endocarditis, and the enlargement usually is secondary to multiple, small septic foci within the spleen. Degrees of splenic enlargement may be seen in the miliary stage of tuberculosis (Fig. 5-60). Disseminated fungal infections including candidiasis and histoplasmosis may also produce splenic enlargement. Splenomegaly is a common finding in patients with typhoid fever.

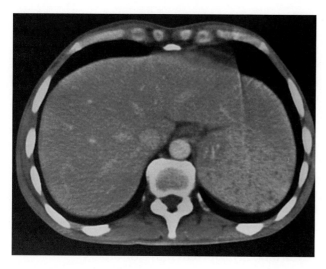

Fig. 5-60 CT image of the splenic region in a patient with acquired immunodeficiency syndrome and tuberculosis. The spleen is enlarged and there are multiple, tiny splenic abscesses.

Erythropoietic disorders

Hereditary spherocytosis is the best known of these disorders. This condition is inherited as an autosomal dominant trait and results in spherocytic changes in the affected individual's red blood cells. Splenomegaly is almost always present and of a mild to moderate degree. Splenomegaly is usually therapeutic in the treatment of this disorder because of the important role of the spleen in erythrocyte destruction.

Splenomegaly may be prominent in early childhood manifestation of sickle cell disease. The older the patient, the less prominent the spleen as a result of progressive atrophy and fibrosis secondary to repeated infarctions.

The thalassemia syndromes, representing an abnormality of hemoglobin production, can result in mild to moderate degrees of splenomegaly. Similar findings are also found in patients with autoimmune hemolytic anemias and idiopathic thrombocytopenic purpura.

Felty's syndrome, although an abnormality of granulocytes rather than erythrocytes, may be included here as an additional example of splenomegaly associated with blood cell abnormalities. The syndrome consists of the triad of rheumatoid arthritis, splenomegaly, and neutropenia. It is most commonly seen in patients with long-standing rheumatoid arthritis. The spleen may be markedly enlarged, possibly relating to the ongoing selective granulocytic destruction occurring within the spleen.

Infiltrative and storage diseases

Lipogenic storage disorders, such as all forms of Gaucher's disease, as well as Niemann-Pick disease, are associated with moderate to massive splenomegaly.

Increased splenic size may also be a feature of the mucopolysaccharidoses, the best known being Hurler's and Hunter's syndromes. Patients with histiocytosis X, particularly with Letterer-Siwe disease, occasionally have splenomegaly as part of the presenting picture.

Although both primary and secondary amyloidosis can involve the spleen, it is more common in the secondary form and frequently causes splenomegaly.

Small or Shrunken Spleen

Sickle cell disease

Sickle cell disease is one of the more common causes of diminished splenic size. In the advanced stages, fibrotic changes as a result of chronic recurrent infarctions lead to a small, shrunken, and often calcified spleen. The extensive fibrosis coupled with diffuse occlusion of the splenic microvasculature results in nonfunction and autosplenectomy.

Essential thrombocythemia

For similar reasons, splenic atrophy may also be seen during the chronic course of essential thrombocythemia. The resultant infarctions are most likely secondary to stagnated aggregates of platelets within the splenic circulation.

Congenital causes

Congenital hypoplasia of the spleen is relatively uncommon but has been seen and described in cases of Fanconi's anemia with associated marrow hypoplasia.

Irradiation

Radiation to the upper abdomen and splenic bed can result in a small, shrunken fibrotic spleen with thickened capsule. Usually this is a delayed response to radiation-induced vascular damage of the spleen.

Thorotrast

Thorotrast, a radioactive contrast agent emitting alpha rays, which had been formerly used as an angiographic contrast agent, is retained within the reticuloendothelial system and may be seen within the liver or spleen (Fig. 5-61). In the spleen, over a period of years, splenic atrophy and fibrosis develop. Although these changes within the liver put patients at a higher risk for malignant disease, the same malignant potential has not been reported for the spleen.

Malabsorption syndromes

Degrees of atrophy of the spleen are, on rare occasion, seen as a complication of some of the malabsorption syndromes. Splenic atrophy has been reported in inflammatory bowel disease, particularly ulcerative colitis, and to a lesser extent in Crohn's disease. It is also

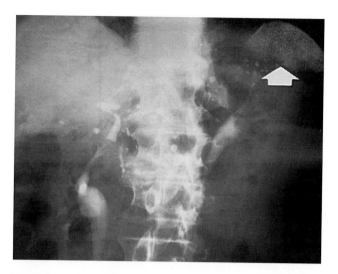

Fig. 5-61   Film obtained during an intravenous pyelogram on patient who had previously received Thorotrast for hepatosplenic imaging. The spleen is small *(arrow)* with fine nodular calcium-like density throughout the spleen.

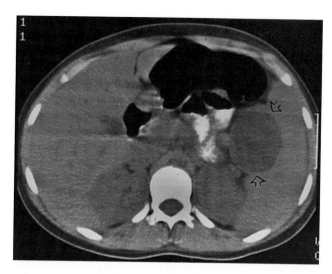

Fig. 5-62   A large splenic epithelial cyst *(arrows)* is seen during a CT examination for patient with diagnosis of appendicitis.

associated with celiac disease. This complication of malabsorption syndromes is relatively uncommon and something of a curiosity. It cannot be directly related to malnutrition because hyposplenism is not seen in starvation. The exact causes of this complication are unknown.

Focal Defects

Cystic lesions

The most common type of splenic cyst is the pseudocyst or so-called acquired cyst of the spleen. These cysts are most commonly found in adults and are presumed to be of the traumatic origin. The cyst wall may be calcified and without an epithelial lining. These account for approximately 80% of splenic cysts. True epidermoid cysts are less common (approximately 20%) and are lined by stratified squamous epithelium. These cysts are believed to be congenital in origin (Figs. 5-62 and 5-63). Calcification can be seen in the wall of both acquired and congenital types of splenic cysts. The cysts can be quite variable in size and generally contain clear fluid, although turbid or bloody contents may also be present. There is no sexual predilection for the congenital type of cyst. Congenital splenic cysts are not thought to represent part of the spectrum of more widespread cystic disease involving the pancreas, kidney, and liver. These usually occur as incidental findings within the spleen of asymptomatic patients. On rare occasions the splenic cyst may be complicated by hemorrhage, rupture, or even infection.

Pancreatic pseudocysts involving the tail of the pancreas occasionally give the appearance of splenic cysts on CT. The cyst may adhere to and indent the

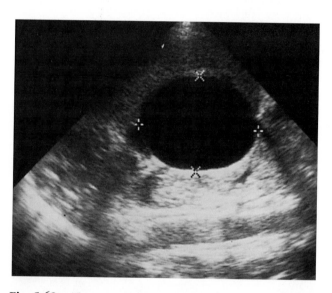

Fig. 5-63   The same patient as in Fig. 5-62 also underwent ultrasound examination of the spleen that demonstrated typical appearance of a large, well-defined splenic cyst.

splenic capsule or actually invade the substance of the spleen.

Echinococcal cysts involving the spleen are uncommon. Less than one third of cases of hydatid disease have splenic involvement.

Primary neoplastic lesions

Hemangiomas are the most common benign neoplasms of the spleen. These are almost always asymptomatic and are incidental findings. It is possible that a large splenic hemangioma or diffuse splenic hemangiomas could lead to splenomegaly, although this is rare. The lesions are usually solitary. Lymphangiomas occur in the spleen and are less common than hemangiomas. Distinguishing between the two can be impossible. It has been suggested that lymphangiomas occur more commonly in the subcapsular region than hemangiomas.

Splenic hamartomas are uncommon and are almost always asymptomatic. Most are solitary. CT demonstration of these lesions may show a well-defined, solitary splenic lesion with homogeneous or mixed cystic components.

Primary malignant lesions of the spleen are rare. These are generally angiosarcomas, and unlike in the liver, there appears to be no direct relationship between Thorotrast and development of splenic angiosarcomas. Patients with these tumors carry a poor prognosis, often having widespread metastatic disease at the time of diagnosis. Primary malignant fibrous histiocytomas of the spleen have been reported but are extremely rare.

Metastatic disease

Surprisingly, apart from lymphomatous involvement, secondary hematogenous metastatic lesions to the spleen are unusual (Fig. 5-64). A number of different explanations have been put forward to explain this scarcity of splenic metastatic disease, although none is fully satisfying. Metastatic lesions to the spleen, although rare, do tend to occur when there is a widespread dissemination of tumor throughout the body. In such patients, splenic involvement is found in less than 4% at autopsy.

Lymphoma

As previously discussed, both Hodgkin's and non-Hodgkin's lymphoma can involve the spleen. The involvement can be diffuse or focal. The focal lesions can be solitary or more commonly multiple. These are usually demonstrated on CT as low-density lesions or on MRI as high-signal lesions on T2-weighted images.

Abscesses

Large solitary focal abscesses of the spleen are fortunately an uncommon condition, since they generally are associated with high mortality. These lesions tend to be poorly encapsulated and have intermediate densities on CT. There is often enhancement of the rim during the contrast phase of CT examination.

More recently, widespread disseminated microabscesses occurring in both liver and spleen have been seen predominantly in immunosuppressed patients (Fig. 5-65). They are commonly due to *Candida albicans* and on occasion tuberculosis. CT appearance demonstrates multiple areas of low attenuation within the spleen and commonly in the liver as well.

Focal infarctions

In any condition in which systemic emboli may occur, such as in cardiac valvular disease, emboli can become lodged within the vasculature of the spleen and

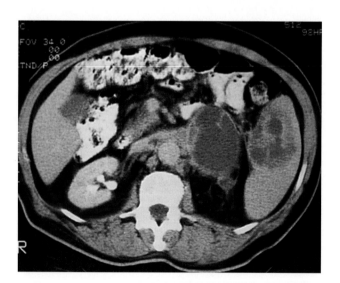

Fig. 5-64   CT scan through the midabdomen demonstrates a cystic neoplastic lesion of the tail of the pancreas. There has also been metastatic spread of the lesion to the spleen.

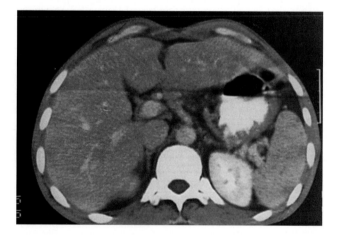

Fig. 5-65   Multiple, tiny splenic abscesses are seen in this immunoimpaired patient. These were found to be tuberculosis.

result in splenic infarctions. These, in the early stage, are hemorrhagic in their appearance but eventually become smaller, fibrotic, and more dense. Quite often, they are associated with left upper quadrant pain and initially there may be some mild splenomegaly. Vascular thrombosis within the spleen and resultant infarctions may also be seen in disease processes such as leukemia, particularly of the chronic myelogenous variety, and are also commonly encountered in patients with sickle cell disease, eventually leading to splenic atrophy. Splenic infarcts secondary to septic emboli may also be encountered as a result of bacterial endocarditis.

Increased Density

On routine CT of the abdomen (particularly unenhanced), the tissue density of the spleen is slightly less than that of the liver. There are relatively few conditions that result in true increased splenic density. The use of the contrast agent Thorotrast in earlier decades has been previously discussed. It is possible for the spleen to demonstrate increased density in cases of hemochromatosis. In a small, shrunken, nonfunctioning spleen having undergone autoamputation, the spleen may appear increased in density (Fig. 5-66). This most commonly occurs as a chronic sequela of sickle cell disease. Splenic trauma with diffuse bleeding throughout the spleen in the acute stage results in increased density in the subcapsular region or possibly diffusely throughout the spleen (Fig. 5-67).

Calcifications

The most common cause of calcification in the spleen is previous histoplasmosis in which small punctate calcifications are identified within a normal-sized spleen. Tuberculosis and brucellosis may also result in calcifications. Phlebolith formation within the spleen with calcification is rare but can occur. The possibility that old focal areas of infarction will calcify must also be a consideration. Old healed abscesses within the spleen, particularly microabscesses, may also lead to residual calcification (Fig. 5-68). Old hematomas readily calcify. Calcification can be seen in the walls of both acquired and congenital cysts. In addition, focal calcifications in abdominal organs, including the spleen, have

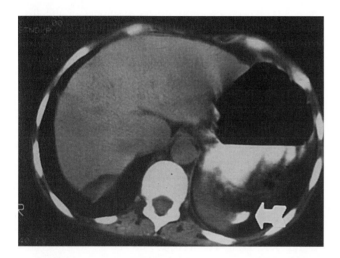

Fig. 5-66   CT scan demonstrates a tiny, calcified shrunken spleen posterior to the stomach *(arrow)* in this patient with sickle cell anemia. The spleen has undergone autoamputation.

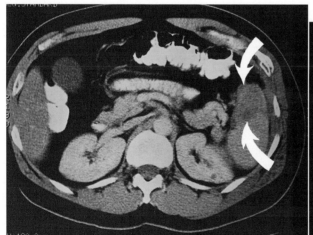
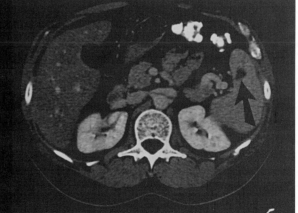

Fig. 5-67   A 50-year-old man who fell off a ladder and injured the left ribs. **A,** CT image at the time of injury shows an ill-defined splenic defect with hazy margins representing a splenic hematoma *(arrows)*. **B,** Images obtained 1 month later show marked interval improvement. Only a small, well-defined cyst remains *(arrow)*.

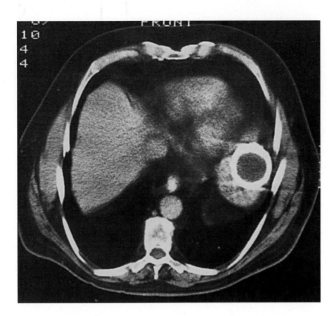

Fig. 5-68 CT scan demonstrates an old splenic abscess that is densely calcified in the wall.

been described in acquired immunodeficiency syndrome patients with disseminated *Pneumocystis carinii* infections.

SUGGESTED READINGS
Liver

Acunas B, Rozanes I, Acunas G, et al: Hydatid cyst of the liver: identification of detached cyst lining on CT scans obtained after cyst puncture, *AJR* 156:751-752, 1991.

Baker ME, Silverman PM: Nodular focal fatty infiltration of the liver: CT appearance, *AJR* 145:79-80, 1985.

Beggs I: The radiology of hydatid disease, *AJR* 145:639-648, 1985.

Bonaldi VM, Bret PM, Reinhold C, et al: Helical CT of the liver: value of an early hepatic arterial phase, *Radiology* 197:357-363, 1995.

Bradley DW, Maynard JE: Etiological and natural history of post-transfusion and enterically transmitted non-A, non-B hepatitis, *Semin Liver Dis* 6:56-63, 1986.

Brown JJ, Naylor MJ, Yagan N: Imaging of hepatic cirrhosis, *Radiology* 202:1-16, 1997.

Brunt PW: Alcohol and the liver, *Gut* 12:222-229, 1971.

Casarella WJ, Knowles DM, Wolff M, et al: Focal nodular hyperplasia and liver cell adenoma: radiologic and pathologic differentiation, *AJR* 131:393-402, 1978.

Choi BI, Han MC, Kim CW: Small hepatocellular carcinoma versus small cavernous hemangioma: differentiation with MR imaging at 2.0 T, *Radiology* 176:103-106, 1990.

Choi BI, Yeon KM, Kim SH, et al: Caroli disease: central dot sign in CT, *Radiology* 174:161-163, 1990.

Dachman AH, Ros PR, Goodman ZD, et al: Nodular regenerative hyperplasia of the liver: clinical and radiologic observations, *AJR* 148:717-722, 1987.

Dodds WJ, Erickson SJ, Taylor AJ, et al: Caudate lobe of the liver: anatomy, embryology, and pathology, *AJR* 154:87-93, 1990.

Egglin TK, Rummeny E, Stark DD, et al: Hepatic tumors: quantitative tissue characterization with MR imaging, *Radiology* 176:107-110, 1990.

Fasel JH, Selle D, Evertsz CJ, et al: Segmental anatomy of the liver: poor correlation with CT, *Radiology* 206:151-156, 1998.

Ferrucci JT: Liver tumor imaging: current concepts, *AJR* 155:473-484, 1990.

Fulcher AS, Turner MA: HASTE MR cholangiography in the evaluation of hilar cholangiocarcinoma, *AJR* 169:1501-1505, 1997.

Furui S, Itai Y, Ohtomo K, et al: Hepatic epithelioid hemangioendothelioma: report of five cases, *Radiology* 171:63-68, 1989.

Grace ND, Powell LW: Iron storage disorders of the liver, *Gastroenterology* 67:1257-1283, 1974.

Han JK, Choi BI, Kim TK, et al: Hilar cholangiocarcinoma: thin-section spiral CT findings with cholangiographic correlation, *Radiographics* 17:1475-1485, 1997.

Heiken JP, Weyman PJ, Lee JK, et al: Detection of focal hepatic masses: prospective evaluation with CT, delayed CT, CT during arterial portography, and MR imaging, *Radiology* 171:47-51, 1989.

Holley HC, Koslin DB, Berland LL, et al: Inhomogeneous enhancement of liver parenchyma secondary to passive congestion: contrast-enhanced CT, *Radiology* 170:795-800, 1989.

Khuroo MS, Zarger SA, Mahajan R: Echinococcus granulosus cysts in the liver: management with percutaneous drainage, *Radiology* 180:141-145, 1991.

LaBerge JM, Laing FC, Federle MP, et al: Hepatocellular carcinoma: assessment of resectability by computed tomography and ultrasound, *Radiology* 152:485-490, 1984.

Landay MJ, Setaiwan H, Hirsh G, et al: Hepatic and thoracic amoebiasis, *AJR* 135:449-454, 1980.

Langer JC, Rose DB, Keystone JS, et al: Diagnosis and management of hydatid disease of the liver, *Ann Surg* 199:412-417, 1984.

Lee MJ, Saini S, Hamm B, et al: Focal nodular hyperplasia of the liver: MR findings in 35 proved cases, *AJR* 156:317-320, 1991.

Lewis E, Bernardino ME, Barnes PA, et al: The fatty liver: pitfalls of the CT and angiographic evaluation of metastatic disease, *J Comput Assist Tomogr* 7:235-241, 1983.

Lewis JW Jr, Koss N, Kerstein MD: A review of echinococcal disease, *Ann Surg* 181:390-396, 1975.

Ludwig J: Drug effects on the liver, *Dig Dis Sci* 24:785-796, 1979.

Markos J, Veronese ME, Nicholson MR, et al: Value of hepatic computerized tomographic scanning during amiodarone therapy, *Am J Cardiol* 56:89-92, 1985.

Matsui O, Kadoya M, Kameyama T, et al: Adenomatous hyperplastic nodules in the cirrhotic liver: differentiation from hepatocellular carcinoma with MR imaging, *Radiology* 173:123-126, 1989.

Matsui O, Kadoya M, Kameyama T, et al: Benign and malignant nodules in cirrhotic livers: distinction based on blood supply, *Radiology* 178:493-497, 1991.

Matsui O, Takashima T, Kadoya M, et al: Liver metastases from colorectal cancers: detection with CT during arterial portography, *Radiology* 165:65-69, 1987.

Mergo PJ, Ros PR, Buetow PC, et al: Diffuse disease of the liver: radiologic-pathologic correlation, *Radiographics* 14:1291-1307, 1994.

Miller WJ, Baron, RL, Dodd GD, et al: Malignancies in patients with cirrhosis: CT sensitivity and specificity in 200 consecutive transplant patients, *Radiology* 193:645-650, 1994.

Mitchell MC, Biotnott JK, Kaufman S, et al: Budd-Chiari syndrome: etiology, diagnosis and management, *Medicine* 61:199-218, 1982.

Murphy BJ, Casillas J, Ros PR, et al: The CT appearance of cystic masses of the liver, *Radiographics* 9:307-322, 1989.

Nadell J, Kosek J: Peliosis hepatis: twelve cases associated with oral androgen therapy, *Arch Pathol Lab Med* 101:405-410, 1977.

Nakeeb A, Pitt HA, Sohn TA, et al: Cholangiocarcinoma: a spectrum of intrahepatic, perihepatic and distal tumors, *Ann Surg* 224:463-475, 1996.

Nelson RC, Chezmar JL: Diagnostic approach to hepatic hemangiomas, *Radiology* 176:11-13, 1990.

Nelson RC, Chezmar JL, Sugarbaker PH, et al: Preoperative localization of focal liver lesions to specific liver segments: utility of CT during arterial portography, *Radiology* 176:89-94, 1990.

Partin JS, Partin JC, Schubert WK, et al: Serum salicylate concentrations in Reye's disease, *Lancet* 1:191-194, 1982.

Perkocha LA, Geaghan SM, Yen TSB, et al: Clinical and pathological features of bacillary peliosis hepatis in association with human immunodeficiency virus infection, *N Engl J Med* 323:1581-1586, 1990.

Rao BK, Brodell GK, Haaga JR, et al: Visceral CT findings associated with Thorotrast, *J Comput Assist Tomogr* 10:57-61, 1986.

Rummeny E, Weissleder R, Stark DD, et al: Primary liver tumors: diagnosis by MR imaging, *AJR* 152:63-72, 1989.

Siegelman ES, Mitchell DG, Semelka RC: Abdominal iron deposition: metabolism, MR findings, and clinical importance, *Radiology* 199:13-22, 1996.

Silverman PM, Kohan L, Ducic I, et al: Imaging of the liver with helical CT: a survey of scanning techniques, *AJR* 170:149-152, 1998.

Soto JA, Barish MA, Yucel EK, et al: Magnetic resonance cholangiography: comparison with endoscopic retrograde cholangiopancreatography, *Gastroenterology* 110:589-597, No. 2, 1996.

Terrier F, Becker CD, Triller JK: Morphologic aspects of hepatic abscesses at computed tomography and ultrasound, *Acta Radiol Diagn* 24:129-137, 1983.

Torres WE, Whitmire LF, Gedgaudas-McClees K, et al: Computed tomography of the hepatic morphologic changes in cirrhosis of the liver, *J Comput Assist Tomogr* 10:47-50, 1986.

Vasile N, Lardé D, Zafrani ES, et al: Hepatic angiosarcoma, *J Comput Assist Tomogr* 7:899-901, 1983.

Wall SD, Fisher MR, Amparo EG, et al: Magnetic resonance imaging in the evaluation of abscesses, *AJR* 144:1217-1221, 1985.

Yang PJ, Glazer GM, Bowerman RA: Budd-Chiari syndrome: computed tomographic and ultrasonographic findings, *J Comput Assist Tomogr* 7:148-150, 1983.

Spleen

Amorosi EL: Hypersplenism, *Semin Hematol* 2:249-285, 1965.

Baron JM, Weinshelbaum EI, Block GE: Splenic rupture associated with bacterial endocarditis and sickle cell trait, *JAMA* 205:112-114, 1968.

Bensinger TA, Keller AR, Merrell LF, et al: Thorotrast-induced reticuloendothelial blockage in man, *Am J Med* 51:663-668, 1971.

Berkman WA, Harris SA, Bernardino ME: Nonsurgical drainage of splenic abscesses, *AJR* 141:356-395, 1983.

Brinkley AA, Lee JK: Cystic hamartoma of the spleen: CT and sonographic findings, *J Clin Ultrasound* 9:136-138, 1981.

Burke JS: Surgical pathology of the spleen: an approach to the differential diagnosis of splenic lymphomas and leukemias, part I, diseases of the white pulp, *Am J Surg Pathol* 5:551-563, 1981.

Castellino RA: Hodgkin disease: practical concepts for the diagnostic radiologist, *Radiology* 159:305-310, 1986.

Dachman AH, Ros PR, Murari PJ, et al: Nonparasitic splenic cysts: a report of 52 cases with radiologic-pathologic correlation, *AJR* 147:537-542, 1986.

Dodds WJ, Taylor AJ, Erickson SJ, et al: Radiologic imaging of splenic anomalies, *AJR* 155:805-810, 1990.

Freeman MH, Tonkin AK: Focal splenic defects, *Radiology* 121:689-692, 1976.

Gebbie DAM, Hamilton PJS, Hutt MSR, et al: Malarial antibodies in idiopathic splenomegaly in Uganda, *Lancet* 2:392-393, 1964.

Gill PG, Souter RG, Morris PJ: Splenectomy for hypersplenism in malignant lymphomas, *Br J Surg* 68:29-33, 1981.

Halgrimson CG, Rustad DG, Zeligman BE: Calcified hemangioma of the spleen (letter), *JAMA* 252:2959-2960, 1984.

Louie JS, Pearson CM: Felty's syndrome, *Semin Hematol* 8:216-220, 1971.

Pearson HA, Spencer RP, Cornelius EA: Functional asplenia in sickle cell anemia, *N Engl J Med* 281:923-926, 1969.

Peters SP, Lee RE, Glew RH: Gaucher's disease: a review, *Medicine* 56:425-442, 1977.

Pryor DS: Splenectomy in tropical splenomegaly, *Br Med J* 3:825-828, 1967.

Radin DR, Baker EL, Klatt EC, et al: Visceral and nodal calcification in patients with AIDS-related Pneumocystis carinii infection, *AJR* 154:27-31, 1990.

Strijk SP, Wagener DJT, Bogman MJ, et al: The spleen in Hodgkin disease: diagnostic value of CT, *Radiology* 154:753-757, 1985.

Svartholm EG, Haglund U: Splenic resection for benign cyst, *Acta Chir Scand* 151:491-494, 1985.

Weed RI: Hereditary spherocytosis: a review, *Arch Intern Med* 135:1316-1323, 1975.

CHAPTER 6

Biliary System and Gallbladder

BILIARY SYSTEM

Examination Techniques

The gallbladder and biliary tree are separated into two sections within this chapter. Obviously, there will be an overlap in discussion of imaging technique. To avoid redundancy, the role of ultrasound, magnetic resonance imaging (MRI), computed tomography (CT) imaging, and radioisotope scanning of the biliary system is discussed in the biliary system section. The role of the oral cholecystogram (OCG) and ultrasound of the gallbladder is discussed and amplified at the beginning of the gallbladder section.

For purposes of discussing radiological problems associated with the biliary tree, the radiological problems are based on conventional imaging of the biliary tree following luminal filling with contrast material, such as in endoscopic retrograde cholangiopancreatography (ERCP), percutaneous transhepatic cholangiography, operative cholangiography, or T-tube injections. However, although these examinations have been among the standard imaging studies for biliary diagnosis for decades, the impact of CT and ultrasound in the last two decades has been significant.

Endoscopic retrograde cholangiopancreatography
ERCP is a routinely performed examination in which the papilla of Vater is endoscopically cannulized and contrast material injected. Depending on the clinical indication, the examination usually requires filling of the pancreatic duct and the biliary system. The success rate for cannulation ranges between 75% and 90% with the chief factor appearing to be the expertise and experience of the endoscopist. However, other causes of failure, such as papillary stenosis, peripapillary duodenal fibrosis and deformity, previous gastric surgery, and severe duodenal inflammatory disease, may also result in unsuccessful cannulation. The examination is a staple part of the workup of the jaundiced patient when obstructive causes are suspected. It can be done regardless of the degree of jaundice or hepatic disease. The common bile duct and gallbladder are usually easily demonstrated. The pancreatic aspect of the examination is discussed in Chapter 4.

The complication rate of ERCP is around 5%, and the mortality rate is 0.1% to 0.2%. The most common complication is cholangitis. Bacteremia is reported in a small percentage of patients. Elevations in the serum amylase level and clinical pancreatitis are reported in 1% to 8% of patients.

Percutaneous transhepatic cholangiography

Percutaneous transhepatic cholangiography (PTC) involves the direct percutaneous injection of contrast into bile ducts within the liver. The first PTC is reported to have been performed in Hanoi in the 1930s. The procedure usually involves the use of the Chiba (named after the Japanese university) skinny needle. Ultrasound, CT, or fluoroscopic guidance is used in this procedure. The success of injecting a bile duct increases in the presence of biliary dilatation, reaching near 100% when the ducts are significantly dilated. With nondilated ducts or strictured ducts, the success rate drops below 90%.

Operative cholangiography

Transcystic duct cholangiography performed intraoperatively following cholecystectomy allows radiological demonstration of the common bile duct in the search for residual stones, confirmation of ductal patency, and exclusion of ductal injury. Contrast material is injected through the cystic duct stump, and filling of the biliary tree is attempted. Because of positioning of the patient and the less than optimal situation of obtaining a radiograph on the operating room table, these examinations leave much to be desired technically. Often there is incomplete filling of the biliary system. Injected air bubbles also cause interpretive difficulties, and leakage around the cystic duct stump is common. Reflux into the pancreatic duct is frequent.

Computed tomography

CT of the liver has emerged over the last decade and a half as a highly sensitive and noninvasive method of detecting biliary ductal distention. In some cases, mild to moderate degrees of distention can be observed before the patient manifests obstructive jaundice. The evaluation of the common bile duct in the region of the pancreatic head is relatively easy, and a fairly accurate measurement can usually be obtained. The usual cause of biliary distention is obstruction. However, in the absence of a mass in the pancreatic head, CT may not always demonstrate the nature of the obstructing process. The presence of biliary distention within the liver and a normal common bile duct in the pancreatic head gives fairly conclusive secondary evidence of obstruction, although the actual obstruction site may not be well demonstrated. Lesions in the porta hepatis, particularly primary bile duct lesions, are extremely difficult to demonstrate on CT. MRI has not been shown to demonstrate any advantage to date in the evaluation of the biliary system.

Ultrasound

The effectiveness of real-time ultrasound in the evaluation of the biliary tree was established in the 1980s. In the hands of a skilled operator, this examina-

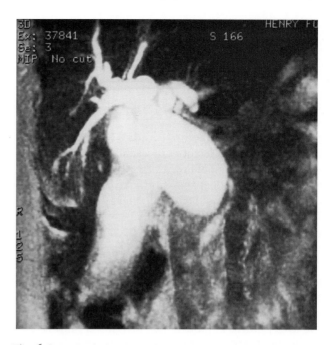

Fig. 6-1   MR cholangiography demonstrates a dilated common bile duct and intrahepatic system. The changes are secondary to a choledochal cyst.

tion can be done quickly, effectively, and accurately. The presence of biliary distention can easily be detected and the diameter of the common bile duct measured. The presence or absence of stones in the gallbladder is accurately evaluated. Stones are typically hyperechoic, resulting in acoustic shadowing. Stones within the common hepatic or common bile duct are also demonstrated but with a lesser degree of sensitivity (between 40% and 70%). In a patient in whom either gallbladder disease or biliary obstruction and distention are suspected, ultrasound is often the initial examination.

Magnetic resonance cholangiography

It has become increasingly apparent that visualization of the biliary and pancreatic ducts during MRI can be achieved. Using imaging sequences that were first developed for vascular imaging, variations of these sequences can now demonstrate moderate anatomic detail of the ductal structures (Fig. 6-1). This is now referred to as magnetic resonance cholangiopancreatography. Advantages over other imaging modalities are the fact that it is noninvasive and does not result in any radiation exposure. Also, it can be performed at the same time that MRI of the liver is being done, so that both the liver parenchyma and ductal structures can be evaluated during the same examination. Finally, the image can be projected in several planes, and coronal images can depict the entire biliary/pancreatic system, which is easily appreciated by clinicians. As further imaging advances are made, this technique will supplant other modalities.

Radioisotope evaluation

Radioisotopes used for imaging the biliary system are cleared from the blood by the hepatocytes and excreted with bile into the biliary system. Scanning the right upper quadrant demonstrates the biliary ducts and gallbladder. These agents are useful in evaluating patency of the cystic duct as well as the common hepatic and common bile duct and are effective in the evaluation of acute cholecystitis. Before the mid-1970s, rose bengal I-131 was the radiopharmaceutical used to demonstrate the biliary system. In the mid-1970s a new series of technetium-labeled radiopharmaceuticals was developed, having the advantage of a short half-life (6 hours) and a relatively low patient radiation dose. These agents are derivatives of iminodiacetic acid (IDA), and a variety of these derivatives have been developed, resulting in the well-known Tc-99m lidofenin (HIDA) and Tc-99m disofenin (DISIDA) scans that allow excellent visualization of the biliary system, even in the presence of mild to moderate jaundice.

Filling Defects

Calculi

Calculi are the most common cause of filling defects within the biliary system. For the most part, they originate within the gallbladder and traverse the cystic duct.

Filling defects in the common bile duct resulting from intraluminal stones are demonstrated with relative ease on ERCP. If the stones are sufficiently large, they will also be seen on CT (Fig. 6-2). However, stones within both the cystic duct and the common bile duct can easily be missed on CT, especially when oral contrast is used and the stone is obscured by opacified bowel. Ultrasound may be helpful in demonstrating common bile duct stones (Fig. 6-3). However, the reliability of the ultrasound examination in this region is much less than in the gallbladder (Fig. 6-4).

Primary stone formation in the common bile duct may occur, usually proximal to an area of narrowing in the duct. The origin of a prestenotic stone may still be the gallbladder, and as a result of obstruction and stasis, these stones accumulate within the common bile duct and increase in size. Certainly, in the postcholecystectomy patient with a documented normal biliary system postoperatively, primary stone formation in the common duct or cystic duct remnant can be seen.

Differentiation of primary from secondary common bile duct stones may be impossible. Occasionally, the configuration of the stone is helpful. Ovoid stones or stone formations that appear to be developing a luminal configuration may suggest the presence of primary stones (Figs. 6-5 and 6-6).

Pseudocalculus

Although a solitary air bubble may mimic a calculus within the common bile duct, the term *pseudocalculus* is reserved for a convex filling defect in the distal common bile duct that has the appearance of the top of a stone (Fig. 6-7). However, no contrast passes lateral or inferior to the convexity. This appearance is secondary to spasm of the sphincter of Oddi and can be confirmed by simply waiting a few minutes for relaxation to occur. If the spasm appears prolonged or the examiner is impatient, a 1-mg intravenous (IV) injection of glucagon

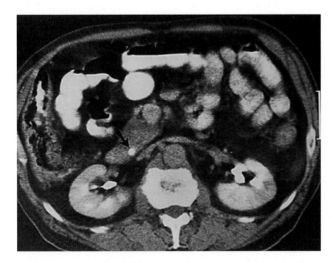

Fig. 6-2   A small, rounded calcified stone *(arrow)* is seen on a CT section through the distal common bile duct and pancreatic head region. The stone is in the common bile duct.

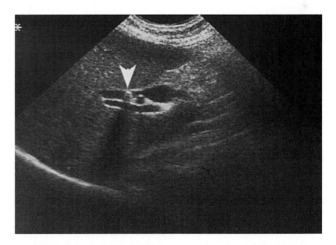

Fig. 6-3   Ultrasound examination of the common bile duct demonstrates a small stone within the duct *(arrow)* casting an acoustic shadow.

will usually result in the relaxation of the sphincter and resumption of a normal-appearing distal common bile duct (Fig. 6-8).

Blood clot

Hemorrhage into the biliary tract can result in a variety of appearances, from an isolated filling defect to several filling defects to a total cast of the lumen. The extent and rate of bleeding determine the appearance. Bleeding into the biliary tree, hemobilia, does not always result in the formation of a blood clot. This finding is becoming more common with the increasing availability of ERCP. The most common causes include trauma, instrumentation, tumor, and vascular abnormalities within the biliary tract. The presence of stones within the common bile duct can also, on occasion, result in bleeding. The etiology of this is unclear, although stones passing through the cystic duct or the distal common bile duct

may result in injured mucosa. The filling defects caused by clot formation are often different from the appearance of stones. They tend to be less defined and more ovoid (Fig. 6-9). There may be some changing of configuration as the filling defect moves. Blood clots almost never result in obstruction.

Benign polypoid lesions

Benign bile duct tumors are uncommon, but when present, most frequently present as small, rounded filling defects on the margin of the duct. These include such benign lesions as adenomas and papillomas, as well as fibromas, neurofibromas, lipomas, hamartomas, and carcinoids (Fig. 6-10). These lesions are usually solitary, although multiple filling defects are present in biliary papillomatosis, a very rare condition in which multiple papillomas are seen. This condition reputedly carries an increased risk of cholangiocarcinoma.

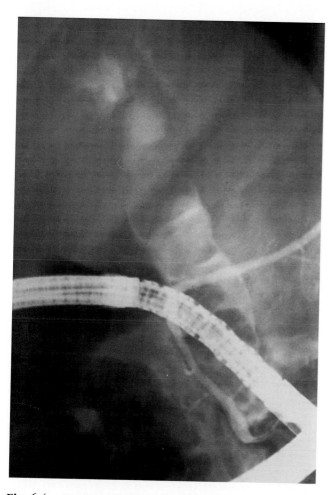

Fig. 6-4 ERCP examination demonstrates a markedly dilated common bile duct filled with multiple, large stones. Ultrasound of this region had failed to reveal the presence of the common bile duct stones. However, the presence of a gas-filled hepatic flexure of the colon seen at the margin of the liver will degrade the ultrasound evaluation of this region.

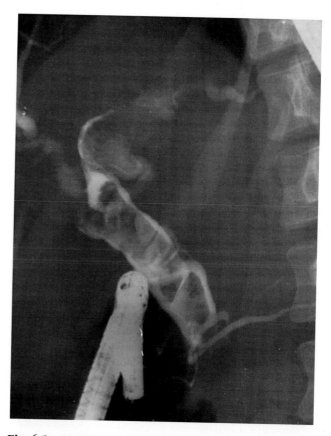

Fig. 6-5 ERCP in a patient 13 years after cholecystectomy demonstrates stones forming an intraluminal cast along the entire length of the common bile duct and common hepatic duct.

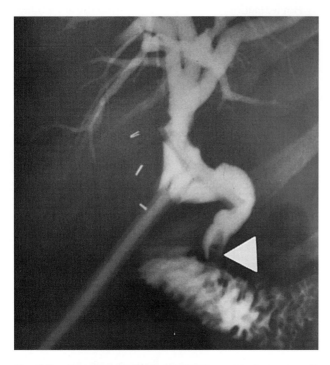

Fig. 6-6   Postoperative T-tube cholangiography shows a small, oval residual stone in the distal common bile duct *(arrowhead)*.

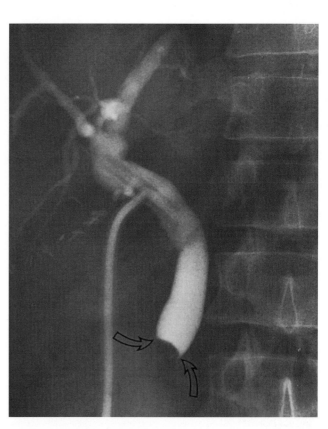

Fig. 6-7   T-tube cholangiogram demonstrates a rounded filling defect in the distal common bile duct *(arrows)*, raising the possibility of an impacted stone.

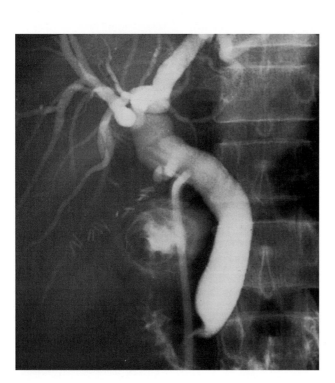

Fig. 6-8   In the same patient as Fig. 6-7 following the administration of IV glucagon, the apparent filling defect in the distal common bile duct has disappeared and represented spasm of the sphincter of Oddi.

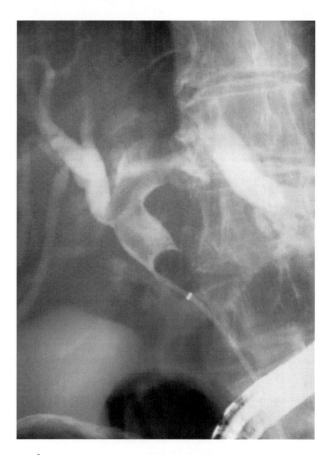

Fig. 6-9   Injection of the bile ducts during an ERCP demonstrates a cast conforming to the bile ducts from a blood clot within the ductal system. The material is soft and pliable and thus conforms to the ductal system without significant obstructive changes.

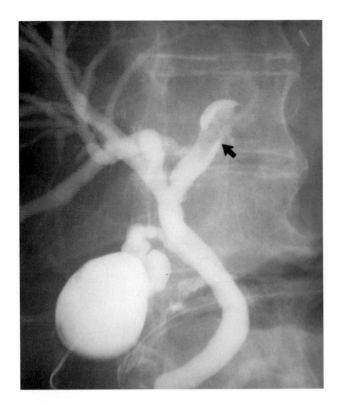

Fig. 6-10   Filling defect *(arrow)* in the left hepatic duct is secondary to an adenoma of the bile ducts.

Parasites

A number of parasitic infestations can affect the biliary system and result in typical filling defects within the common bile duct. The most common is the roundworm, *Ascaris lumbricoides.* The problem is worldwide, with the greatest prevalence in developing nations and rural areas where overcrowding and unsanitary environments are common. The ingested ova hatch in the small bowel and usually make that site their habitation. The worm is capable of ascending the small bowel and reaching the duodenum. This proximal migration can result in some of the worms passing into the common bile duct, leading to degrees of biliary obstruction and possible secondary infection. Often this is accompanied by pancreatitis, either as a secondary effect or as a result of worm migration into the pancreatic duct. Linear intraluminal filling defects are demonstrated on contrast studies of the common bile duct.

Liver flukes, most commonly seen in the Far East, are occasionally being seen in North America and Western Europe with the increase in worldwide travel. The cysts are ingested, usually with raw fish. The larvae hatch in the duodenum and migrate to the liver and biliary system where they can produce biliary obstruction and recurrent cholangitis. There is an increased incidence of cholangiocarcinoma in chronic infestation.

Hydatid echinococcal cysts of the liver can also occasionally communicate with the biliary tree and discharge daughter cysts into the biliary system, resulting in filling defects.

Inspissated bile and sludge

When conditions exist that produce stasis in the biliary system, the bile may congeal and produce a sludgelike deposit, mostly in the gallbladder but sometimes in the bile ducts. This appears as an intraluminal cast within the ducts that conforms to the internal lumen of the duct. Its appearance is similar to that of a blood clot. Although it is a rare filling defect, it is sometimes seen in patients who have had extensive biliary surgery, cholangitis, or liver transplantation. These individuals seem to be more susceptible to biliary stasis and resultant formation of biliary sludge. Treatment of this defect is usually accomplished at ERCP, when the endoscopist can often remove the cast by use of an inflatable balloon. Diagnosis is often made at that time, since the bile cast is a soft greenish black material.

Air

Small air bubbles, resulting in filling defects within the biliary system, are a common and troublesome finding during ERCP, PTC, and operative cholangiography examinations. Generally the defects are small, round, and mobile and therefore can be distinguished from stones when patients are positioned in dependent and nondependent positions. However, in examinations in which patient positioning is a problem, such as operative cholangiography and occasionally ERCP studies, a small, rounded filling defect caused by an air bubble inadvertently injected with contrast material cannot be distinguished from a stone. Reinjection is often necessary to clear up the issue. However, the problem may be avoided entirely if adequate precautions are observed during the contrast filling phase to exclude the possibility of injecting air.

Ductal Narrowing

Postinflammation

Chronic pancreatitis is one of the most frequent causes of common bile duct narrowing. This narrowing occurs as a result of changes in the pancreatic head, consisting of edema, chronic inflammation, and eventually fibrosis resulting in a mass effect. The combination of mass and cicatrization about the intrapancreatic portion of the common bile duct results in a smooth, tapered narrowing. Approximately 25% of these patients have sufficient narrowing to induce obstructive jaundice. When the stricture is the result of mass effect secondary to inflammation and edema and less due to cicatrization, the severity of the stricture may not be permanent and some degree of relief may be observed as the pancreatic inflammatory process subsides. Prolonged strictures, resulting mostly from fibrotic changes about the common bile duct in the intrapancreatic portion, can result in permanent liver damage if unrelieved. These patients eventually go on to develop cirrhosis. This type of stricture is not very amenable to dilatation, and the definitive treatment is choledochoduodenostomy or a choledochojejunostomy.

The configuration of smooth, narrow tapering over a 2- to 4-cm segment of the distal common bile duct in its intrapancreatic portion is benign in most cases. However, occasionally malignancy presents in such a manner. In a patient with no clinical or radiological evidence of pancreatitis or gallstone disease, the physician should be suspicious.

Other causes of stricture resulting from inflammation and fibrosis include trauma caused by difficult stone passage, ischemic and inflammatory damage that can occur as a result of hepatic artery chemotherapy infusion, as well as external penetrating and blunt trauma. Recurrent biliary infections may also result in stricture formation. Sclerosing cholangitis is discussed separately.

Postsurgery

Another important cause of benign strictures is accidental injury to the bile duct during cholecystectomy. The inadvertent placement of a ligature or a hemostat around the common bile duct or common hepatic duct is the most common injury. Most frequently the trauma involves the common hepatic duct, and depending on the degree of injury and the severity of the stricture, symptoms may appear weeks or years after the injury. Acutely, the patient may be jaundiced or experience intermittent attacks of cholangitis. Ductal stones develop above the stricture in about 25% of these patients. Long-term, unrelieved strictures eventually lead to obstructive biliary cirrhosis and liver failure.

Careful fundal to ductal dissection by the surgeon to clearly identify the common hepatic and common bile ducts, as well as routine use of intraoperative cholangiography, reduces the incidence of these injuries.

Cholangitis

Several different conditions produce what can be termed a cholangitis appearance to the bile ducts (Box 6-1). This consists of multiple areas of narrowing of the ductal structures, often involving both intrahepatic and extrahepatic systems. The areas of narrowing can be of varying lengths and severity, even in the same patient or duct. The intervening portions of ducts can show a mild degree of dilatation, particularly as the disease becomes progressive. The development of cholangitis can also predispose patients to the later occurrence of cholangiocarcinoma. Cholangiocarcinoma is a well-known complication of sclerosing cholangitis from inflammatory bowel disease but also can occur with parasitic cholangitides.

Sclerosing cholangitis Sclerosing cholangitis is a progressive, inflammatory process involving all or parts of the bile duct system. Frequently it involves the biliary system diffusely with both extrahepatic and intrahepatic involvement. The inflammation results in diffuse thickening of the bile duct walls. Quite commonly the degree of severity varies segmentally (Fig. 6-11). The disease appears to be more common in men by a 2:1 ratio.

Several conditions are associated with sclerosing cholangitis, with ulcerative colitis being the most frequently observed. At least one half of patients with

---

Box 6-1   Causes of "Sclerosing Cholangitic" Appearance of the Bile Ducts

ULCERATIVE COLITIS

IDIOPATHIC CAUSES

ASCENDING (INFECTIOUS) CHOLANGITIS
Postoperative
Immunosuppressed (AIDS, transplants)
Parasitic

OTHER
Retroperitoneal fibrosis
Crohn's disease
Riedel's thyroiditis

CHOLANGIOCARCINOMA

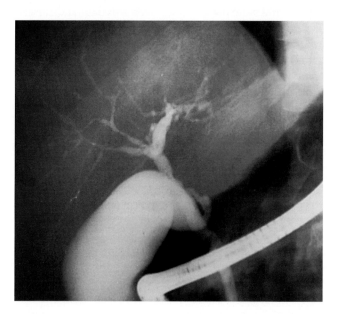

Fig. 6-11   ERCP in a 32-year-old patient with ulcerative colitis and sclerosing cholangitis demonstrates intrahepatic areas of segmental narrowing.

sclerosing cholangitis have associated inflammatory bowel disease. Conversely, sclerosing cholangitis eventually develops in 3% to 10% of patients with ulcerative colitis. The relationship is not understood. However, some regression in the severity of the disease has been reported in patients with ulcerative colitis who have had total colectomies.

Other conditions associated with sclerosing cholangitis include Crohn's disease, Riedel's thyroiditis, and retroperitoneal and mediastinal fibrosis. This incidence with these conditions is much less compared with that of ulcerative colitis.

The imaging diagnosis is best obtained by either ERCP or PTC. Although the small sclerosed ducts are difficult to aspirate with the percutaneous transhepatic approach, the use of the Chiba skinny needle in recent years has made the success rate somewhat higher.

Diffuse or localized areas of alternating narrowing and relative dilatation are seen involving both the intrahepatic and extrahepatic biliary system. The differential considerations include a slow-growing scirrhous type of bile duct carcinoma as well as the possibility of congenital cystic disease when the strictures are segmental. In addition, cholangiocarcinoma may develop as a complication of sclerosing cholangitis and the neoplasm's appearance is difficult to distinguish from the cholangitis. It should be noted that a secondary bile duct sclerosis can occur above chronic partial obstructions of benign causes. The appearance will be similar to primary sclerosing cholangitis, and a clear limitation of the changes in the extrahepatic system should at least raise the suspicion of this possibility. These changes are postulated to result from the chronic recurrent cholangitis associated with partial obstruction.

Ascending cholangitis As previously discussed, chronic recurrent ascending cholangitis proximal to a long-term partial obstruction of the common hepatic or common bile duct results in proximal bile stasis, dilatation, potential development of primary stone formation, and bacterial cholangitis. Both intrahepatic and extrahepatic ducts can be involved in a secondary sclerosing (ascending) cholangitis. The resultant changes in the biliary system can be indistinguishable from primary sclerosing cholangitis (Fig. 6-12). These are usually seriously ill patients with a biliary system that in the worst scenario is filled with pus at the height of the infectious process. Numerous small pericholangitic abscesses may form and make the diagnosis somewhat easier. If untreated, the condition is usually fatal. Treatment and multiple recurrences of the infectious process are usually the scenario for the sclerosing ductal changes. Although the treatment of the septic process is primary, the definitive treatment consists of relieving the distal obstructive process.

Occasionally, tiny common bile duct diverticula are encountered that may be indicative of previous ascending cholangitis (Fig. 6-13).

Recently, nonbacterial types of ascending cholangitis have been described in patients with acquired immunodeficiency syndrome (AIDS), with a radiological picture similar to primary sclerosing cholangitis. Biliary *Cryptosporidium,* although uncommon, is being encountered with more frequency with the increasing number of AIDS patients. Biliary cytomegalovirus and moniliasis, although extremely uncommon, may produce similar pictures in the immunocompromised patient.

Parasitic cholangitis Although rare in developed countries, parasitic migration into the biliary system is one of the most common causes of cholangitis in the world. Intestinal parasites such as *Ascaris lumbricoides* and *Clonorchis sinensis* migrate from the intestinal tract into the biliary system. Echinococcal cysts have been known to rupture into the biliary system and produce cholangitis by a seeding process into the bile ducts.

Ascaris lumbricoides is the most common cause of cholangitis in the world and infects a large proportion of the world's population. This large roundworm migrates up from the intestinal tract. It is easily recognizable as a long, tubular filling defect within the extrahepatic ducts. *Clonorchis sinensis* is a flat worm

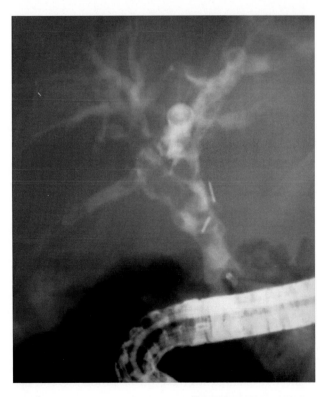

Fig. 6-12   Areas of narrowing with filling defects in the ducts are secondary to ascending cholangitis with pus present within the ducts.

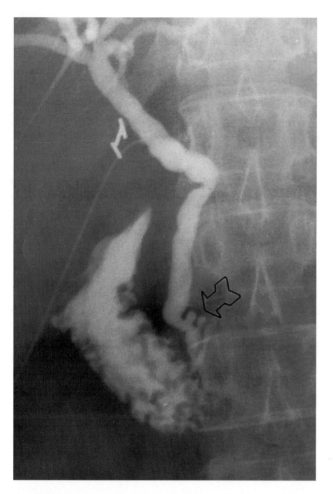

Fig. 6-13   Cholangiogram demonstrates several small diverticula *(arrow)* in the distal common bile duct associated with slight narrowing and irregularity but no obstruction.

Box 6-2   **Biliary Tract Abnormalities in Liver Transplantation**

Leak
Stricture at anastomosis
Attenuated intrahepatic ducts (rejection)
Multifocal strictures (duct ischemia)

only 1 to 2 cm in length. This parasite is most common in Southeast Asia. When it migrates into the biliary system, it tends to settle into the intrahepatic ducts. Unlike ascariasis, the abnormalities in the intrahepatic ducts are more severely involved by *Clonorchis.* Like sclerosing cholangitis with inflammatory bowel disease, the parasitic cholangitides are associated with an increased incidence of cholangiocarcinoma.

Liver transplant rejection

Several different conditions affect the biliary system of the transplanted liver. This can occur from one third to one half of all transplanted patients, and thus represents a major diagnostic challenge for the clinician and radiologist (Box 6-2). Some of these conditions such as leakage are not discussed here. However, a number of conditions in the transplanted liver eventually produce some narrowing of the bile ducts.

During liver transplant rejection, edema and cellular infiltration of the liver parenchyma occur. These pro-

cesses can be seen with both acute and chronic rejection, although the biliary changes may be more pronounced with acute rejection. Imaging of the biliary radicles during rejection shows attenuation of the radicles and sometimes splaying (Fig. 6-14). The changes may become quite pronounced, depending on the severity of the condition. Strictures of the extrahepatic biliary system may also be seen. The most common site of narrowing is the anastomosis site in the common bile duct. The cause for stenosis at the anastomosis may just be scarring or sometimes focal ischemia. When strictures occur in a multifocal distribution after transplant, the most likely cause is ischemia. When liver transplantation is performed for sclerosing cholangitis, the potential exists for recurrence of the cholangitis. The appearance is similar to what is seen typically with sclerosing cholangitis.

Extrinsic obstructive processes

Stricture of the intrapancreatic portion of the common bile duct is a well-known result of both acute and chronic pancreatitis involving the pancreatic head. This has been discussed previously. However, metastatic spread in the porta hepatis or the peripancreatic or periduodenal region can also, on occasion, produce sufficient extrinsic compression to cause bile duct narrowing and obstruction. Tumors from the gastrointestinal tract, lung, or breast are most commonly involved.

Lymphomatous nodes, although large and bulky, seldom result in sufficient extrinsic pressure to seriously narrow the common hepatic or common bile duct except when accompanied by desmoplastic changes.

Mirizzi syndrome and Mirizzi-like syndrome are unusual conditions that result in degrees of biliary obstruction. Mirizzi syndrome classically refers to a stone impacted in the neck of the gallbladder or the cystic duct, with the mass of the stone and accompanying inflammatory changes causing compression and narrowing of the adjacent common bile duct (Fig. 6-15). Malignant masses arising from the neck of the gallbladder or the cystic duct region can result in a Mirizzi-like picture as a result of contiguous spread, involvement of the common bile duct, and biliary narrowing and obstruction (Fig. 6-16).

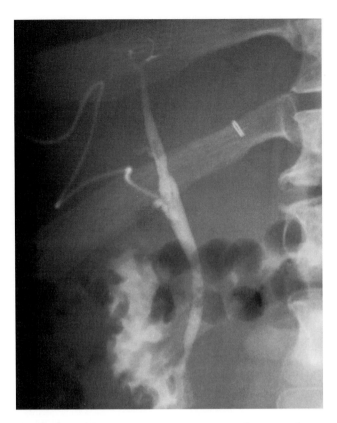

Fig. 6-14 Markedly attenuated intrahepatic ducts are due to edema in this liver transplant patient with rejection.

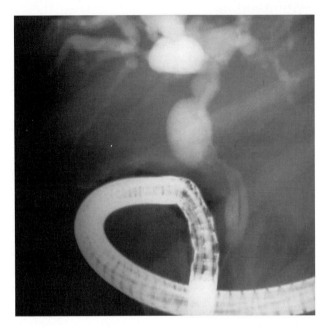

Fig. 6-15 Narrowing of the midextrahepatic ducts is from a stone impacted in the neck of the gallbladder with inflammatory changes (Mirizzi syndrome).

Cholangiocarcinoma

This lesion is uncommon but associated with high mortality. It occurs most often in adults 50 to 70 years old. Five percent of the patients have associated ulcerative colitis, almost always pancolonic in its distribution. These patients do not always have sclerosing cholangitis, but the risk of malignancy increases with the presence of sclerosing cholangitis (Box 6-3). There is also increased risk in any condition that results in chronic bile stasis, including Caroli's disease, choledochal cysts, and widespread cystic disease of the liver. There is also an increased risk with chronic parasitic infections of the biliary system, with biliary papillomatosis, and in certain environmental circumstances, such as are encountered in the chemical industry.

The most common presentation of cholangiocarcinoma is a short area of biliary stenosis (Box 6-4). This is occasionally accompanied by marked desmoplastic changes, and on rare occasion the lesion can resemble sclerosing cholangitis. Approximately half of the tumors are located in the region of the bifurcation of the main biliary ducts (Klatskin's tumors) (Fig. 6-17). Morphologically, these lesions can be focally stenotic (most common), as well as polypoid or diffusely scirrhous in nature. CT and ultrasound are often unable to demon-

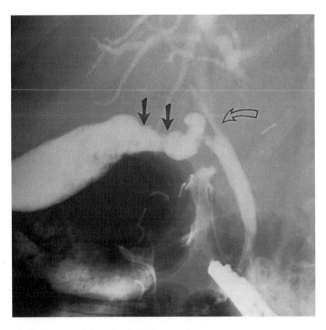

Fig. 6-16 ERCP demonstrates a lesion arising from the neck of the gallbladder (*arrows*) narrowing the gallbladder neck, cystic duct, and the adjacent common hepatic duct (*curved arrow*).

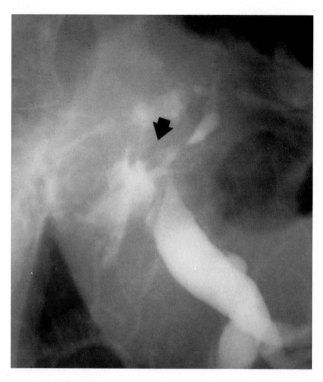

Fig. 6-17 Cholangiography demonstrates narrowing of the ducts at the bifurcation, representing a sclerosing cholangiocarcinoma (arrow). This is called a Klatskin tumor.

Box 6-3 Precursor Conditions for Cholangiocarcinoma

Sclerosing cholangitis
Choledochal cyst
Parasitic cholangitis
Biliary papillomatosis

Box 6-4 Radiographic Appearance of Cholangiocarcinoma

Focal stricture
Polypoid lesion
Diffuse narrowing (scirrhous)

Box 6-5 Bile Duct Stricture/Narrowing: Location vs. Etiology

PANCREATIC

Pancreatic carcinoma
Pancreatitis
Cholangiocarcinoma

SUPRAPANCREATIC

Adenopathy (metastases)
Cholangiocarcinoma
Mirizzi syndrome (stone impacted in cystic duct)
Gallbladder neoplasm

INTRAHEPATIC

Cholangiocarcinoma
Liver metastases
Primary hepatic neoplasm

---

strate the tumor, although the secondary effects of biliary obstruction are readily identified using these modalities. ERCP is helpful, but in cases with high-grade obstructive lesions, PTC is superior in that it is able to show the proximal extent of the lesion. The value of MRI in this lesion is debatable. There is some suggestion that the tumor may be more visible on certain MRI protocols. However, at this point MRI does not occupy a primary or even secondary place in the imaging workup.

The most common lesion pattern is a short, irregular stricture, although smooth margins are not infrequent. The polypoid form has the best prognosis while the scirrhous has the worst. Only a small number of patients are candidates for any form of surgical resection. For the remainder, once the diagnosis has been firmly established, biliary drainage is the goal. This can be accomplished by stenting the narrowed segment either from below (ERCP) or from above (PTC).

Adjacent malignant lesions

Malignant lesions arising in the tissues adjacent to the biliary system (Box 6-5), such as the liver in the case of hepatoma, or occasionally hepatic metastatic lesions, can result in biliary stenosis caused by compression or invasion (Fig. 6-18). A similar pattern can be seen with cancer of the pancreatic head. Moreover, cancer of the ampulla of Vater commonly constricts the distal common bile duct, leading to proximal distention. The bile ducts can be divided into pancreatic, suprapancreatic, and intrahepatic regions. If the pancreatic portion of the common duct is involved, the most likely process would be arising from the pancreas, such as pancreatic carcinoma or pancreatitis. Above the pancreas, but still in the extrahepatic ducts, the most likely cause of narrowing is enlarged lymph nodes from either an abdominal or an extraabdominal tumor. Involvement by gallbladder disease, either malignant or inflammatory, can also produce narrowing. Intrahepatic involvement of the ducts is produced by hepatic neoplasms, usually metastatic.

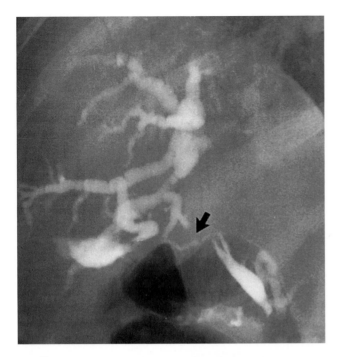

Fig. 6-18   Cholangiogram in a patient with known breast cancer and disseminated metastatic disease demonstrates obstruction of the biliary system at the level of the common hepatic duct *(arrow)* as a result of metastatic disease in the porta hepatis.

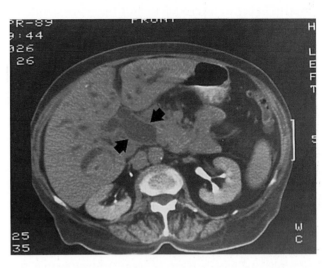

Fig. 6-19   A patient with pancreatic carcinoma presenting with biliary obstruction. A CT section through the region of the common bile duct demonstrates a grossly dilated common bile duct *(arrows)* and intrahepatic system.

Ampullary and periampullary processes

Carcinoma of the ampulla of Vater is often a nonspecific entity that includes lesions arising from the distal common bile duct, the pancreatic duct, and the adjacent duodenum. The appellation is more regional than histological, and in many instances it is impossible to differentiate these tumors histologically. True periampullary carcinomas are relatively rare. Carcinomas of the pancreatic head are three to four times more common (Fig. 6-19). Whereas the survival rate with pancreatic carcinoma is usually not reckoned beyond a year, true periampullary lesions can hold a much better prognosis, with 5-year survival rates as high as 40% in patients with negative nodes. In this patient group jaundice resulting from common bile duct obstruction is one of the most common presenting symptoms along with weight loss and anorexia. A palpable gallbladder (Courvoisier's gallbladder) is seen in at least 25% of the patients.

Other assorted ampullary and periampullary processes that may result in biliary duct obstruction include polyps arising in the periampullary region. These are uncommon, but adenomas, particularly the villous type, are the most frequently encountered lesion (Fig. 6-20). Carcinoids of the periampullary region have also been described, along with most of the other benign tumors of the GI tract.

Duodenal diverticula are a common and mostly innocuous finding on upper gastrointestinal (UGI) exami-

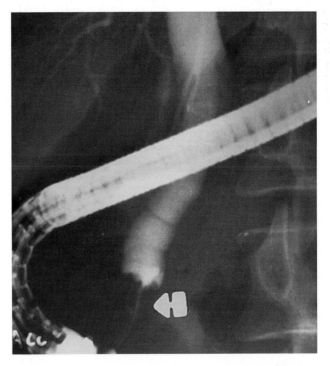

Fig. 6-20   ERCP examination demonstrates some dilatation of the common bile duct with narrowing distally *(arrow)*. The finding was persistent and proved to be a villous adenoma of the duodenum with extension into the distal common bile duct.

nations. Most of the diverticula occur in the juxtaampullary region, and the ampulla may actually empty into the diverticulum. In most instances this provides little or no problem. However, under certain circumstances the anatomical arrangement becomes important. If the ampulla empties into the diverticulum and there are duodenal inflammatory changes involving the diverticulum, the possibility of inflammatory and edematous changes resulting in some obstruction to the outflow of bile and pancreatic secretions is increased. This is uncommon. Moreover, if the diverticulum is sufficiently large and bulky, it may present a mechanical difficulty by impressing the distal common bile duct.

When the papilla is located within a diverticulum, the risk of papillary injury during cannulation is increased.

Biliary atresia

Biliary atresia is defined as luminal obliteration of either the intrahepatic or the extrahepatic bile ducts during the neonatal period. It is the most common cause of jaundice and liver-related death in neonates. It may be congenital, although there is some suspicion that the lesions are caused by intrauterine, biliary, or hepatic infections and inflammation resulting in sclerosing changes within the ductal system.

The symptoms usually develop shortly after birth, and without liver transplantation the life expectancy depends on the degree of biliary patency present. Life expectancy in general is approximately 2 years.

Of interest is the ongoing problem of trying to sort out the confusion surrounding the two neonatal conditions, biliary atresia and neonatal hepatitis. Even with liver biopsies a clear differentiation may not be possible. It is this interesting observation that has led some to suggest that biliary cirrhosis and neonatal hepatitis may be manifestations of the same disease process.

Ductal Dilatation

Obstruction

The radiological problems of biliary stenosis and bile duct dilatation clearly overlap, with one commonly leading to the other. Our classification in this and the following section is at best arbitrary, choosing to emphasize the primary pathophysiological process. It should be noted that the most common cause of biliary duct distention is obstruction, many of the causes of which have been previously discussed. The problem of a dilated biliary ductal system is viewed in this section from the perspective of the dilated ducts as the primary problem instead of as the sequela of some other problem such as stenosis.

Choledochal cysts

Choledochal cysts are not true cysts but rather cystic dilatations of the biliary tree. The condition is uncommon, although the Japanese report a higher incidence than the rest of the world. The changes in the biliary tree are thought to be congenital, but evidence suggests that some cases may be acquired as a result of an anomalous configuration of the pancreaticobiliary junction and subsequent reflux of pancreatic secretions into the bile duct. Whether the dilatation is congenital or acquired, it appears that it is a progressive process and it is interesting to note that choledochal cysts are only infrequently encountered in infancy.

The original classification of choledochal cysts divided them into three categories (Fig. 6-21). The first and most common presentation (80% to 90%) is manifested as a cystic dilatation of the entire common bile duct (type 1A). A subtype of this (type 1B) is focal dilatation of the common bile duct (Fig. 6-22). Another subtype (type 1C) is fusiform dilatation of the common bile duct (Fig. 6-23). In the type 1 form of choledochal cysts, the lesion is solitary and limited and neither the cystic duct nor the intrahepatic system is involved. The cystic dilatation can be fusiform or saccular in configuration.

In type 2 (about 2% of all cases) a well-defined diverticulum with an ostium is seen arising from the common bile duct. The remainder of the biliary tree is usually normal. If the diverticulum becomes sufficiently large, it may begin to extrinsically compress, narrow, and obstruct the common bile duct.

Type 3 choledochal cyst is a choledochocele, in which there is cystic dilatation of the intraduodenal portion of the common bile duct and protrusion into the duodenal lumen (2% to 5% of all cases).

In recent years two categories have been added. These are type 4A, which consists of multiple intrahepatic and extrahepatic segmental cystic dilatations (Fig. 6-24), and an extremely uncommon type, type 4B, which is limited to extrahepatic segmental cystic dilatations. The condition designated as type 5, which is a pattern of multiple intrahepatic cystic dilatations with sparing of the extrahepatic system (also known as Caroli's disease), is discussed separately.

Every medical student is familiar with the clinical triad of right upper quadrant pain, mass, and jaundice, which is said to represent the classic findings of choledochal cysts. As is frequently the case, the classic findings occur in only a minority of patients (22% to 40%). Right upper quadrant pain or discomfort is the most common symptom and is frequently attributed to the gallbladder, misdirecting the initial workup. Other clinical presentations include cholangitis and pancreatitis. Gallstones are found in a higher number of patients than expected who present as adults, and acute cholecystitis or gallstone-related pancreatitis can occasionally be the presenting problem. In many instances the correct diagnosis is not made preoperatively.

Imaging methods of choice include ERCP and PTC,

which permit the morphology of the ductal systems to be seen in detail. Ultrasound, CT, and radionuclide scans may also be helpful, but in many cases it is impossible to rule out an obstructing process as the cause of ductal dilatation.

Caroli's disease

Caroli's disease, also designated as type 5 choledochal cystic disease, is a condition usually limited to the intrahepatic ductal system and manifested as segmental saccular dilatations within a nonobstructed system. For some unknown reason, portions of the ductal system are spared in some patients. The process results in stasis and all the attendant complications associated with biliary stasis, including infection and stone formation. It is these complications that usually cause patients to seek medical attention. Liver function and portal blood flow are generally well preserved.

The disease is rare and is probably seen with considerably more frequency in written and oral board examinations than in actual practice. The course of the process is linked to the predisposition to develop bacterial cholangitis, as well as a definite increased risk for cholangiocarcinoma. These patients have an approximately 100 times increased risk for the development of this cancer.

Some controversy exists as to the etiology of Caroli's disease. Some believe that it is but one manifestation of a more generalized disease process that includes renal tubular ectasia (medullary sponge kidney), congenital hepatic fibrosis, and intrabiliary sacculations. Renal tubular ectasia, as well as renal cystic disease, is seen in almost 80% of reported cases. There is also an increased incidence of pancreatic cyst formation.

Ultrasound and CT demonstrate multiple intrahepatic cysts (Figs. 6-25 and 6-26), but differentiation from polycystic disease may not be possible without luminal contrast studies, such as ERCP or PTC. These studies clearly demonstrate the ductal origin of the cystic structures and provide a better opportunity to evaluate potential complications.

Papillary stenosis

Periampullary fibrosis or papillary stenosis can occur as a result of chronic inflammatory changes in the ampullary region. The difficult passage of a gallstone may account for some of the stenotic changes observed. It may also be possible that some of the stenosis could be iatrogenic as a result of previous failed sphincterotomies or repeated cannulations. This is one of the more common causes of mild diffuse dilatation of the bile ducts without any other underlying etiology apparent. Often these patients have mild abnormalities in their liver function test, but the degree of jaundice is typically minimal. The diagnosis is made at ERCP and really is one of exclusion, although some will measure intraductal pressures. Treatment can also be done by the endoscopist, and sphincterotomy is usually all that is necessary for treatment.

Cholangitis

Recurrent bacterial cholangitis can result in changes in the intrahepatic ductal system that can produce dilatation in its initial stages. Numerous sacculations and strictures are the usual pattern in chronic disease, and the changes begin to resemble sclerosing cholangitis (Fig. 6-27). Chronic recurrent cholangitis is uncommon in North America and Europe. However, in the Far East it is among the most common causes of abdominal emergency leading to hospital admission. The extrahepatic ducts can also be involved. The most important etiological factor is the antecedent presence of intrabiliary parasitic disease that results in an increased incidence of stone formation, obstruction, and subsequent infection.

Postcholecystectomy

It has been asserted that the common bile duct can become mildly dilated following cholecystectomy. The issue is controversial, and postsurgical common bile duct dilatation is not accepted by everyone. The literature reports the results of studies supporting both perspectives. However, episodic right upper quadrant pain is seen in 5% to 40% of postcholecystectomy patients. In such symptomatic patients there is an increased incidence of mild common bile duct dilatation.

Miscellaneous

Pneumobilia

By far the most common cause of pneumobilia is previous diverting surgery for biliary obstruction, such as choledochojejunostomy or choledochoduodenostomy (Box 6-6). In patients who have had previous sphincterotomies during ERCP, air may reflux from the duodenum into the biliary system. Any condition that undermines the competence of the sphincter of Oddi, whether it be traumatic, inflammatory, neoplastic, or iatrogenic, can result in air in the biliary system. On plain abdominal films the air is seen as linear branching lucencies, and during UGI studies barium may also be seen within the biliary system. The air collections within the biliary system are generally centralized as a result of the centripetal flow of bile. This observation helps distinguish air in the biliary system from air in the portal venous system, which is carried peripherally.

One of the more interesting causes of air in the biliary system is biliary-enteric fistula. This condition is discussed in more depth in the gallbladder section, since the fistulous connection is almost always between the gallbladder and the adjacent bowel. Most cases involve the duodenum, although fistulous connection from the

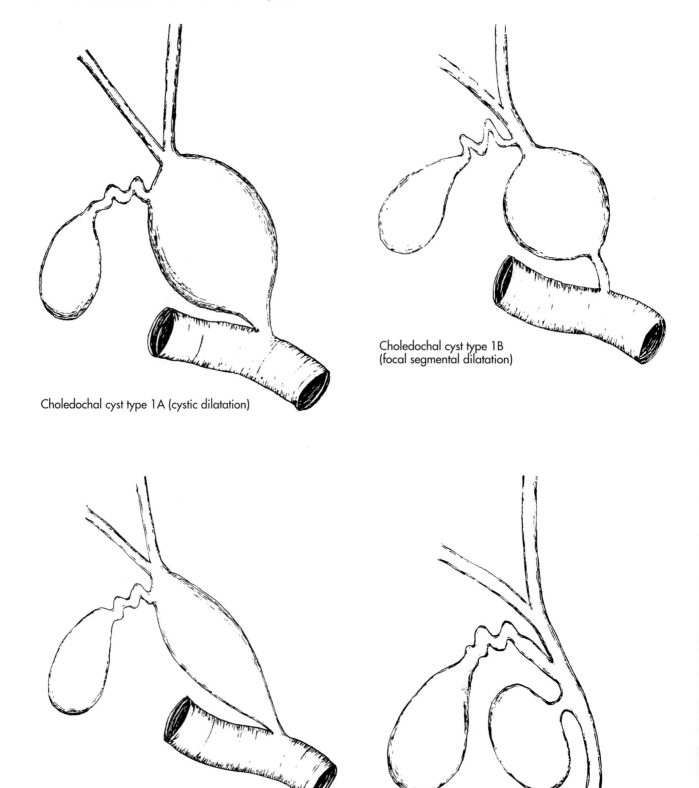

Choledochal cyst type 1A (cystic dilatation)

Choledochal cyst type 1B
(focal segmental dilatation)

Choledochal cyst type 1C (fusiform dilatation)

Choledochal cyst type 2
(well-defined diverticulum)

Fig. 6-21   Classification of choledochal cysts.
Continued

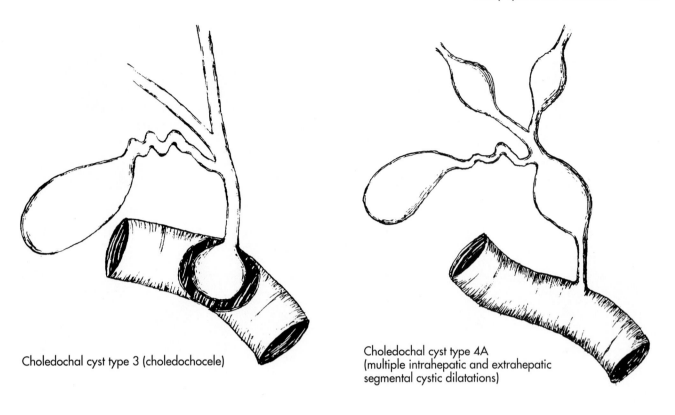

Choledochal cyst type 3 (choledochocele)

Choledochal cyst type 4A
(multiple intrahepatic and extrahepatic
segmental cystic dilatations)

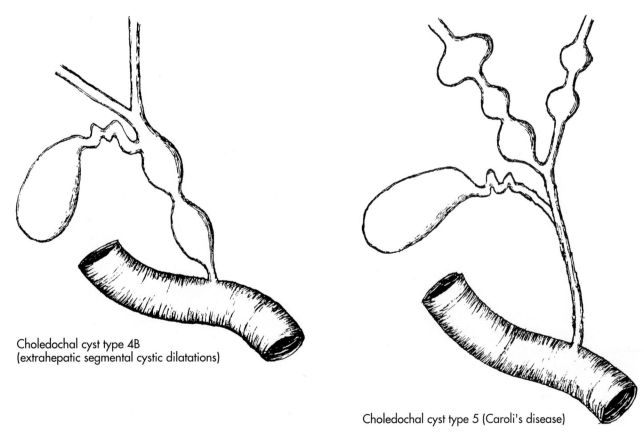

Choledochal cyst type 4B
(extrahepatic segmental cystic dilatations)

Choledochal cyst type 5 (Caroli's disease)

Fig. 6-21, cont'd   For legend see opposite page.

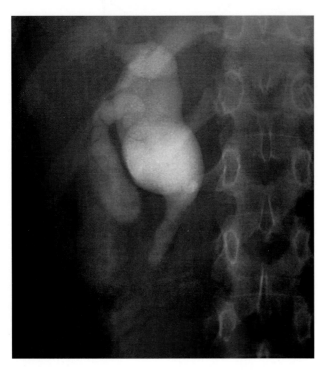

Fig. 6-22 Choledochal cyst. Cholangiogram demonstrates focal dilatation involving part of the common bile duct and common hepatic duct.

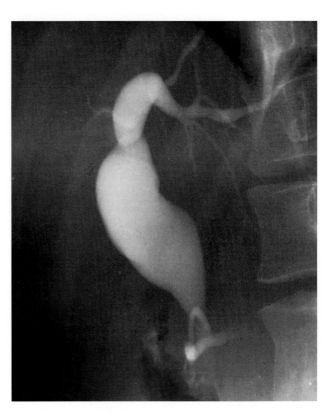

Fig. 6-23 Choledochal cyst. Retrograde cholangiogram demonstrates fusiform dilatation of the entire common bile duct.

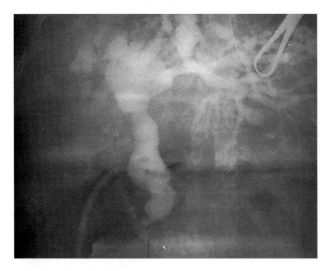

Fig. 6-24 T-tube cholangiogram demonstrates multiple biliary cystic changes throughout the extrahepatic and intrahepatic system, consistent with Caroli's disease.

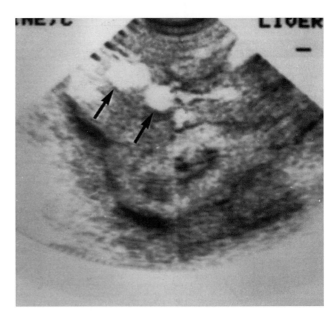

Fig. 6-25 Ultrasound examination of the liver in a patient with Caroli's disease demonstrates multiple cysts (arrows).

gallbladder to the colon can occur (Fig. 6-28). Even less common is a fistulous connection to the stomach. These conditions most commonly result from chronic chole-cystic inflammation combined with erosion of a stone through the gallbladder wall and communication with the adjacent bowel lumen. In about half the cases a permanently open fistulous tract remains and air can be seen within the biliary tree. The next most common cause is peptic ulcer disease, usually from the duodenal bulb. The common bile duct is in close apposition to the proximal duodenum, and ulcers in that location may perforate into the duct. Other unusual causes of biliary-enteric fistula include Crohn's disease and neoplasms.

In most inflammatory conditions of the duodenum, even the more severe peptic processes, the biliary system is unaffected. However, reflux of air into the biliary tree has been seen on rare occasion in patients with severe involvement of the duodenum with Crohn's disease. Whether this is due to distortion, deformity, and subsequent incompetence of the sphincter of Oddi or is a result of fistulous connections between the duodenum and common bile duct is not clear.

Occasionally a periampullary neoplastic process suf-ficiently affects the sphincter of Oddi to induce incom-petence and reflux of air.

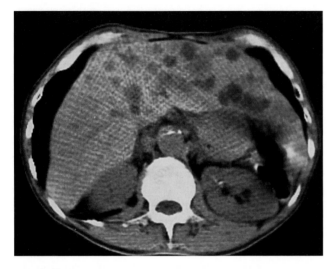

Fig. 6-26   CT of a patient with Caroli's disease demonstrates multiple cystic changes more prominently seen in the left lobe of the liver. Although most of the cysts seem discrete, some give the appearance of being part of the branching biliary system, suggest-ing this diagnostic possibility.

Box 6-6   Causes of Air in the Biliary System
PRIOR SURGERY OR SPHINCTEROTOMY
FISTULA, BILIARY-ENTERIC   Ulcer   Gallstone erosion   Crohn's disease   Carcinoma
EMPHYSEMATOUS CHOLECYSTITIS/CHOLANGITIS

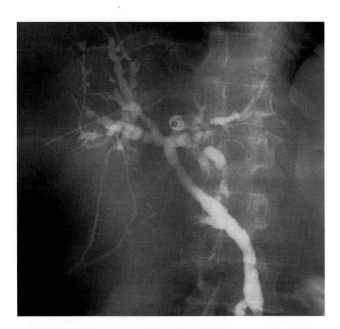

Fig. 6-27   PTC in a patient with infectious cholangitis demon-strates multiple strictures and sacculations of the intrahepatic system.

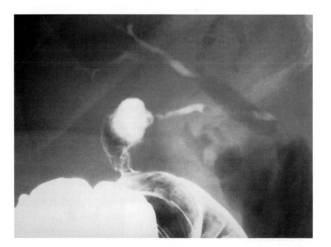

Fig. 6-28   Film from a barium enema demonstrates barium filling of a small, tubular structure adjacent to the colon and just superior to the hepatic flexure that proved to be a small, contracted gallbladder continuous with the colon as a result of a fistulous connection.

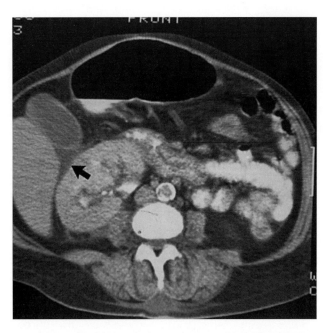

Fig. 6-29 CT section through the lower portion of the gallbladder in a patient with severe inflammation and gangrene of the gallbladder wall and a pericholecystic bile collection *(arrow)*.

Rarely, biliary air may be seen in asymptomatic patients with no evidence of current disease or history of previous disease or surgery. This finding may be related to anomalous pancreaticobiliary duct relationships.

Bile peritonitis and biloma

Leakage of bile from either the gallbladder or the biliary ductal system can result from several conditions. Focal bile leakage after biliary surgery or after PTC is not uncommon, although serious consequences associated with these leaks are much less common. Abdominal trauma, particularly penetrating trauma, is another important cause of bile leakage. Serious free spillage of bile into the peritoneal cavity can result in bile peritonitis with the clinical picture of an acute surgical abdomen. If the bile leakage is sequestered and loculated, usually in the right upper quadrant of the abdomen, a biloma develops. Bilomas that mature for a few weeks usually are round and have a thin capsule. Patients present with abdominal tenderness and a mass in the right upper quadrant in most cases. However, the biloma can occur in the midabdomen or left upper quadrant in about one third of the cases. If the biloma ruptures, the clinical presentation is more dramatic, similar to that of frank bile peritonitis. Additionally, a biloma can decompress itself by eroding into an adjacent hollow viscus and possibly setting up a fistulous connection between the bowel and biliary system.

Gallbladder perforation is also a known complication of acute cholecystitis in approximately 10% of cases (Fig. 6-29). The spillage of infected bile (which is almost always the case in this complication of acute cholecystitis) into the peritoneal cavity results in a fulminating peritonitis that requires immediate surgical intervention. Approximately half the patients with acute cholecystitis and perforation of the gallbladder form a biloma that usually becomes infected as well. This may present several days to weeks after the perforation as a pericholecystic abscess.

GALLBLADDER

Examination Techniques

Oral cholecystogram

In February 1924 a method for opacifying the gallbladder was reported by Graham and Cole in the *Journal of the American Medical Association*. The original contrast agent used was the sodium salt of tetrabromophenolphthalein. In the ensuing decades, more efficient and safer cholecystographic agents have been developed. Iopanoic acid (Telepaque), a triiodobenzene ring compound, was introduced in the 1950s and along with variations has been the standard oral cholecystographic agent.

Being mostly lipid soluble, orally administered iopanoic acid is readily absorbed from the gut into the portal bloodstream where it is bound to serum albumin and transported to the liver. In the hepatocyte the bound cholecystographic agent undergoes conjugation in a manner similar to bilirubin. It is then excreted into the biliary ductal system where it ultimately collects in the gallbladder. In the fasting, fat-restricted patient, gallbladder contractility is diminished and the contrast agent remains within the gallbladder where concentration can occur as a result of water absorption. In most patients the gallbladder is sufficiently opacified for imaging 18 to 24 hours following the ingestion of the contrast agent (Fig. 6-30).

Not all of the ingested contrast agent is absorbed. Some passes through the small bowel into the colon and appears as dense flecks of contrast sprinkled throughout the lower bowel. Not all conjugated contrast is retained in the gallbladder. In the bowel, the conjugated excreted contrast agent is seen as a homogeneous, hazy, luminal opacity. It has also been estimated that a sizeable amount (up to one third) of conjugated agent is excreted through the kidneys. As a result, renal toxicity is a known but rare complication of oral cholecystography.

For years the usual dosage regimen has consisted of 3 gm (6 tablets) of the oral contrast agents. Approximately 30% of patients have faint or no opacification of the gallbladder following this dose regimen. Two thirds of these patients demonstrate gallbladder visualization following the administration of a second 3-gm dose. Unfortunately, this two-dose schedule is incorrectly

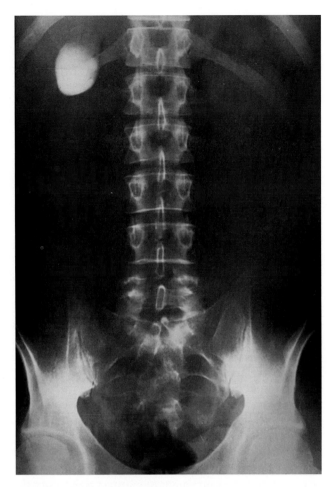

Fig. 6-30   Normal opacification of the gallbladder following the ingestion of oral cholecystographic contrast material.

referred to as a double-dose examination in many radiology departments and occasionally results in a patient's receiving 6 gm (12 tablets) of oral contrast agent at the same time. This may actually reduce the chances of opacification because of the significant diarrhea this dosage often causes. The correct application of this regimen, which is now routinely used by many institutions, is to administer 6 gm of the contrast agent to the patient divided into 3-gm doses over a 2-day period. This is done while a fat-restrictive diet is observed.

In a diseased or obstructed gallbladder, little or no opacification occurs. In a diseased nonobstructed gallbladder the reason for nonopacification may relate to the inability of the sick gallbladder to concentrate the bile and hence the contrast agent. On the other hand, inflammatory changes involving the wall of the gallbladder, in particular the mucosal surface, resulting in edema and hyperemia, may impair the integrity of the gallbladder mucosa. This increases its permeability to the contrast agent, and some of the contrast may escape the gallbladder via absorption through the mucosal surface with vicarious excretion through the kidneys.

Although the failure to opacify the gallbladder following a repeat-dose examination is presumptive evidence of gallbladder disease, there may be other causes of nonopacification not directly related to gallbladder pathology, and these causes must be excluded (Box 6-7). Some of them include the following:

- *Problems with patient compliance.* Most commonly the problem of patient compliance is a result of the patient's failure to understand the instructions for the ingestion of the tablets and dietary restrictions. These problems are best avoided by a careful explanation to the patient accompanied by a simple set of written instructions and the phone number of a person within the department who may be reached if the patient has questions or concerns.
- *Failure to reach the absorbing surface.* Unless the contrast reaches the absorbing surfaces of the small bowel in adequate amounts, insufficient absorption will occur and poor opacification will be the result. This can occur for a number of reasons. Diverticula anywhere in the gut proximal to these absorbing surfaces can sequester contrast, greatly diminishing flow distally. These diverticula can be located in the esophagus, the gastric fundus, the duodenum, or the jejunum. Patients with or without diverticula who are sick, immobile, and limited to the supine position may also sequester the contrast material in the fundus of the stomach. Gastric outlet obstruction, of any cause, whether inflammatory or neoplastic, can result in lack of presentation of the contrast to the small bowel. A patient with constant vomiting may lose much of the contrast before it reaches the small bowel. Patients with gastric atony or gastrocolic fistulas can also be expected to present some difficulty in achieving opacification of the gallbladder.
- *Absorbing surface abnormalities.* Absorbing surface abnormalities are a relatively uncommon cause of nonopacification, even among patients with known inflammatory bowel disease and malabsorption syndromes that affect the absorbing surface of

the small bowel. Occasionally a patient with Crohn's disease or extensive small bowel resection who has a normal gallbladder can show nonopacification at oral cholecystogram (OCG) because of inadequate absorption. Patients with severe acute pancreatitis and accompanying malabsorption may fall into the same category.

• *Hepatic abnormalities.* Because the contrast agent must undergo conjugation within the hepatocyte before being excreted into the biliary system, the presence of normal hepatic function is necessary to undertake OCG examination. Patients with elevated bilirubin levels (above 2 mg/dl), whether from primary hepatocellular disease or from biliary ductal obstructing processes, are not candidates for OCG examination. Diminished opacification or nonopacification occurs in these patients not only because of the impairment of the intrahepatic capacity to transport the contrast agent but also because the contrast agent molecule competes with bilirubin for the hepatobiliary-excretion mechanisms.

The use of the OCG fell off dramatically during the 1980s with the widespread use of ultrasound in the evaluation of the gallbladder. In recent years its use increased modestly for a period concomitant with the use of biliary lithotripsy to evaluate for stone size, number, and calcification.

Despite the decrease in the number of OCGs being performed in the United States, physicians should remember that this is a simple, safe, inexpensive, and very accurate method for examining the gallbladder. Its sensitivity in detecting gallstones approaches that of ultrasound, while the cost of ultrasound ranges from 1½ to 2 times that of an OCG. The sensitivity for detection of gallstones with OCG is said to be around 94%, compared with 98% for ultrasonography.

A significant limitation of the OCG is that diagnostic information is limited to the gallbladder. However, in a patient with a clinical history and symptoms that are most consistent with gallstone disease, an OCG may still be considered a reasonable first step in the evaluation of the patient. Filming procedure for the OCG includes upright, oblique, and compression views of the gallbladder.

Ultrasound

Ultrasound has the advantage of being noninvasive and not using ionizing radiation. It is highly accurate in detecting gallstones. It can provide additional valuable information regarding gallbladder wall thickness and pericholecystic abnormalities, as well as an evaluation of the liver and pancreas (Fig. 6-31).

With the widespread use of real-time ultrasound, this method of imaging has become the primary diagnostic modality for gallbladder and biliary pathology. When the

OCG is contraindicated, ultrasound is an effective alternative. This applies in jaundiced patients with abnormal bilirubin levels, as well as in patients with known allergies to iodinated contrast material. Any patient with known structural abnormalities, such as high small bowel obstruction or gastric outlet obstruction, will predictably have an unsuccessful OCG examination. In these instances ultrasound should always be considered the first choice.

In any instance in which the OCG examination is not conclusive or there is nonopacification of the gallbladder, ultrasound is indicated.

Radioisotope studies

Direct radionuclide imaging of the biliary system and gallbladder may be obtained using technetium-99m–labeled derivatives of iminodiacetic acid (HIDA, DISIDA, Mebrofenin), which are excreted directly into the biliary tract and can demonstrate patency with a high degree of sensitivity. Its most obvious use is in the evaluation of cystic duct patency in patients with signs and symptoms of acute cholecystitis.

Following the administration of the radionuclide, concentration can be detected in the liver within 5 to 10 minutes. Usually by 40 to 60 minutes the biliary system, including the gallbladder, common bile duct, and possibly the cystic duct, may be seen, with some activity already present within the adjacent small bowel loops. Cholecystokinin (CCK) or an analog may be given before the examination to contract and empty the gallbladder and thus possibly promote filling during the study. This maneuver should be considered in patients in whom normal dietary stimulation of the gallbladder is ineffective.

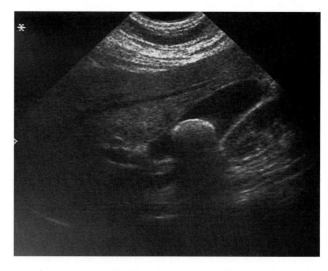

Fig. 6-31 Ultrasound examination of patient with a large, solitary gallstone casting a prominent acoustic shadow.

In some instances the efficiency of gallbladder contraction and emptying can be determined using the same agent by measuring uptake over the gallbladder before and after intravenous injection of CCK. There is an assumption that some patients who have no evidence of stones or inflammation but have symptoms similar to those seen in gallstone disease suffer from biliary dyskinesia, which can give identical symptoms. This diagnosis is somewhat controversial.

Nonvisualization of the gallbladder after 1 hour is usually indicative of cystic duct obstruction. Delayed gallbladder visualization beyond 1 hour after the common bile duct and the adjacent bowel have already been identified does not rule out the possibility of acute cholecystitis, although such a finding would be unusual. More commonly, delayed visualization of the gallbladder is associated with chronic cholecystitis. Generally speaking, the longer the delay, the greater the likelihood of chronic cholecystitis.

Computed tomography and magnetic resonance imaging

CT cannot be considered a primary examination technique for gallbladder evaluation at this time. If gallstones are calcified, they may be detected on CT scanning depending on the location of the stones and the thickness of the slices. Most stones, being composed of cholesterol, tend to blend into the bile environment within the gallbladder and are often not seen. However, pericholecystic fluid or masses can be well demonstrated on CT. MRI has not played any significant role to date in the evaluation of gallbladder disease.

Dilated Gallbladder

Physiological causes

Patients undergoing prolonged fasting or starvation accumulate increased amounts of bile within the gallbladder, with resultant distention of the organ. These people also have an increased risk of stone formation. A similar picture is encountered in patients receiving prolonged hyperalimentation. After bone marrow transplantation, patients commonly show some distention of the gallbladder on ultrasound and CT of the abdomen. Often this is accompanied by sludge or stone formation. The exact cause of these findings is not clear at this time.

Courvoisier's gallbladder

Progressive, painless enlargement of the gallbladder with late development of jaundice has long been recognized as a high-probability sign for pancreatic cancer with secondary involvement and narrowing of the distal common bile duct (Fig. 6-32). Other lesions, such as carcinoma of the ampulla of Vater or the peripapillary duodenum, can result in a similar clinical presentation. Additionally, benign processes, such as villous adenomas or carcinoids involving the region of the papilla, have been noted to result in Courvoisier's sign. The general clinical significance of the Courvoisier's gallbladder is that a palpable nontender gallbladder in a jaundiced patient is more likely to be related to a neoplastic process than to an inflammatory process or a stone. Progressive, slow obstruction of a normal gallbladder results in a considerable amount of painless distention. Conversely, distention in chronic disease is less likely, even with significant obstruction, because of gallbladder wall thickening and fibrosis. Distention secondary to stones is commonly intermittent, incomplete, and painful. Inexplicably, some patients with complete cystic duct obstruction who do not present in the acute stage go on to manifest one of several conditions associated with chronic aseptic cystic duct obstruction. These include porcelain gallbladder, milk of calcium bile, cholesterol impregnation of the gallbladder wall and mucosal surface (strawberry gallbladder), and hydrops of the gallbladder.

Hydrops

In most instances patients with gallstone obstruction of the gallbladder neck or cystic duct present with acute cholecystitis. These patients frequently have a distended, painful gallbladder. The treatment of acute cholecystitis is variable, depending on the condition of the patient and operative risks. Most commonly, early surgery is favored. However, in a small number of individuals who have chronic obstruction of the cystic duct, the gallbladder can become distended and surprisingly large. It contains a clear or mucoid, milky aseptic bile. This is the condition known as hydrops of the gallbladder. Some of

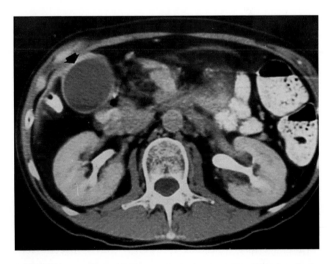

Fig. 6-32   CT of a patient with known carcinoma of the pancreas and marked passive dilatation of the biliary system and gallbladder (arrow).

these patients have little or no history of gallbladder disease, and the finding can be incidental. However, most patients have degrees of right upper quadrant discomfort and possibly biliary colic. These patients are almost never jaundiced unless some intervening process results in common bile duct obstruction. Complications of hydrops of the gallbladder include gallbladder empyema (when the gallbladder content becomes infected), perforation, or, rarely, infarction. While radionuclide imaging is the examination of choice in suspected acute cholecystitis, ultrasound has been found to be a superior method of evaluation in the chronic situation, with remarkably easy and quick identification of the dilated, distended gallbladder. If the obstructing stone can be demonstrated in the gallbladder neck or cystic duct, the diagnosis is complete.

Neuromuscular abnormalities

Gallbladder atony and enlargement are common among patients with diabetes mellitus, occurring in up to half of the patients with insulin-dependent diabetes. The incidence may be higher in patients with peripheral vascular disease or diabetic neuropathy. Additionally, patients with diabetes have a decreased ability to empty the gallbladder, with resultant increased bile stasis and increased risk of stone formation. The increased size of the gallbladder relates to contractile abnormalities of the muscular wall of the gallbladder secondary to neuromuscular changes associated with the disease.

Postvagotomy patients may demonstrate increased gallbladder size. An increased incidence of gallstone formation in this group has also been observed. Truncal vagotomies are more frequently associated with increased gallbladder volume, and selective vagotomies less so.

Small, Shrunken Gallbladder

Chronic cholecystitis

The term *chronic cholecystitis* has meant different things to different people in various specialties. In a few patients obstruction of the cystic duct results in hydrops of the gallbladder with intermittent or persistent symptoms. These patients may be said to have chronic cholecystitis. However, more frequently chronic cholecystitis refers to the presence of chronic inflammatory changes in the gallbladder wall with associated thickening of the wall. The gallbladder is small and often contracted and in 95% of the cases contains numerous stones. This pattern is probably the most commonly encountered form of gallbladder inflammation seen at surgery. These patients frequently have intermittent biliary colic resulting from intermittent cystic duct obstruction. Typically the pain is severe, in the right upper abdomen, possibly radiating to the back or shoulder. The pain has a tendency to escalate shortly

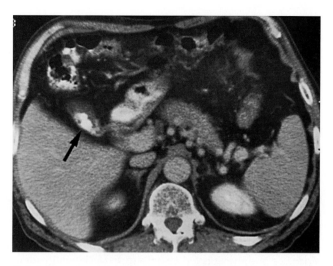

Fig. 6-33 CT examination through the inferior aspect of the liver demonstrates a small, contracted gallbladder containing several calcified stones *(arrow)*.

after the onset of symptoms and diminish slowly over the next few hours, as opposed to acute cholecystitis in which the pain continues to increase and is prolonged beyond 5 or 6 hours.

The diagnosis of chronic cholecystitis may be suggested on CT or ultrasound studies in which a small, contracted gallbladder is demonstrated with a thickened wall and gallstones (Fig. 6-33). Small amounts of pericholecystic fluid may be seen, although this is more common in acute cholecystitis. The diagnosis can also be suggested by biliary scintigraphy when the gallbladder is seen to fill in a delayed fashion either spontaneously or with pharmacological assistance, such as the administration of 2 mg of IV morphine to induce spasm of the sphincter of Oddi.

Cystic fibrosis

Gallbladder changes are seen in approximately one third of patients with cystic fibrosis. A small, hypoplastic gallbladder is not uncommon among this group. In addition, the bile is somewhat thicker than normal and it is assumed that some impairment of bile flow is present, accounting for the increased incidence of gallstones. These changes are unusual in infancy and are usually seen during the teen years.

Hyperplastic cholecystoses

The term *hyperplastic cholecystoses* refers to two conditions that lead to thickening of the gallbladder wall and in advanced conditions to diminished size or lack of distensibility of the gallbladder (Fig. 6-34). The two diseases are adenomyomatosis and cholesterolosis. This is discussed in further detail in a later section. It should be noted here that both conditions limit the size and distensibility of the gallbladder when they begin to diffusely involve the gallbladder.

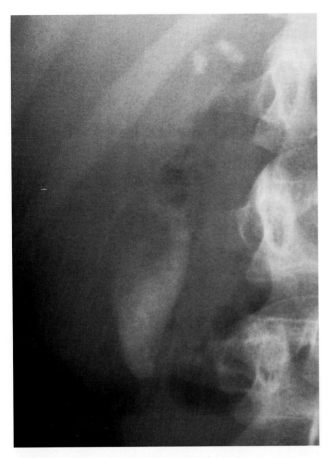

Fig. 6-34 Small, poorly functioning gallbladder as seen in cholesterolosis.

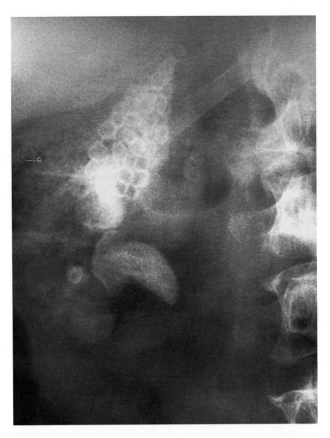

Fig. 6-35 Right upper quadrant coned-down view of supine abdomen of a patient with numerous faceted gallstones filling the entire gallbladder. Adjacent to this can be seen prominent renal calcifications.

Filling Defects

Artifacts and spurious filling defects

One of the more common problems encountered with the OCG examination is that of spurious lucencies projected over the gallbladder and mimicking gallstones. These are usually air bubbles in the adjacent hepatic flexure of the colon or the duodenal bulb. If multiple positional views are routinely obtained, this is usually not a serious problem. Routine compression views also diminish the potential of mistaking overlying air bubbles for gallstones.

Occasionally a tiny, persistent filling defect in the neck of the gallbladder can be seen, representing a slight invagination of the cystic duct into the neck of the gallbladder lumen.

Calcification in the anterior ribs, liver, right kidney, lymph nodes in the right upper quadrant, pancreatic head, and abdominal wall projecting over the gallbladder can be occasionally mistaken for calcified stones. Supine, upright, and compression views as a routine part of the examination should deal with the problem. In some instances fluoroscopy may be required to sort out some of these calcifications.

Gallstones

It is estimated that approximately 20 million people in the United States have gallstones. Of these an estimated 500,000 annually undergo cholecystectomy. Unfortunately, the estimates of the prevalence of gallbladder disease depend to a large extent on the method by which information is gathered and the type of imaging techniques used. Many of the epidemiological studies have produced incidences based on interviews or questionnaires regarding a history of gallbladder surgery or reported findings of gallstones on previous imaging studies. The figures thus obtained are, at best, loose estimates of the prevalence of the disease. Realistically, we probably do not know with certainty what the incidence is and have probably underestimated it. We do know, however, that most removed gallstones (80%) are composed of cholesterol, while the remainder contain a variety of calcium salts. Approximately 15% of gallstones are sufficiently calcified to be seen on plain films of the abdomen (Fig. 6-35). Stones that are predominantly pigmented tend to occur in patients with hemolytic types of anemias such as sickle cell disease. Cholesterol stone formation is more common in females than males, slightly more common in whites, and much more common in native American Indians. Moreover, there is a relationship between obesity and the incidence of gallstone formation, particularly in young women. Other etiological factors include chronic liver disease, the use of certain types of antilipidemic agents, and hyperalimentation.

Most gallbladder stones are never diagnosed. Many patients with stones are asymptomatic, while others have vague nonspecific symptoms. Only a fraction of patients come to cholecystectomy. Interestingly, the heightened attention to alternative therapies for the treatment of cholelithiasis has brought about a renewed interest in the composition as well as the pathophysiological processes that lead to the formation of gallstones. Gallstone pharmacological dissolution, as well as biliary lithotripsy or combinations of both therapies, has been used in the contemporary treatment of gallstones.

As previously mentioned, 15% of gallstones can be diagnosed on the basis of plain films of the abdomen. Plain film diagnosis of cholesterol stones with fissured interiors containing gas is a rare occurrence and a curious phenomenon of gallstone formation (Fig. 6-36). When present, this is usually manifested by cross-shaped or stellate thin lucencies in the right upper quadrant. This has been referred to as the Mercedes-Benz sign and is pathognomonic of gallstones (Fig. 6-37).

The principal methods of imaging gallstones are ultrasonography and OCG. The sensitivity for the detection of stones is quite high in both examinations and slightly higher for ultrasound. Both have certain advantages and some limitations. The OCG requires some patient preparation and the use of ionizing radiation. On the other hand, it demonstrates not only gallbladder morphology but also function. Ultrasound does not demonstrate function but is highly sensitive in the detection of stones and can give additional information regarding the surrounding organs. Little or no patient preparation is necessary for ultrasound examination.

On OCG examination with opacification of the gallbladder, noncalcified stones show as filling defects of varying number and size (Fig. 6-38). A single stone may be present or the gallbladder may be distended with numerous stones. Stones may be sandlike, rounded, or faceted. On ultrasound examination the presence of acoustic shadowing in the dependent portion of the gallbladder is typical of gallstones. The composition of the gallstone does not appear to be a factor in the degree of acoustic shadowing present. On occasion, gallstones

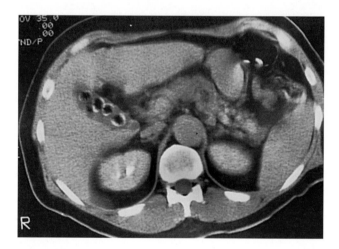

Fig. 6-37 CT through the liver demonstrates numerous gallstones, calcified in their rim with internal fissures and gas collections resulting in the Mercedes-Benz sign seen on plain film.

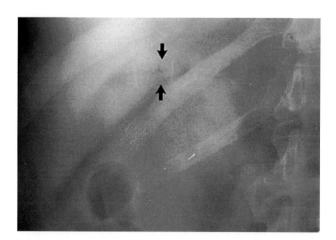

Fig. 6-36 A coned-down view of the right upper quadrant demonstrates a subtle stellate lucency (arrows) representing gas within a large, fissured gallstone (the Mercedes-Benz sign).

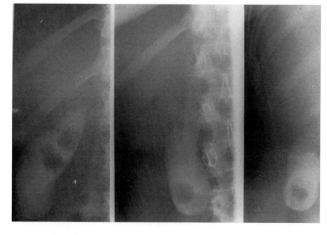

Fig. 6-38 Gallstones. OCG demonstrates good opacification of the gallbladder that has at least two rounded mobile lucencies within it.

float, particularly pure cholesterol gallstones. The layering out process can be observed in both ultrasound and OCG studies. A striking finding on OCG occurs when multiple small stones layer out and form a radiolucent band across the gallbladder lumen (Fig. 6-39).

New approaches to gallstone therapy have led to a mild resurgence in use of the OCG. Methods for chemical stone dissolution and biliary lithotripsy have been major topics for discussion, both in the medical literature and in the lay media in the last decade. Initially, oral bile salts were used in an attempt to dissolve gallstones. Success was limited and not always reproducible, and recurrence was common. Newer, direct-dissolving agents have been developed, the most noteworthy of which is methyl *tert*-butyl ether (MTBE). Dissolution of gallstones using MTBE does require the direct application of the chemical to the gallstones, which in turn requires a percutaneous transhepatic route or endoscopic cannulation of the cystic duct. Infusion and aspiration of MTBE follow, resulting in complete

dissolution of the stones in 30% to 60% of patients. Stone recurrence is a problem following MTBE treatment, more so in patients with multiple stones.

Length of hospital stay is often greater for MTBE treatment than for laparoscopic cholecystectomy, particularly if the transhepatic percutaneous route is undertaken. A small number of patients (5% to 10%) experience complications related to transhepatic puncture or cystic duct perforation.

The first extracorporeal shock-wave lithotripsy (ESWL) treatments were undertaken in the mid-1980s following success in renal stone therapy. The goal of ESWL is to shock gallstones into tiny fragments that can pass through the biliary system into the gut or be dissolved more easily by MTBE. Focused shock waves, generated by either electromagnetic or piezo-ceramic techniques, are used to produce a high-pressure shock effect over an area of several centimeters. The tissue damage to the gallbladder and adjacent organs is minimal and, with the exception of the occasional case of mild pancreatitis, appears to be of little consequence. The amount of fragmentation appears to depend on the number, size, and composition of the stones. Best results are obtained in patients with a limited number of small, noncalcified stones. The recurrence rate of gallstones after complete clearance is significant, ranging between 10% and 15%. Combining ESWL with powerful dissolving agents like MTBE appears to give a slightly higher rate of success. The unresolved question is the relative cost of different therapies with the advent of laparoscopic surgery. In general, the enthusiasm for ESWL seen during the 1980s has waned significantly. Clearly, in symptomatic patients for whom surgery is contraindicated, it does represent an encouraging alternative.

Nonadenomatous polyps

The most common cause of polypoid (nonmobile) filling defects within the gallbladder is cholesterol polyps (Fig. 6-40). These polyps arise from a condition of the gallbladder known as cholesterolosis, in which deposits of cholesterol and cholesterol precursors are found within the gallbladder wall. The typical OCG and ultrasound findings are similar to those of a gallstone, with the exceptions that the lesion is fixed on the gallbladder wall and there is no acoustic shadowing on ultrasound. The morphological changes can be either a focal buildup forming a discrete cholesterol polyp or diffuse surface deposition over the gallbladder mucosa, giving rise to an unusual surface texture and pattern sometimes referred to as strawberry gallbladder.

Cholesterolosis and its manifestations are part of a larger group of conditions often referred to as the hyperplastic cholecystoses, first described by Jutras in 1960. Under the same heading, he also included adenomyomatosis and several rare and unusual conditions. The valid-

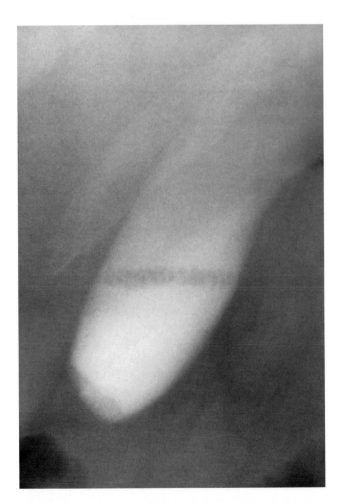

Fig. 6-39   OCG on a patient in the upright position demonstrates numerous tiny cholesterol stones layering out, forming a linear radiolucent band across the lumen of the gallbladder.

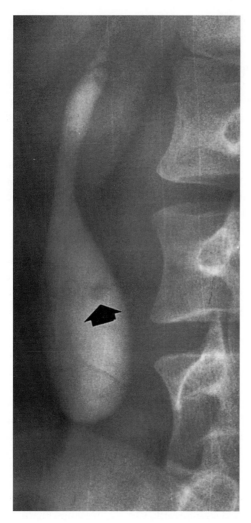

Fig. 6-40   OCG on a patient with a single, nonmobile filling defect within the gallbladder *(arrow)* found to represent a solitary cholesterol polyp.

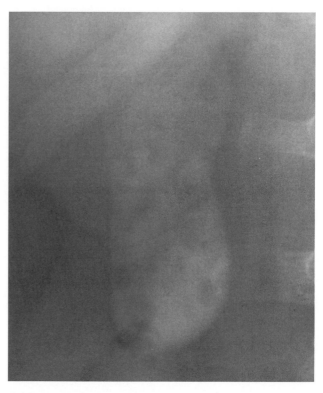

Fig. 6-41   Multiple filling defects within the gallbladder from papillomatosis.

ity and significance of the latter conditions have been questioned, and for the most part cholesterolosis and adenomyomatosis are considered the only two important conditions under the hyperplastic cholecystoses classification. Jutras used the term *hyperplastic cholecystoses* to describe a group of gallbladder disorders that had common functional abnormalities such as hyperconcentration, hyperexcretion, and hypercontractibility. Adenomyomatosis is discussed in more detail in upcoming sections.

Other nonadenomatous polypoid lesions of the gallbladder are rare. These include such lesions as lipomas, leiomyomas, fibromas, hemangiomas, and neurofibromas. Carcinoid tumors of the gallbladder have been reported. On rare occasion, granular cell myoblastomas (also a rare finding in the esophagus) have also been described in the gallbladder. Papillomas of the gallblad-

der, and of the biliary tree as well, have been reported and produce multiple filling defects (Fig. 6-41).

In addition to the above, an unusual but troublesome filling defect in the gallbladder is seen on rare occasion as a result of a gallstone adherent to the gallbladder mucosa.

Adenomatous polyps

True epithelial adenomas are uncommon. When present, they can occur as either sessile or pedunculated filling defects. They can occur in any portion of the gallbladder, and multiplicity is a frequent finding. The possibility that gallbladder adenomas represent a definite precursor to carcinoma, such as in the colon, still lacks convincing scientific support. However, the presence of carcinoma-in-situ in some reported cases of gallbladder adenomas does make it a real possibility.

Carcinoma

An estimated 6000 people in the United States each year die as a result of gallbladder carcinoma. The incidence is higher in females and among Native American Indians and Hispanics.

Gallbladder carcinoma continues to be one of the more dismal malignant neoplasms, with a 5-year survival rate between 2% and 4%. If the patient is symptomatic, the prognosis is always grave. On the other hand,

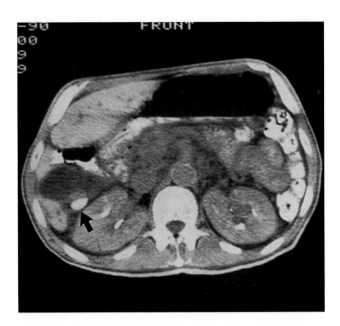

Fig. 6-42   CT section through the region of the gallbladder in a patient with carcinoma of the gallbladder demonstrates perforation of the gallbladder with pericholecystic fluid and gallstones *(arrow)* seen outside the confines of the gallbladder.

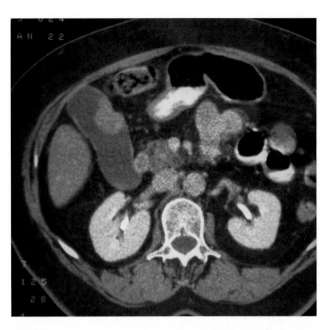

Fig. 6-43   CT demonstrates a soft-tissue mass in the wall of the gallbladder in this patient with gallbladder carcinoma.

patients who are asymptomatic and whose lesions are discovered fortuitously have a higher 5-year survival rate. The etiology of gallbladder cancer is poorly understood. It must include the possibility of malignant degeneration of gallbladder adenomas. The development of gallbladder cancer in patients with calcified gallbladder walls (porcelain gallbladders) is thought to be extremely high, ranging between 20% and 30%.

The relationship between gallstones and the development of gallbladder cancer remains controversial. However, like gallstone disease, gallbladder cancer is more common among women. Moreover, 80% of patients with gallbladder cancer do have gallstones (Fig. 6-42). The size of the stones has also been suggested as a factor because patients with larger stones have an increased association with gallbladder cancer. The most common presentation of this cancer is a large mass in or around the gallbladder. This is easily demonstrated with CT or ultrasound (Fig. 6-43). The effect of the tumor as it involves adjacent bowel, such as the duodenum or the hepatic flexure of the colon, can be seen with barium studies. The presence of calcium within the gallbladder wall, in cases of porcelain gallbladder, is nicely shown on CT examination. Intraluminal masses arising from the wall may also be seen on ultrasound examination of the gallbladder (Fig. 6-44).

The correct diagnosis, particularly in advanced disease, is often difficult to make because of the marked contiguous spread of disease to the adjacent structures such that the actual site of origin cannot be determined.

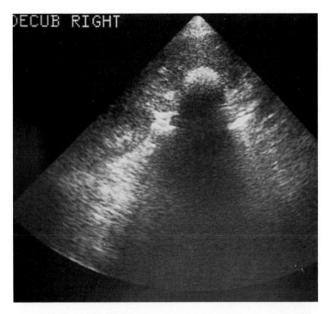

Fig. 6-44   Ultrasound of a patient with porcelain gallbladder demonstrates marked acoustic shadowing. There was also a mass associated with the gallbladder, found to be gallbladder carcinoma.

Metastatic disease

Metastatic disease is an uncommon cause of filling defects within the gallbladder. The most common metastatic lesion is melanoma. The known predisposition of melanoma to metastasize to the GI tract is also known to include the gallbladder in approximately 15% of cases with GI metastatic disease (Fig. 6-45). These metastatic lesions may be solitary or multiple. They are usually identified on ultrasound or OCG as irregular polypoid lesions. In most cases, there is accompanying metastatic disease in the liver.

Thickened Wall

Thickening of the gallbladder wall is an imaging abnormality that can be identified by either ultrasound or computed tomography. It may represent either an actual or an apparent thickening and is related to the underlying condition. The actual thickness of the gallbladder wall is itself a nonspecific finding, and it is difficult to relate a specific measurement of the wall to the underlying disease entity (Box 6-8).

Cholecystitis

Thickening of the gallbladder wall can be identified in either acute or chronic cholecystitis. This can be related to inflammation of the gallbladder wall with infiltration by inflammatory cells, as well as edema. Adjacent edema or fluid can accentuate the appearance of the wall

thickening. The presence of stones with gallbladder wall thickening is pathognomonic of cholecystitis. It becomes more difficult to diagnose without the presence of gallstones (Fig. 6-46).

Cholecystitis in the absence of gallstones is thought to occur in approximately 5% of cases, although the incidence appears to be higher in children. The signs and symptoms are identical to acute cholecystitis caused by gallstones. However, the lack of stones tends to make the diagnosis difficult because the demonstration of the gallstones on imaging is often the central diagnostic feature. The difficulty in correctly diagnosing acalculous cholecystitis is not limited to any one imaging method. There may be faint or no opacification on OCG examination. Ultrasound has also proved to have less than an ideal sensitivity in detecting this condition, with a reported range of 60% to 70%. The diagnostic criterion in the absence of gallstones is often the thickness of the gallbladder wall, which has proved to be more nonspe-

---

Box 6-8 Gallbladder Wall Thickening Identifiable by Ultrasound or CT

Cholecystitis (acute or chronic)
Hyperplastic cholecystoses
Ascites
Edema (congestive heart failure, chronic renal failure, liver failure)
Carcinoma

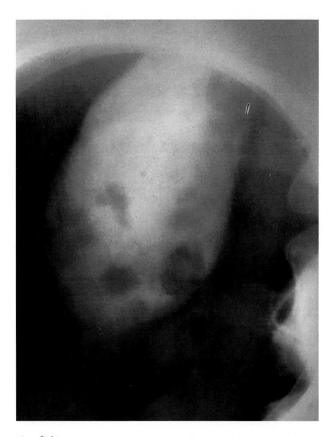

Fig. 6-45 OCG on a patient with known malignant melanoma demonstrates multiple, irregular nonmobile filling defects that proved to be metastatic lesions to the gallbladder.

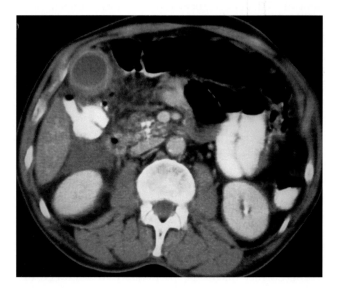

Fig. 6-46 CT at the level of the gallbladder shows marked thickening of the wall with some enhancement in the patient with acute cholecystitis.

cific than previously realized (Box 6-9). The etiology of acalculous cholecystitis is not clear. It has been suggested that patients in the recovery phase from previous trauma, surgery, or severe systemic diseases may be more susceptible to acalculous cholecystitis.

It has been suggested that radionuclide imaging may be more useful in the diagnosis of acalculous cholecystitis because the diagnosis does not hinge on the presence of stones (Box 6-10). However, this has not proved to be the case, and the diagnostic sensitivity is similar to that of ultrasound.

Acute acalculous cholecystitis is considered a more dangerous process than acute calculous cholecystitis with respect to morbidity and mortality. This most likely relates to difficulties in making an early diagnosis.

Adenomyomatosis and cholesterolosis

Adenomyomatosis and cholesterolosis are hyperplastic cholecystoses that can result in some thickening of the gallbladder wall. Adenomyomatosis is the most interesting part of Jutras' classification of hyperplastic cholecystoses. It occurs as a result of poorly understood hyperplastic changes involving the mucosa and muscular wall of the gallbladder and the formation of intramural sinuses, known as the Rokitansky-Aschoff sinuses, which are characteristic of this disease. Involvement of the gallbladder may be diffuse or segmental. There appears to be an increased association with gallstones. The focal fundal type of adenomyomatosis shows char-

acteristic changes involving the gallbladder fundus with round, smooth polypoid filling defects quite frequently accompanied by filling of Rokitansky-Aschoff sinuses with contrast material (Fig. 6-47). Involvement of the gallbladder may also be segmental, with a well-defined narrowed waist within the body of the gallbladder in which marked wall thickening, including sinus formation, may be demonstrated (Fig. 6-48). Diffuse involvement is also well known, with narrowing and irregularity of the gallbladder lumen, possible focal filling defects, and filling of multiple, intramural sinuses.

The diagnosis of segmental or diffuse adenomyomatosis is relatively easy using OCG or ultrasound. Focal adenomyomatosis is somewhat more difficult to diagnose and can be missed. This is supported by the pathological examination of gallbladders in which focal changes are seen more frequently than demonstrated on imaging studies.

Ultrasound demonstrates gallbladder wall thickening and on occasion may demonstrate sinus formation.

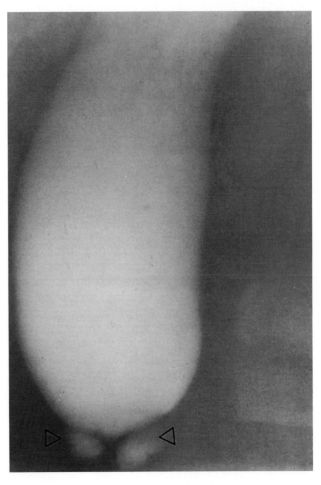

Fig. 6-47 OCG of a patient with adenomyomatosis showing filling of prominent intramural sinuses *(arrowheads)* at the tip of the gallbladder fundus.

Box 6-9 Sonographic Findings of Acute Cholecystitis

Cholelithiasis
Gallbladder wall thickening
Pain over gallbladder (Murphy's sign)
Intramural sonolucency
Pericholecystic fluid/abscess
Gas in lumen

Box 6-10 Causes of False-Positive Biliary Scintigraphy for Acute Cholecystitis

Prolonged fasting
Failure to obtain delayed views
Chronic cholecystitis
Pancreatitis
Systemic illnesses
Gallbladder neoplasm

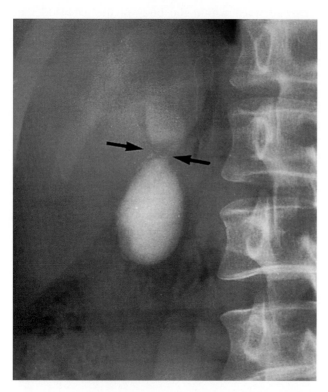

Fig. 6-48   OCG of a patient with segmental adenomyomatosis of the gallbladder, demonstrating focal narrowing *(arrows)* of the body of the gallbladder.

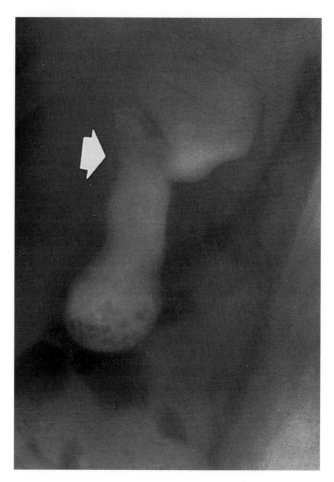

Fig. 6-49   OCG of a patient with right upper quadrant pain demonstrates numerous small gallstones and some deformity of the gallbladder. There is a faint suggestion of filling of intramural sinuses *(arrow)*.

Segmental involvement of the gallbladder is easily demonstrated using ultrasound.

OCG findings in this condition generally include good function and opacification of the gallbladder. There may be filling of the intramural sinuses with contrast material. Quite often this is incomplete, and the addition of a fatty meal or the use of cholecystokinin enhances the demonstration of the Rokitansky-Aschoff sinuses (Figs. 6-49 and 6-50).

Adenomyomatosis represents a benign proliferation of normal tissues and cannot be considered a neoplastic process. There is no evidence that it is premalignant. Many of the patients are asymptomatic. Treatment of symptomatic patients is still somewhat controversial. However, there is evidence to suggest that symptomatic patients who receive cholecystectomy frequently experience abatement of symptoms.

Cholesterolosis has been described in the previous section. In this condition, cholesterol deposits form in the wall of the gallbladder. Often they present as small polyps and are seen as filling defects. Sometimes the deposition is in a diffuse fashion, with an irregular thickened gallbladder mucosa developing, which can be seen with cross-sectional imaging as a thickened wall.

Miscellaneous causes

On occasion, the presence of neoplastic infiltration of the gallbladder wall causes the appearance of wall thickening. This is not a common presentation, however.

When ascites or pericholecystic fluid is present, the gallbladder wall may have the appearance of thickening on ultrasound or CT. Sometimes this is just a spurious finding, however. Any medical conditions that result in edema can cause gallbladder wall thickening because edema develops in the wall of the gallbladder. This is apparent in hypoalbuminemia or other causes of low protein, including liver failure. Patients in chronic or acute renal failure may also develop wall thickening,

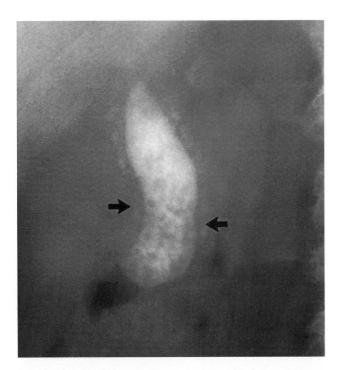

Fig. 6-50   Following ingestion of a fatty meal, the intramural sinuses of Rokitansky-Aschoff faintly seen in Fig. 6-49 are well demonstrated *(arrows)*.

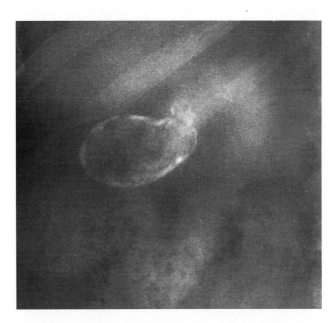

Fig. 6-51   Porcelain gallbladder with segmental calcification throughout the wall.

and this can also be apparent in congestive heart failure as well.

Calcifications

Stones
As previously mentioned, approximately 15% of gallstones contain sufficient calcium to be radiopaque on plain films. CT, being more sensitive to smaller amounts of calcium, yields a somewhat higher percentage. Radiopaque gallstones commonly have calcium in their outer rim. However, calcification can vary in its pattern. Some stones have an irregular, mottled calcification, while others have a laminated appearance. Some stones have a small, central calcified nidus around which radiolucent cholesterol layers accumulate.

Porcelain gallbladder
Porcelain gallbladder is a name given to a gallbladder that has undergone chronic inflammation and subsequent calcification in its wall (Fig. 6-51). The wall is usually thickened and the gallbladder often small and contracted. The cystic duct is always obstructed. The relationship between porcelain gallbladder and gallbladder carcinoma is striking, with gallbladder carcinoma developing in 20% to 30% of patients with porcelain gallbladder. Conversely, it should be noted that the majority of patients with gallbladder carcinoma do not have antecedent porcelain gallbladder.

A small, contracted calcified gallbladder, seen as a rounded, ringlike density in the right upper quadrant, can easily be mistaken for a large gallstone on a plain film of the abdomen (Fig. 6-52).

Milk of calcium bile
Yet another manifestation of chronic cholecystitis and obstruction of the cystic duct is the condition known as milk of calcium bile. This represents a situation in which the bile contained within the obstructed gallbladder becomes radiopaque because of the high concentration of calcium carbonate and its resultant precipitation. This interesting condition can easily be demonstrated by obtaining upright, supine, and decubitus views of the gallbladder in which the fluid character of the radiopacity can be demonstrated (Fig. 6-53). Although the gallbladder is commonly small and contracted, on some occasions the appearance can simulate a contrast-filled gallbladder seen during OCG examination or ERCP.

Miscellaneous

Emphysematous cholecystitis
Emphysematous cholecystitis is a rare condition in which bubbles and streaks of gas appear within the wall and possibly the lumen of the gallbladder (Fig. 6-54). There may be collections of gas in the pericholecystic region as well. The cause of the gas is almost always related to the presence of gas-forming organisms in-

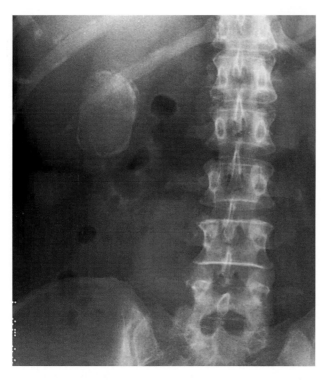

Fig. 6-52 An oblong calcification in the right upper quadrant was initially thought to represent a large calcified gallstone but proved to be a porcelain gallbladder.

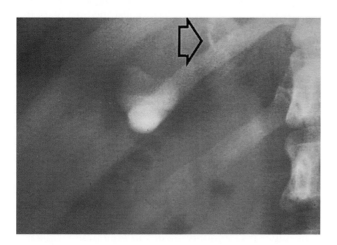

Fig. 6-53 A patient with chronic cystic duct obstruction and milk of calcium bile. Note the layering of the milk of calcium bile in the fundus of the gallbladder on this upright view. Also seen is the calcified stone *(arrow)* obstructing the gallbladder neck and cystic duct.

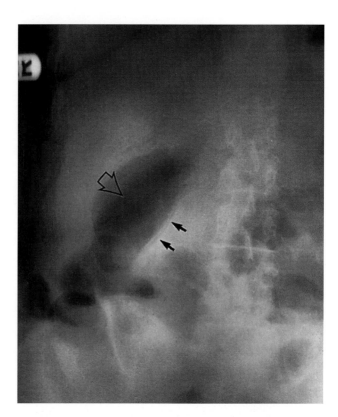

Fig. 6-54 A patient with emphysematous cholecystitis with air seen within the gallbladder lumen *(open arrow)* and the gallbladder wall *(small arrows)*.

> **Box 6-11 Characteristics of Emphysematous Cholecystitis**
>
> Elderly patients, usually men
> Diabetes in approximately half of cases
> High incidence of perforation
> *Clostridium welchii,* a common organism

volved in the infectious and inflammatory processes occurring in or around the gallbladder. The condition is most commonly seen in patients with diabetes mellitus and, unlike most gallbladder inflammatory processes, is more commonly seen in men (Box 6-11).

On plain films of the abdomen the most important diagnostic criterion is intramural gas in the gallbladder wall. Occasionally, mottled collections of gas can be seen around the gallbladder fossa. The radiological finding of gas confined to the gallbladder lumen or the biliary tree without intramural or pericholecystic gas should lead one away from the diagnosis of infection and toward consideration of benign causes of pneumobilia. Moreover, those patients are seldom ill in contrast to the severe toxic state of patients with emphysematous cholecystitis. Clinically, patients with emphysematous cholecystitis present with sudden and rapidly progressive right upper quadrant pain accompanied by fever and elevated white blood cell counts. Treatment and diagnosis must be prompt because the mortality rate is significantly higher than that of the usual acute cholecystitis. The ongoing inflammatory and infectious processes can quickly lead to gangrenous changes within the gallbladder wall, perforation, and catastrophe. The treatment is prompt cholecystectomy.

Gallstone ileus

Gallstone ileus (Box 6-12) is a misleading name of a condition in which the most striking finding is intestinal obstruction. The obstruction results from the erosion of a gallstone (usually larger than 2.5 cm) into the adjacent duodenum, forming a cholecystoduodenal fistula. The stone passes distally until it reaches the narrowest portion of the small bowel in the distal ileum where it becomes lodged, resulting in intestinal obstruction. The condition is much more common in women and generally seen in the older age category.

If the stone is somewhat smaller, it may pass through the gut without resulting in obstruction. The patient may not be left with a cholecystoduodenal fistula, since many of these seal off. However, deformity in both the gallbladder and duodenum is seen on UGI and OCG examinations. Approximately 10% of cholecystoenteric fistulas are between the gallbladder and the adjacent hepatic flexure of the colon. In this instance most stones pass through the colon without causing obstruction. On rare occasions there may be erosion of a gallstone into the adjacent stomach, possibly leading to pyloric obstruction.

In over half of the cases of patients presenting with small bowel obstruction as a result of gallstone ileus, air can be seen within the biliary tree. The absence of air in the biliary tree does not exclude the diagnosis. The presence of a calcified stone in the right lower quadrant may be helpful. Lacking this, diagnosis may be extremely elusive, which accounts for the higher mortality rate seen in this condition than is normally associated with other causes of small bowel obstruction. The erosion of a gallstone into the colon is unlikely to lead to obstruction and may be the preferable site for fistulous communication. On the other hand, residual cholecystocolonic fistula is not a happy proposition to contemplate, with gram-negative coliform organisms ascending the biliary system.

Abdominal CT undertaken for evaluation of possible gallstone ileus should be performed without oral con-trast to increase the possibility of detecting the obstructing stone.

Postcholecystectomy syndrome

Although most patients with symptoms relating to gallstones are cured following cholecystectomy, approximately 5% to 40% have persistence of symptoms or recurrent symptoms. These patients fall within a somewhat confusing category known as the postcholecystectomy syndrome.

Residual common bile duct stones may account for symptoms in a small percentage of patients. However, the routine use of operative cholangiography during cholecystectomy has significantly reduced the incidence of residual stones.

Additionally, intraoperative trauma and resultant injury to either the ductal system or the sphincter of Oddi may be implicated in a small number of patients. In most instances a clear anatomical cause for the symptoms will not be found. Nonbiliary causes such as duodenal or gastric ulcer or pancreatitis should also be considered as potential sources of the symptoms.

There is an increasing tendency to implicate changes in the papilla of Vater in postcholecystectomy syndrome. It is postulated that patients with underlying, unrecognized papillitis or papillary stricture most likely undergo cholecystectomy as a result of their symptoms. Frequently, the pathological changes at the sphincter are not anatomical but physiological, and manometry of this segment, as well as a careful ERCP examination of the biliary tree with delayed images to evaluate for biliary emptying, can be helpful. The common bile duct in symptomatic postcholecystectomy patients tends to be mildly dilated.

VARIATIONS AND ANOMALIES

Phrygian Cap

Normal anatomic variations within the gallbladder, representing either folding of the gallbladder on itself or intraluminal septations, do occur and should not be confused with disease. A fold or septation near the gallbladder fundus is a relatively common finding and represents the well-known "Phrygian cap" (Fig. 6-55), referring to the hats worn by slaves in the ancient Greek province of Phrygia in Asia Minor. This finding is of no clinical consequence.

The size and configuration of the gallbladder can vary considerably from patient to patient. There may also be a variation in the position of the gallbladder. In most patients the gallbladder is located in the subhepatic fossa. In a few particularly tall, slender individuals, the gallbladder is vertically oriented with its fundus in the lower abdomen. In such individuals the gallbladder is frequently on a long mesentery and may be located in ectopic locations (Fig. 6-56). In addition, herniations into the lesser sac through the foramen of Winslow have been reported. Conversely, a small number of people have the gallbladder in an intrahepatic position (Fig. 6-57). Patients with small left lobes of the liver frequently will have a malpositioned gallbladder.

Ectopic Gallbladder

Rarely, the gallbladder is congenitally absent. When this occurs, there is a high incidence of common bile duct stones. This congenital anomaly is also associated with other malformations seen within the cardiovascular system and the GI system. Of course, agenesis of the gallbladder is very difficult to distinguish radiologically from any condition in which the gallbladder fails to function or in which there is obstruction of the cystic duct.

Duplications and Septations

Duplication of the gallbladder and cystic duct has been reported and is extremely rare. Occasionally an apparent double gallbladder can be seen on OCG when a long, slender gallbladder is found to have turned upon itself, giving the appearance of two well-opacified gallbladders. Often these are just septations that may be occurring within the gallbladder

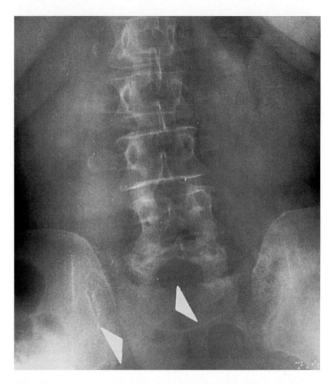

Fig. 6-56 A patient with OCG shows relatively faint opacification of the gallbladder that is located at the pelvic inlet *(arrowheads)*.

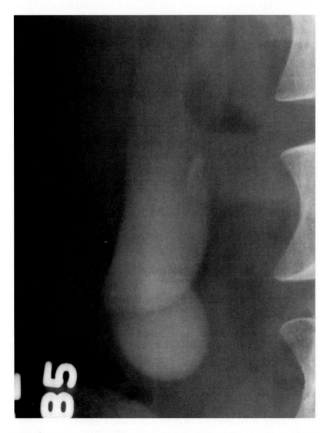

Fig. 6-55 Bandlike narrowing across the fundus of the gallbladder is a "Phrygian cap" deformity and is of no clinical significance.

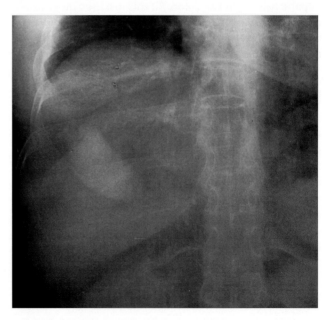

Fig. 6-57 OCG shows good opacification in a patient with an intrahepatic gallbladder.

because of abnormalities in recanalization of the lumen (Fig. 6-58).

With a long, tortuous gallbladder that may be on a mesentery, the potential for torsion of the gallbladder increases. This is unusual but is almost always associated with the aforementioned condition. Clinically, the pre-

sentation is that of severe acute cholecystitis. The potential for gangrenous changes and perforation is greatly increased. Other uncommon causes of gallbladder deformity are pericholecystic adhesions and adhesive bands. These are thought to be congenital in nature and probably of little clinical significance.

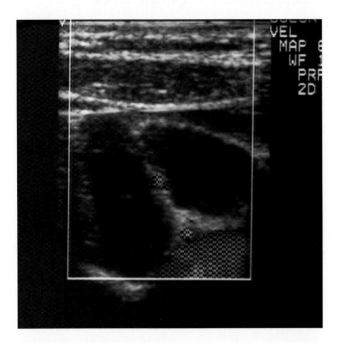

Fig. 6-58 Ultrasound demonstrates two distinct gallbladder lumens because of a duplication.

Anomalous Ductal Insertions

Of great clinical concern is the presence of anomalous position of some of the ducts, since the potential for injury during surgery or interventional procedures is greatly increased. As noted previously, the bile ducts form as a bud from the ventral pancreas and gradually arborize as they branch into the liver. It is not uncommon to see unusual branching patterns of the ducts. Sometimes the major left or right branches are seen to insert quite low into the extrahepatic ducts (Fig. 6-59). It is in these situations that the likelihood of injury during surgery is greatly increased. Some ducts have even been known to drain into the gallbladder or cystic duct.

SUGGESTED READINGS

Berk RN, Armbuster TG, Saltzstein SL: Carcinoma in the porcelain gallbladder, *Radiology* 106:29-31, 1973.

Bucceri AM, Brogna A, Ferrera R: Common bile duct caliber following cholecystectomy: two-year sonographic survey, *Abdom Imag* 19:251-258, 1994.

Chan YL, Chan ACW, Lam WWM, et al: Choledocholithiasis: comparison of MR cholangiography and endoscopic retrograde cholangiography, *Radiology* 200:85-91, 1996.

Chen RC, Liu MH, Tu HY, et al: Value of ultrasound measurement of gallbladder wall thickness in predicting laparoscopic operability prior to cholecystectomy, *Clin Radiol* 50:570-578, 1995.

Crittenden SL, McKinley MJ: Choledochal cyst—clinical features and classification, *Am J Gastroenterol* 80:643-647, 1985.

Delius M, Ueberle F, Gambihler S: Destruction of gallstones and model stones by extracorporeal shock waves, *Ultrasound Med Biol* 20:251-258, 1996.

Fromm H: Gallstone dissolution therapy: current status and future prospects, *Gastroenterology* 91:1560-1567, 1986.

Hall-Craggs MA, Allen CM, Owens CM: MR cholangiography: clinical evaluation in 40 cases, *Radiology* 189:423-427, 1993.

Haller JO: Sonography of the biliary tract in infants and children, *AJR* 157:1051-1058, 1991.

Huntington DK, Hill MC, Steinberg W: Biliary tract dilatation in chronic pancreatitis: CT and sonographic findings, *Radiology* 172:47-50, 1989.

Jutras JA: Hyperplastic cholecystoses, *AJR* 83:795-827, 1960.

Kim OH, Chung HJ, Choi BG: Imaging of the choledochal cyst, *Radiographics* 15:69-88, 1995.

Koehler RE, Melson GL, Lee JKT, et al: Common hepatic duct obstruction by cystic duct stone: Mirizzi syndrome, *AJR* 132:1007-1009, 1979.

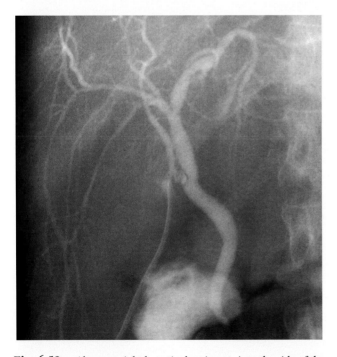

Fig. 6-59 Aberrant right hepatic duct inserts into the side of the cystic duct. It was narrowly missed at surgery and was evident only during the cholangiogram.

Kumar A, Aggarwal S: Carcinoma of the gallbladder: CT findings in 50 patients, *Abdom Imag* 19:304-310, 1994.

Larsen CR, Scholz FJ, Wise RE: Diseases of the biliary ducts, *Semin Roentgenol* 11:259-267, 1976.

LaRusso NF, Wiesner RH, Ludwig J, et al: Primary sclerosing cholangitis, *N Engl J Med* 310:899-903, 1984.

Li-Yeng C, Goldberg HI: Sclerosing cholangitis: broad spectrum of radiographic features, *Gastrointest Radiol* 9:39-47, 1984.

Malet PF, Baker J, Kahn MJ, et al: Gallstone composition in relation to buoyancy at oral cholecystography, *Radiology* 177:167-169, 1990.

Mall JC, Gharemani CG, Boyer JL: Caroli's disease associated with congenital hepatic fibrosis and renal tubular ectasia, *Gastroenterology* 66:1029-1035, 1974.

Miller WJ, Sechtin AG, Campbell WL, et al: Imaging findings in Caroli's disease, *AJR* 165:333-340, 1995.

Moliver CL, Saltzstein EC: Common bile duct distensibility after cholecystectomy, *Southern Med J* 84:719-721, 1991.

Mujahed Z: Factors interfering with the opacification of a normal gallbladder, *Gastrointest Radiol* 1:183-185, 1976.

Poppel MH, Jacobson HG, Smith RW: *The Roentgen aspects of the papilla and ampulla of Vater,* Springfield, Ill, 1953, Charles C Thomas.

Reinhold C, Bret PM, Guibaud L, et al: MR cholangiopancreatography: potential clinical applications, *Radiographics* 16:309-331, 1996.

Rizzo RJ, Szucs RA, Turner MA: Congenital abnormalities of the pancreas and biliary tree in adults, *Radiographics* 15:49-68, 1995.

Rooholaminia SA, Tehrani NS, Razavi MK, et al: Imaging of gallbladder carcinoma, *Radiographics* 14:291-310, 1994.

Sackmann M, Delius M, Sauerbruch T, et al: Shock-wave lithotripsy of gallbladder stones, *N Engl J Med* 318:393-397, 1988.

Savader SJ, Benenati JF, Venbrux AC, et al: Choledochal cysts: classification and cholangiographic appearance, *AJR* 156:327-331, 1991.

Schuster DM, Pedrosa MC, Robbins AH: Magnetic resonance cholangiography, *Abdom Imag* 20:353-361, 1995.

Sheng R, Campbell WL, Zahko AB, et al: Cholangiographic features of biliary strictures after liver transplantation for primary sclerosing cholangitis: evidence of recurrent disease, *AJR* 166:1109-1116, 1996.

Steinberg HV, Torres WE, Nelson RC: Gallbladder lithotripsy, *Radiology* 172:7-11, 1989.

van Sonnenberg E, Hofmann AF, Neoptolemus J, et al: Gallstone dissolution with methyl-tert-butyl ether via percutaneous cholecystostomy: success and caveats, *AJR* 146:865-867, 1986.

Taourel P, Bret PM, Reinhold C, et al: Anatomic variants of the biliary tree: diagnosis with MR cholangiopancreatography, *Radiology* 199:521-527, 1996.

Wastie ML, Cunningham IGE: Roentgenologic findings in recurrent pyogenic cholangitis, *AJR* 119:71-77, 1973.

Wedmann B, Borsch G, Coenen C, et al: Effect of cholecystectomy on common bile duct diameters: a longitudinal prospective ultrasonographic study, *J Clin Ultrasound* 16:619-624, 1988.

Weltman DI, Zeman RK: Acute diseases of the gallbladder and biliary ducts, *Radiol Clin North Am* 32:933-954, 1994.

Wiot JF, Felson B: Gas in the portal venous system, *AJR* 86:920-929, 1961.

Colon and Rectum

The colon and rectum are two of the more common sites for disease in the gut, with a wide spectrum of disease processes encountered on a daily basis in medical practice. However, the steady increase in the incidence and mortality resulting from colorectal cancer (CRC) has focused both the medical and lay communities' attention on early detection and potentially effective screening strategies for this disease. With the advent of colonoscopy and the refinement of air-contrast barium enemas (ACBE), there has been some improvement in overall survival and mortality rates in the last 40 years. However, until recently there has been relatively little detailed analysis of the screening strategies put forth at various times by various groups. In recent years, more careful scrutiny has shown most screening strategies to be either not efficient or not very cost effective.

As a result, the question of an efficient and cost-effective method of screening may be considered, to some extent, not entirely answered at this time. It appears that the barium enema, whose demise was announced by our gastroenterology colleagues in the late 1970s and early 1980s, is still quite useful. Indeed, the barium enema could be a better and more cost-effective method of examining the colon than previously realized and will undoubtedly play a role in future screening strategies. However, before we see that, many questions regarding screening for colorectal cancer remain to be answered. Among the choices or combination of choices for screening, what is the most cost-effective method? Or, even more fundamental, does any form of widespread screening for colorectal cancer actually reduce mortality in the population, such as has been shown with mammography for breast cancer, or the Pap test for cervical cancer? At this point there is accumulating data suggesting that this may be the case. Thus the U.S. Preventive Services Task Force has recommended that screening for colorectal carcinoma be performed for all persons over 50 years of age with annual fecal occult blood tests (FOBT), while the American Cancer Society and the World Health Organization recommend yearly FOBT and flexible sigmoidoscopy (FS) every 3 to 5 years. While the intent is commendable, screening that does not examine the entire colon is a curious proposition, given that at least 50% of lesions will be proximal to the area of examination. The American College of Physicians, in considering the evaluation of the entire colon as a necessity for appropriate screening, has proposed screening strategies to include FS, colonoscopy, and ACBE at 10-year intervals. There is considerable evidence that the most efficient and least cost-effective method of screening is colonoscopy. Additionally, there is evidence that the most cost-effective method is a combination of ACBE and FS.

EXAMINATION TECHNIQUES

Double-Contrast Barium Enema

Although the number of barium enemas has declined over the last decade, there appear to be a renewed interest and increased use of the double-contrast barium enema (DCBE). The DCBE study remains one of the mainstays in the diagnostic evaluation of the colon. It is an effective and relatively inexpensive method for evaluation of the entire colon. Good double-contrast technique is also reliable for excellent evaluation of the rectum. The detection rate for CRC varies somewhat from study to study but is probably about 94%. The ability to detect small polyps (less than 1 cm) is less than with colonoscopy, while ACBE has been shown to be the equal of colonoscopy in detecting larger polyps (greater than 1 cm). The risk of perforation is considerably less than with colonoscopy (10 to 25 times). The examination can be done quickly and requires no sedation, no extended time off work, and no accompanying person to drive the patient home.

The three types of contrast enemas used today are the DCBE, the single-contrast barium enema (SCBE), and the water-soluble contrast enema. It is beyond the scope of this book to instruct in the technique and mechanics of performing these examinations. However, it is important to discuss certain general principles regarding how a radiologist decides which type of examination to use in a given clinical situation.

The DCBE is, for all practical purposes, considered the standard radiological examination of the colon (Fig. 7-1). However, there are still very good indications for both the SCBE and the water-soluble contrast enema. The issue, of course, rests on preexamination diagnostic goals. In patients with bleeding, mild to moderate degrees of diarrhea, nonspecific abdominal pain, or a risk for polyp or cancer development, the DCBE study will be used. These patients require an efficient bowel preparation, for which a variety of commercially prepared products are available. The polyethylene glycol electrolyte solution for colonic lavage is becoming popular. It is the same preparation commonly used for colonoscopy. The tendency of this type of bowel preparation to leave the colon clean but wet can be dealt with by the administration of bisacodyl suppositories at appropriate intervals before the examination (Figs. 7-2 and 7-3). The use of all bowel preparations should be made with some knowledge of the patient's current clinical status and the diagnostic questions to be addressed. In some instances, particularly in inflammatory bowel disease or bowel obstruction, colonic bowel preparation may require modification or, in some cases, be totally omitted.

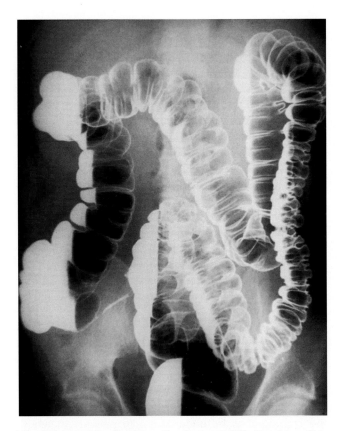

Fig. 7-1   A right decubitus film from a DCBE. Decubitus films with compensation filtration are the most important overhead views in this examination.

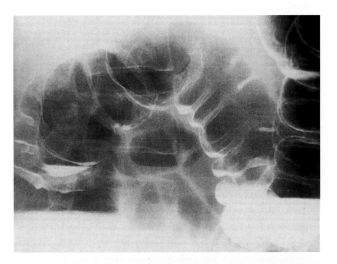

Fig. 7-2   Air-contrast examination in which residual fluid makes coating of the ascending and transverse colon ineffectual. Lesions can easily be missed under these circumstances. Rotating the patient and washing the area with barium can result in additional coating.

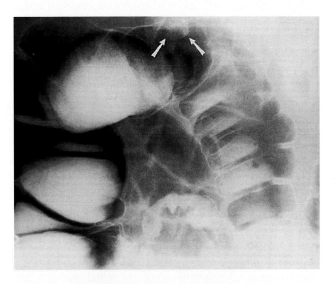

Fig. 7-3   Same patient as shown in Fig. 7-2. Because of the wetness and poor coating of the right colon, the patient was rotated and additional barium was allowed to wash over the area, demonstrating a rounded polyp on the superior margin of the hepatic flexure *(arrows)*.

Double-contrast technique consists of administering a high-density, low-viscosity barium into the colon followed by air insufflation and the demonstration of the entire mucosal surface of the rectum and colon. In the well-prepared patient, this is a sensitive examination detecting cancer in approximately 94% of cases. It is also able to detect early mucosal inflammatory changes. The guiding principle in the performance of this, like all radiological procedures, is to achieve a high-quality examination that results in maximum information about the state of the patient's colon. Having said this, it should also be a high priority of the examining radiologist to attempt to achieve this goal with certain well-founded patient concerns in mind.

The technologist who prepares the patient for the examination will, no doubt, explain the examination in detail and do much to allay most of the patient's concerns. Nevertheless, it is not advisable for the physician practicing radiology to first meet the patient while that patient is on the fluoroscopic table with a rectal tube in place. Despite the acknowledgment that it is an efficient examination for the detection of disease, the barium enema over the decades has achieved a notorious reputation among lay people as a well-devised

form of medical torture. With this in mind, it is the wise radiologist who will endeavor to use every psychological and physical advantage in attempting, to some extent, to debunk this reputation, while at the same time not sacrificing the efficiency of the examination.

The psychological state of the patient is often crucial to the successful completion of the study, and this is particularly the case in the more difficult examinations. Thus, it is not unreasonable to greet the patient before the examination, elicit a brief history, explain the examination, and address whatever concerns the patient has regarding the study. It is also important that the radiologist not lose sight of patient anxiety, discomfort, and embarrassment that are commonly associated with this procedure. All of these issues can be addressed during the course of the examination. The number of films, fluoroscopic time, and overall radiation exposure should be kept to the minimum necessary to achieve an efficient examination. The radiologist should strive to ensure that the amount of time the patient spends on the fluoroscopic table is as short as possible. Concerns with patient dignity and modesty should be dealt with by making sure the patient is properly draped at all times. Many radiologists have perfected the procedure to the point where they are able in many instances to remove the rectal tip relatively early in the examination. This results in a significant decrease in patient discomfort and an increased patient tolerance for the remainder of the study. Indeed, there are also excellent diagnostic reasons for early removal of the rectal tip, since low rectal lesions can be missed if the tip or balloon obscures the lesion (Figs. 7-4 and 7-5).

For similar reasons, some radiologists prefer the tableside fluoroscopic examination to remote control facilities. In some cases the patient will need to be talked through the difficult parts of the examination, and being beside the patient with a hands-on directive approach can sometimes make the difference between success and failure. A spectral voice emanating from a loudspeaker somewhere in the room while the table moves and the overhead tower arcs above the patient will do little to allay the anxieties of many patients. Of course, controversy and disagreement exist on this issue while the number of remote units in use continues to grow. Nevertheless, whether tableside or remote fluoroscopic technique is used, it is clear that the patient is the center of the radiological practice, and it is reasonable therefore to expect that radiologists practice patient-centered rather than machine-centered radiology. Moreover, there is perhaps no other area in radiology where this can be practiced with such gratifying results as fluoroscopy.

Single-Contrast Barium Enema

In most large medical centers, approximately 85% of barium enema studies are double-contrast examinations. However, 15% of the patients will have well-defined reasons for using the SCBE. Before the study, the radiologist should carefully review the goals of the study to establish the technique to be undertaken. In patients in whom colonic obstruction must be excluded, a single-contrast examination will suffice to address the question. In many cases these patients have undergone incomplete bowel preparation or none at all.

In questionable cases of diverticulitis, some radiologists prefer the single-contrast examination, feeling that the radiological findings of diverticulitis are better demonstrated with a single-contrast study. This is based on the supposition that dilute barium will flow more readily into intramural or paraluminal tracts or abscesses than will the more viscous double-contrast barium.

In instances where patients are impaired and cannot move or roll to the extent required for a successful DCBE study, a single-contrast study should be seriously considered. This is particularly the case in older, debilitated, severely mentally retarded, or extremely ill patients. Although a double-contrast examination has been shown to be more sensitive for the detection of both inflammatory and polypoid processes, a bad double-contrast examination is worse than a bad single-contrast examination. This is a good rule of thumb to remember, and, given a choice in a situation where a very limited or poor DCBE is possible, one should opt for the single-contrast study.

Water-Soluble Contrast Enema

There is an increasing but limited role for the water-soluble contrast enema. This is almost entirely for the

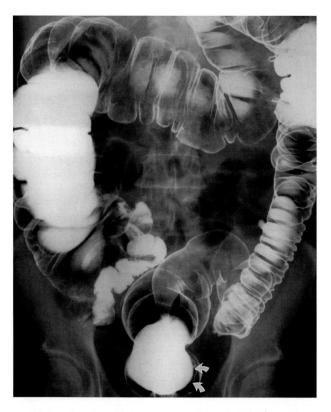

Fig. 7-4 DCBE overhead film. A rectal carcinoma is obscured by the barium pool and the retained rectal tip and balloon. A subtle edge of the mass is all that is visible *(arrows)* on this study.

evaluation of a patient with suspected perforation. Quite frequently these patients have experienced recent trauma, instrumentation, or surgery. The water-soluble contrast enema may also be used in the evaluation of a colon in which the potential for perforation may be high. This includes patients with colonic dilatation and particularly a cecum that may be acutely dilated to a preperforation state.

Additionally, a limited examination to rule out colonic obstruction can be performed with water-soluble contrast, since many of these patients require a computed tomography (CT) examination of the abdomen within the next few hours or days. Retained colonic barium causes severe CT artifacts, making the examination useless and resulting in delays in the workup in such patients.

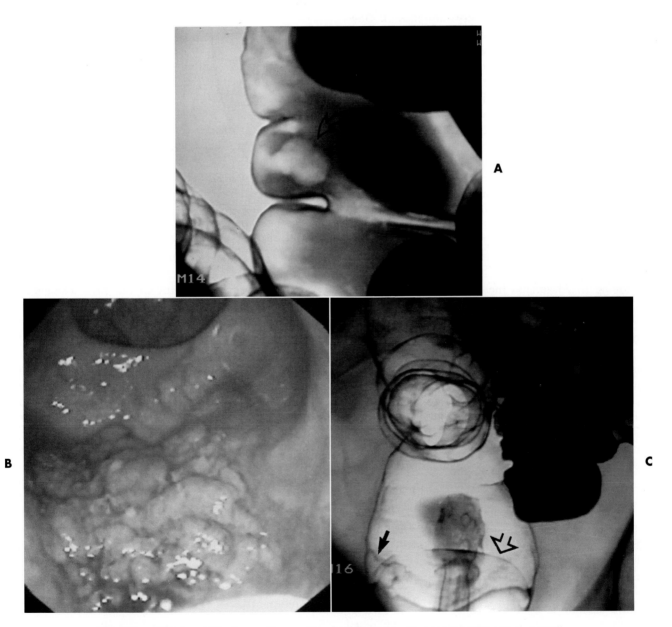

Fig. 7-5   Digital spot film from a 51-year-old male evaluated for Hemoccult-positive stool. A small pedunculated polyp is seen in the ascending colon (**A**). On colonoscopy, a rectal carcinoma is also discovered (**B**). Review of films with image processing (**C**) demonstrates the irregular margin of the rectal lesion *(closed arrow)* mostly obscured by the rectal balloon *(open arrow)*.

Computed Tomography and Magnetic Resonance Imaging

The role of CT continues to become more important in colonic diagnosis. The ability of CT imaging to detect bowel wall thickening makes it somewhat more sensitive in the detection of diverticulitis than is the barium enema. In addition, paraluminal abscesses are readily identified with CT. The ability to evaluate adjacent structures is clearly an added dimension of the examination. Although the occasional dramatic demonstration of a colonic malignancy with CT is encountered (Fig. 7-6), there is no direct role at the moment for CT in the primary evaluation of colonic polyps and masses. However, this will probably change over the next decade with the refinement of CT colonography, or what has sometimes been loosely referred to as "virtual colonoscopy," a name probably best avoided. Three-dimensional (3D) intraluminal images are generated using thin-section helical CT scans of the abdomen and pelvis following colonic insufflation of air or carbon dioxide gas. This must be preceded by a thorough bowel preparation. Software permitting volume and perspective techniques is used to achieve a progressive 3D passage through the colonic lumen evaluating the mucosal surface along the way. The technique is still in the embryonic stage with many technical difficulties to be overcome. However, the early work is startling and dramatic, holding exciting possibilities for the near future.

Although CT is able to demonstrate bowel wall thickening to advantage, the evaluation of superficial inflammatory disease within the colon or adjacent small bowel requires additional examinations, either colonoscopy or barium studies.

The role of magnetic resonance imaging (MRI) in colorectal imaging is extremely limited at this time. However, there are increasing interest and activity in the use of MRI in evaluating rectal tumors for staging purposes. Although there is some evidence to suggest that MRI may be slightly superior to CT in evaluating the extent of tumor invasion of pelvic structures, it apparently is less reliable in the detection of abnormal nodes.

Ultrasound

Except for abscess detection, there is a relatively little role for conventional ultrasound in the evaluation of colonic abnormalities. Although some early success has been reported using conventional ultrasound to examine water-filled colons, its potential as a routine method of colon evaluation is questionable. However, the use of endoscopic sonography in the evaluation of rectal disease has increased in most medical centers with clinical research indicating that it is as accurate as, if not more accurate than, CT in the detection of disease,

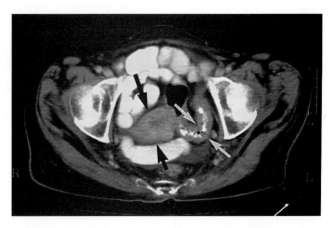

Fig. 7-6   CT scan on 35-year-old female with breast cancer looking for metastatic disease. Scan reveals thickening of the sigmoid colon *(white arrows),* which proved to be primary carcinoma of the colon. The other mass in the pelvis *(black arrows)* is the uterus.

evaluation of the extent of disease, and determination of the absence or presence of affected regional lymph nodes. This is a safe examination with no significant complications reported to date.

SOLITARY FILLING DEFECT

The radiological problems of the colon and rectum will be discussed as they relate to standard intraluminal contrast examinations of the colon. Other imaging techniques will be included as part of the relevant discussion of the radiological problem under consideration.

Filling defect is a term historically rooted in the development of the SCBE and suggests displacement of barium by a space-occupying entity. Hence, for a focal area, a thinner barium column is presented for the x-ray beam to penetrate, resulting in less attenuation and producing a focal lucency. The term is used frequently when describing polypoid lesions on double-contrast studies, although technically these are usually not filling defects in the strict definition.

The radiological problem of an intraluminal filling defect presents a wide variety of diagnostic possibilities and can be divided into benign neoplastic, malignant neoplastic, and a wide assortment of miscellaneous causes (Box 7-1). Inflammatory causes of a solitary filling defect are rare.

Adenoma

Most adenomatous polyps are solitary. However, in the presence of carcinoma, the incidence of multiple adenomatous polyps increases. Approximately 25% of patients with colorectal cancer have one or more adenomatous polyps elsewhere in the large bowel. There is also a suggestion that the presence of multiple hyperplastic polyps may be associated with an increase in the number of adenomas. Moreover, the chance for multiplicity clearly increases with age.

Adenomatous polyps histologically fall within the classification of tubular, tubulovillous, and villous adenoma. The villous adenoma tends to have the greatest malignant potential, while the tubular adenoma has the least. Adenomatous polyps are primarily tubular adenomas and frequently are smooth surfaced or lobulated. They may be sessile or pedunculated, having a stalk of varying lengths (Figs. 7-7 and 7-8). The stalk is usually composed of normal mucosal tissue and is often associated with larger polyps. Progressive peristaltic activity results in stretching of the base of the polyp and, over a prolonged period, elongation into a well-defined stalk. The villous adenoma has the typical frondlike papillary surface, often described by pathologists as being "velvety." They are almost always sessile, and the amount of lobulation may be considerably more than is seen with the tubular adenoma. Moreover, the superficial "carpet lesions" of colon are almost always villous adenomas or superficial carcinomas (Fig. 7-9). These surface characteristics, so familiar to radiologists, hold true for polyps greater than 1 cm but are less reliable for smaller lesions. The classic presentation of a villous adenoma is that of a patient presenting with watery diarrhea as a result of fluid and electrolyte loss from the large surface area of the lesion. In truth this classic clinical presentation is, as with many "classic presentations," uncommon, but will eventually be encountered (Fig. 7-10).

The frequency of adenomatous polyps in the general population has been found to vary markedly from study to study. Autopsy studies may provide the most consistent data, placing the incidence between 10% and 30% of the population. The incidence increases significantly with age.

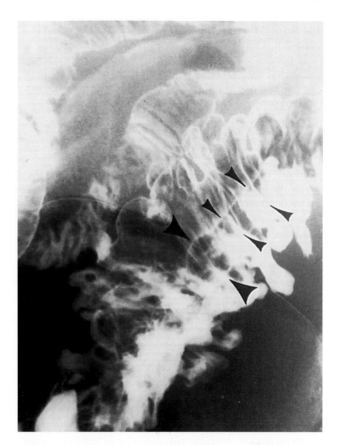

Fig. 7-7   DCBE in a patient with severe diverticular disease of the sigmoid colon. A polyp on a long stalk is present *(arrowheads)* but is obscured by the multiple diverticula.

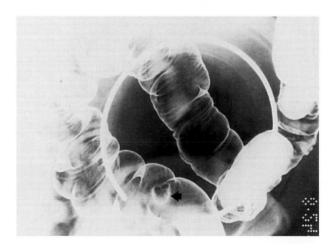

Fig. 7-8   A sessile sigmoid polyp *(arrow)* is demonstrated on a DCBE.

Various studies have indicated that most adenomatous polyps are found in the rectosigmoid region. It has been estimated that as many as 50% of adenomas occur in this area, although in recent years some research has suggested a so-called proximal migration of colonic polyps. This may represent a combination of an increasingly aging population and improvements such as colonoscopy and DCBE in examining the colon.

It is now widely accepted that the great majority of colorectal cancers result from malignant transformation of benign adenomatous polyps, the adenoma-carcinoma sequence. Estimations of the risk of malignant degeneration are imprecise; however, the well-differentiated tubular adenomas have a smaller risk than the more volatile villous adenomas. The incidence of cancer is 0.01% in polyps less than 5 mm and about 1% in polyps 1 cm or smaller. In polyps greater than 2 cm, the incidence increases to 30% to 40%. The time progression of adenoma to carcinoma evolution is estimated at between 10 and 15 years, although startling exceptions are encountered from time to time (Fig. 7-11).

Most adenomas are asymptomatic. By far the most common presentation is rectal bleeding, either occult or overt. Additionally, polyps can act as the lead point for intussusception, although this is unusual in the colon. The classic association of large villous adenomas with loss of fluid and electrolytes (especially potassium) is infrequently encountered.

The detection rate of polyps is higher with double-contrast technique than with single-contrast technique. However, a high kilovoltage, full-column technique, using fluoroscopic manipulation and compression, may have an equally high yield for polyps greater than 1 to 2 cm. Polyps less than 1 cm are detected with less frequency in both types of studies, although the ability to detect smaller polyps appears to be significantly higher in double-contrast studies than in single-contrast studies.

The radiographic appearance of polyps on full-column, single-contrast studies is often that of the traditional filling defect. The demonstration on double-contrast studies is somewhat more complex, since this technique provides the ability to literally see through the colon, observing both mucosal surfaces at the same time. As a result, the polyp can be seen profiled, en face, or tangentially, resulting in different well-known appear-

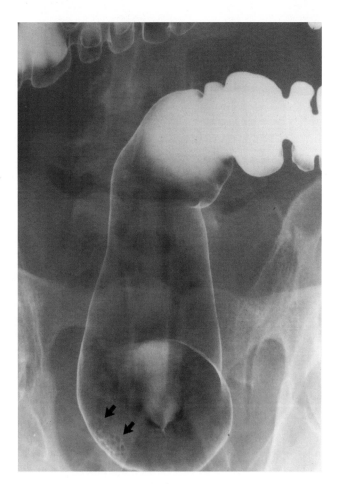

Fig. 7-9 Focal nodularity (carpet lesion) of the rectum *(arrows)* proved to be villous adenoma.

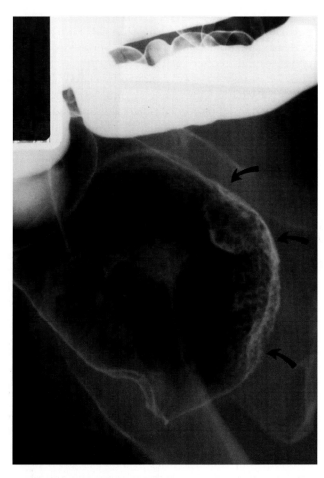

Fig. 7-10 Large carpet lesion of the anterior rectum *(arrows)* in a patient presenting with diarrhea and incontinence. Lesion proved to be large villous adenoma.

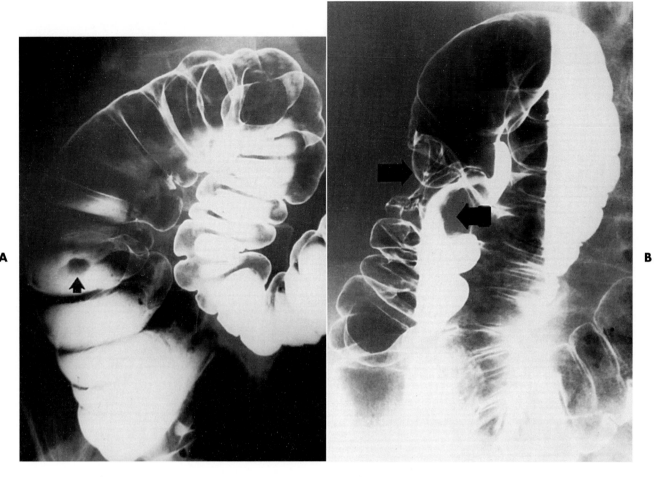

Fig. 7-11   **A,** Barium enema discloses a 1.5-cm pedunculated polyp in the ascending colon *(arrow).* **B,** In the same patient, a DCBE obtained less than 2 years later reveals an annular carcinoma at the site of the polyp on the earlier examination.

ances, such as the Mexican hat sign or the bowler hat sign (Fig. 7-12). Evaluation of the polyp should include size, the presence or absence of a stalk or pedicle, description of the surface features, and the presence or absence of ulceration. With respect to size, it should be remembered that at least a 25% magnification distortion, on average, should be figured into the final estimation of the polyp size.

Interestingly, the polyp that often provides the most difficulty in radiological diagnosis during DCBE is the polyp on a long stalk (Fig. 7-13). Because it shifts position with the various views, it may be misinterpreted as residual stool. Occasionally, these polyps can be quite large, reminding us that the interpretation of double-contrast studies must, by necessity, include a meticulous evaluation of the various lines and contours of the colon. There is a dictum in gastrointestinal (GI) radiology that double-contrast radiology of the colon is an excellent examination, with the only difficulties being lesions that are extremely tiny or those that are extremely large. This can, on occasion, become an embarrassing reality.

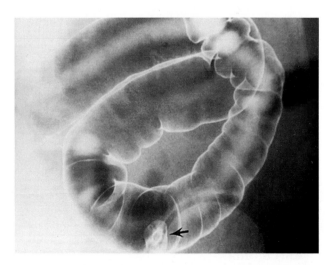

Fig. 7-12   Sigmoid spot film demonstrates a polyp *(arrow)* with a central "ring shadow" representing barium coating of the short stalk of the polyp. This configuration is sometimes known as the Mexican hat sign.

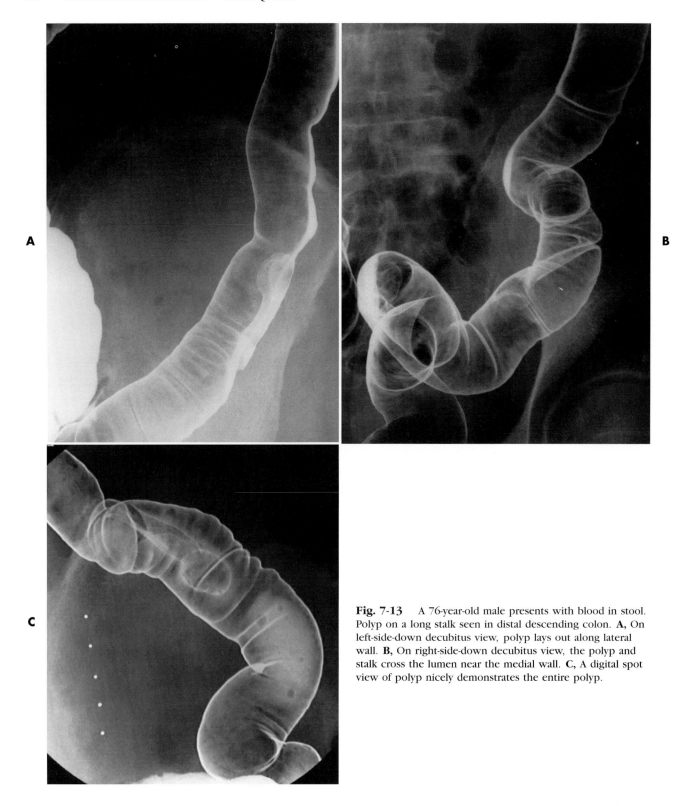

Fig. 7-13   A 76-year-old male presents with blood in stool. Polyp on a long stalk seen in distal descending colon. **A,** On left-side-down decubitus view, polyp lays out along lateral wall. **B,** On right-side-down decubitus view, the polyp and stalk cross the lumen near the medial wall. **C,** A digital spot view of polyp nicely demonstrates the entire polyp.

Carcinoma

In 1996, 134,000 new cases of colorectal carcinoma were diagnosed. Around 55,000 deaths were attributable to this disease in 1996. It is estimated that approximately 130,000 to 135,000 new cases of colorectal carcinoma will have been diagnosed in 1998. In 1992, the estimate was between 150,000 and 160,000. The rate has leveled off and is beginning to decline. Mortality rates have also declined in recent years, after several decades of stability, falling approximately 1.5% to 1.9% per year between 1990 and 1994. It still remains the most common newly diagnosed malignancy behind cancer of the prostate, breast, and lung. The incidence of colon cancer is approximately 2½ times that of rectal cancer. Only lung cancer exceeds colorectal cancer in terms of cancer deaths. However, for any given patient, survival depends on how early the lesion is diagnosed. The Duke's classification, on which the staging of colorectal carcinoma is based, reflects both the extent of tumor involvement and the prognosis. Duke's stage A represents lesions confined to the bowel wall and has an 85% 5-year survival rate. Duke's stage B represents lesions that have extended through the bowel wall, and these are associated with a 70% 5-year survival rate. With Duke's stage C representing metastatic lesions to regional lymph nodes, the survival rate falls to 33%. Distant metastatic disease, Duke's stage D, has a 5% 5-year survival rate. It has been estimated that as many as 40% to 50% of patients have hepatic metastatic disease at the time of diagnosis.

In an attempt to define a universally more applicable and orderly process across the world, the American Joint Committee on Cancer introduced the tumor-node-metastases (TNM) classification for colorectal malignancies (Box 7-2). The classification attempts to classify the extent of the primary lesion (T), extent of spread to regional nodes (N), and the presence or absence of distant metastatic lesions (M). Individual cases are assigned according to the extent of disease based on TNM values and are further grouped into five stages, 0 to IV.

The TNM classification is in common usage at institutional tumor boards or conferences all over the country and most of the world and is crucial in the uniform randomization of patients for various ongoing therapeutic trials.

Colorectal carcinoma continues to be mainly a disease of Western industrialized nations. It is a disease of older people, with the median patient's age at diagnosis in the 60s.

The etiological and epidemiological data associated with this disease are ponderous and cannot be addressed in detail. It is clear that the issues and controversies surrounding the possible etiologies are becoming more openly discussed in the lay media as the nation becomes more conscious of nutrition and health. The controversy surrounding suspected etiologies and associated risk factors includes dietary intake, with particular emphasis on increasing the ingestion of dietary fiber and decreasing the ingestion of animal fats. Recent observations have been put forth suggesting that intake of vitamin C or aspirin on a regular basis may confer some degree of protection. In 1997, there were reports that vitamin E bestowed some protection from the disease. These are interesting possibilities but require considerable further investigation.

There are, however, some things about which we are more certain, and one is that most colorectal cancers

---

Box 7-2 American Joint Committee on Cancer (AJCC) Tumor Node Metastases Staging System

STAGE 0

Carcinoma in situ—T_{is}, N0, M0

STAGE I

Tumor invading submucosa—T1, N0, M0
Tumor invading muscularis propria—T2, N0, M0

STAGE II

Tumor penetrates beyond muscularis propria into subserosal but not peritoneum—T3, N0, M0
Tumor penetrates into peritoneum or directly invades other structures or organs—T4, N0, M0

STAGE III

Any degree of bowel wall penetration with regional lymph node spread
N1 1-3 pericolic or perirectal lymph nodes involved
N2 4 or more lymph nodes involved
N3 Metastatic disease in any lymph node along a vascular trunk
Any T, N1 or N2 or N3, M0

STAGE IV

Tumor invasion of bowel wall with or without lymph node involvement, but distant metastatic disease
Any T, any N, M1

---

progress through the adenoma-to-cancer route. A few may arise de novo from dysplastic changes within the mucosal surface, although this is felt to be uncommon in patients without inflammatory bowel disease (IBD). We know that with IBD, in particular, ulcerative colitis carries a higher risk for the development of colorectal cancer. We know that certain familial polyposis syndromes carry an extremely high if not absolute certain risk of cancer. We also know that colorectal cancer can run in certain families with sporadic manifestation, and that in approximately 25% of new cases there is a family history of colorectal cancer. Furthermore, it has been estimated that individuals who are first-generation relatives of patients with colorectal cancer have a 10% to 15% increased risk above that of the general population.

Hereditary nonpolyposis colorectal cancer (HNPCC) has been recognized in recent years as a disease of autosomal-dominant inheritance in which colon cancers arise via the recognized adenoma-to-cancer mechanism, but the marked colonic polyposis of familial polyposis (hundreds or thousands of polyps) does not occur. The definition of HNPCC has recently been standardized. Families must have at least three relatives with CRC, one of whom must be a first-degree relative of the other two.

CRC must involve at least two generations and one must occur before age 50. It should also be noted that these families may be further divided as being at risk for only CRC (Lynch syndrome I) or other cancers (particularly of the female genital tract) in addition to CRC (Lynch syndrome II). It is estimated that HNPCC may account for as many as 5% to 6% of colorectal cancers (Box 7-3).

The clinical presentation of colorectal carcinoma is, to a large extent, dependent upon the site of the lesion. During early stages of growth, the patient may be asymptomatic, or there may be undetected occult bleeding (Fig. 7-14). The most insidious lesions usually arise from

the right side of the colon. This occurs because the wider luminal diameter, greater distensibility of the right colon, and more liquid nature of the colonic content on the right side delay the onset of obstructive symptoms and allow the lesion to become larger and invasive before the diagnosis is finally made (Fig. 7-15). Patients with right-sided lesions often present with bleeding. They may experience crampy, nonspecific right-sided abdominal pain. However, by far the most common presenting problem is iron deficiency anemia as a result of chronic blood loss. Tumors on the left side, in the descending and sigmoid colon, tend to present earlier. This is a result of the smaller luminal diameter of the colon in this region and the firmer colonic content. Changes in the luminal diameter, secondary to tumor growth, will most commonly result in obstruction. However, an interesting but not uncommon exception should be mentioned regarding left-sided lesions. Some tumors in the sigmoid or descending colon that are slow growing can attain significant size without resulting in the expected obstruction. Because of the indolent nature of the lesion, its physical

---

Box 7-3   Risk Factors of Colorectal Cancer

Habitation in an industrialized region of the world
Diet
Familial polyposis
Family history of hereditary nonpolyposis colorectal cancer
Chronic ulcerative colitis
First generation family member with colorectal cancer
Presence or history of colonic adenomatous polyps

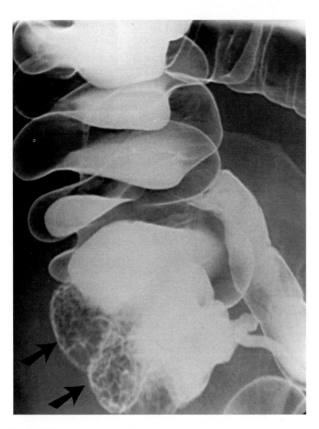

Fig. 7-14   A 53-year-old patient presents with Hemoccult-positive stool. ACBE demonstrates superficial spreading carcinoma of the cecum *(arrows)*.

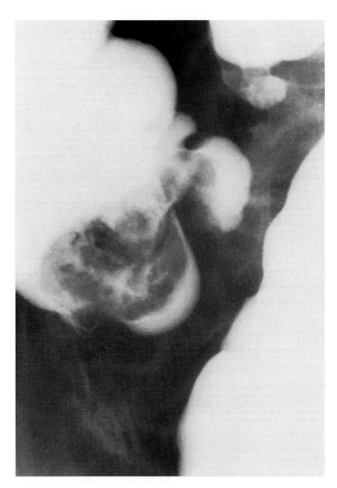

Fig. 7-15   Single-contrast examination of the colon reveals a large, lobulated cecal mass representing an adenocarcinoma. The mass is ulcerated on its surface and is nonobstructing.

contours to some extent can be molded by the fecal stream, assuming a form of "flap valve" configuration. Thus, it is possible to find a distal lesion with complete retrograde obstruction on barium enema, with no physical or radiological evidence of antegrade obstruction (Fig. 7-16). Lesions in the rectum commonly present with bright red bleeding and changes in bowel habits. Generally, lesions in the distal colon are detected earlier and survival is somewhat better. Approximately 50% of lesions are found distal to the mid-descending colon. On rare occasions, colonic adenocarcinoma can perforate, and the patient may present with a pericolic abscess. Also seen infrequently are lesions with ischemic changes immediately proximal to the malignancy (Fig. 7-17).

Given the impact of this disease in terms of the morbidity and mortality, a complete examination of the colon is required. Although flexible sigmoidoscopy can examine up to 50 cm, this still results in approximately half of the lesions being undetected. Colonoscopy permits direct examination of the mucosal surface of the entire length of the colon. However, the examination is incomplete in 10% to 30% of attempts (Fig. 7-18). Colonoscopy is a relatively expensive undertaking, although it can be of considerable value because it

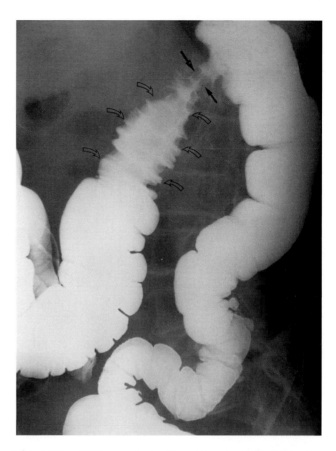

Fig. 7-17   SCBE on patient with carcinoma of the distal transverse colon *(black arrows)* and evidence of fold thickening proximal to the lesion *(open arrows)*, which proved to be ischemic changes.

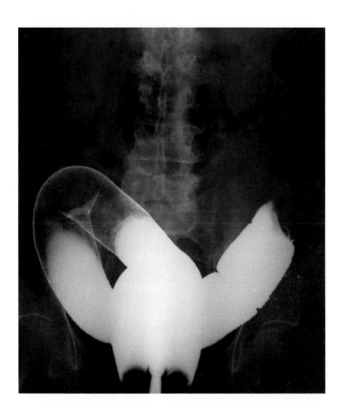

Fig. 7-16   A 68-year-old female presents with GI bleeding, but no evidence of bowel obstruction. ACBE demonstrates obstructing lesion at junction of sigmoid and descending colon. The retrograde obstruction is complete. However, note the radiological evidence of complete lack of antegrade obstruction.

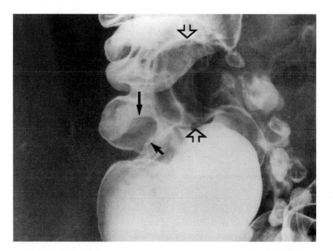

Fig. 7-18   A 65-year-old female presents with Hemoccult-positive stool. Colonoscopy is incomplete and the right colon is unexamined. An ACBE demonstrates a lesion arising in *(open arrows)* and around *(closed arrows)* the ileocecal valve.

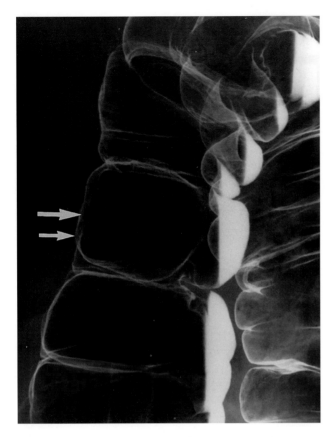

Fig. 7-19   A 70-year-old female with family history of carcinoma of the colon. An ACBE demonstrates an focal area of marginal irregularity in the ascending colon *(arrows)*. Biopsy revealed it to be superficial spreading carcinoma.

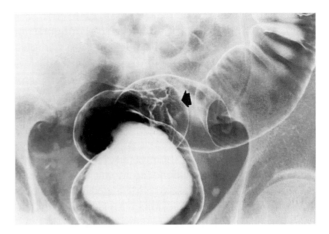

Fig. 7-20   Spot film from a DCBE reveals a focal area of raised, irregular mucosa with radiation toward a small, central mound *(arrow)*. Biopsy revealed villous adenoma with malignant degeneration.

Box 7-4   Radiological Presentations of Colorectal Cancer

COMMON

Annular lesions
Polypoid lesions

LESS COMMON

Infiltrative lesions with little mass effect
Superficial surface (carpet lesions)

---

permits removal of polyps and the retrieval of tissue specimens for pathological diagnosis.

The DCBE is a relatively low-cost examination with a high rate of detection for colorectal cancers (approximately 94%) and an extremely low rate of incomplete examinations. Moreover, this examination is considerably safer than instrumentation, having one tenth the incidence of bowel perforation associated with colonoscopy.

Problems associated with DCBE relate to bowel preparation and coexistent diverticular disease. Both of these factors can render the examination less sensitive. The presence of extensive diverticular disease in the sigmoid region results in such significant bowel distortion that it may be virtually impossible to identify a polypoid lesion. It is possible that single-contrast compression views of this area would be much more useful in detecting polypoid lesions in this situation. Additionally, residual stool can be troublesome. Double-contrast examinations ought to include decubitus views, which can often sort out these problems. Other areas of difficulty include the ileocecal region and the wall of the ascending colon, where subtle or occult lesions can hide

(Fig. 7-19). The majority of missed colorectal carcinomas on double-contrast examination have been shown to be errors of perception. The importance of meticulous and careful analysis of double-contrast views of the colon cannot be overstated. Interpretation of these studies is an exercise in self-discipline and concentration.

The radiological findings of colorectal cancer can include a number of configurations (Box 7-4), from round polypoid filling defects to encircling, constricting lesions. They can also be seen as raised, ulcerated masses or as irregular, villous-appearing lesions (Fig. 7-20). The more subtle lesions may be manifested as distortions in the normal haustral pattern or bowel wall contours (Figs. 7-21 and 7-22).

Frequently CT evaluation of the abdomen reveals a soft-tissue mass adjacent to or within the colonic lumen (Fig. 7-23). One should take care not to misinterpret a prolapsed ileocecal valve or stool as a cecal mass (Figs. 7-24 and 7-25). There may be evidence of extension of the tumor beyond the wall, or involvement of adjacent organs, such as lymph nodes or the liver. Ultrasonography may demonstrate a large hypoechoic mass with some central echoes representing thickened bowel wall

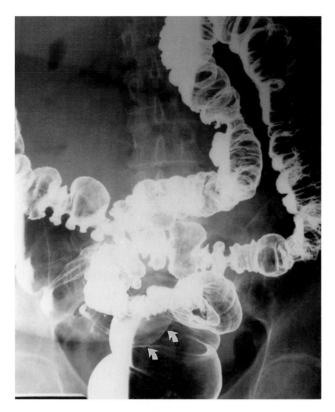

Fig. 7-21   A polypoid lesion of the rectum *(arrows)* seen clearly only on the left decubitus film.

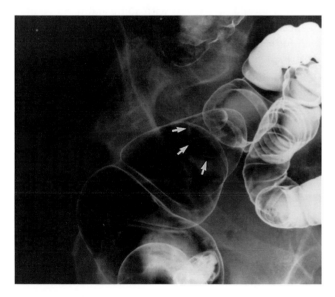

Fig. 7-22   A 58-year-old male presents with Hemoccult-positive stool. A very subtle polypoid carcinoma is seen in the sigmoid as an abnormal margin *(arrows)*.

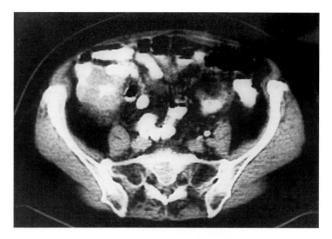

Fig. 7-23   CT of the pelvis in an anemic patient reveals a mass within the cecum with extension beyond the cecal wall posteriorly. There is no evidence of obstruction, and the lesion proved to be an adenocarcinoma.

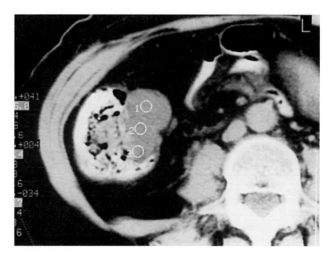

Fig. 7-24   CT scan on a patient with vague abdominal complaints. A cecal mass was diagnosed *(circles),* and a barium enema was obtained for further evaluation (see Fig. 7-25).

and the central lumen, respectively. This is nonspecific and certainly can be seen in other conditions, such as lymphoma, Crohn's disease, or intussusception. Transrectal endosonography has been shown to be a potentially useful technique in the evaluation of the spread of rectal carcinoma into the perirectal soft tissues. Early reports suggest that it is more accurate than CT in evaluating the extent of invasion.

One of the more unusual lesions under the category of rectal carcinomas is the cloacogenic carcinoma (Fig. 7-26). This is a rare tumor seen at the anorectal junction and arising from remnants of the cloacal membrane. The lesion is aggressive, and in over half of the patients lymphatic spread will have occurred at the time of diagnosis. The tumor is variable in its radiological presentation. It is most commonly seen on the anterior rectal wall and has all the appearances of a typical bulky rectal adenocarcinoma. Additionally, well-defined submucosal masses or mucosal plaques may be seen.

Synchronous colorectal cancer lesions are uncommon and occur in no more than 1% to 2% of cases. It

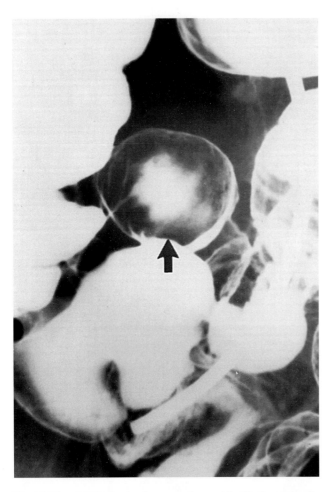

Fig. 7-25 DCBE obtained on a patient with CT diagnosis of a cecal mass (see Fig. 7-24) shows a normal cecum. Reflux into the terminal ileum demonstrates some focal dilatation without evidence of obstruction or disease *(arrow)*. This fluid-filled terminal ileum, partially prolapsed through the ileocecal valve, accounts for the CT findings.

is said that metachronous lesions, which is a second lesion discovered subsequently and unrelated to the previous lesion, can occur in approximately 5% of patients.

Lipoma

Lipomas of the colon are not common but do represent the next most common benign tumor of the large bowel after adenomas. They are mostly solitary lesions and can occur anywhere within the colon, although the right side appears to be the most frequent site.

The lesion is usually asymptomatic, but erosions or ulcers on the mucosal surface overlying the lipoma can result in bleeding. The lipoma, in general, is 1 to 3 cm in size and rarely exceeds 4 cm. It shows the typical

radiological findings of a submucosal lesion with a smooth surface and a right or obtuse angle formed with the adjacent mucosal surface. Occasionally, there can be some pedunculation of the lipoma. Because of the softness of the tumor, it is known that these lesions, particularly the larger ones, can change shape with compression, and this can be a helpful method of differentiating them from other neoplasms. The old diagnostic trick of performing a water enema to demonstrate the lipoma (which is less than water density) is virtually useless. CT of a sufficiently large lesion (greater than 2 cm) can definitively demonstrate the lipoma as a fatty tumor. Lipomatous infiltration of the ileocecal valve is not considered a neoplastic process.

Stromal Cell Tumor (Leiomyoma)

Although common in the more proximal GI tract, these benign mesenchymal tumors are relatively uncommon in the colon (Fig. 7-27). They also present as a submucosal mass with the usual radiological findings (Fig. 7-28). The patients are mostly asymptomatic. Bleeding from ulceration on the stretched mucosal surface over the stromal cell tumor may result in the patient's presenting with rectal bleeding or anemia. On rare occasion, the stromal cell tumor may act as a lead point for an intussusception. However, intussusception in adults should be viewed with some alarm, since most of these are the result of malignant lesions.

Another rare mesenchymal tumor that has been described in the colon is the hemangioma. These are often located distally in the colon and are almost always multiple. An interesting sidelight to this neoplasm is the occasional demonstration of calcified phleboliths on plain films. These patients most commonly present with bleeding.

Carcinoid Tumor

Approximately 85% to 90% of all carcinoid tumors of the GI tract occur in the appendix and are benign. The ileum is the next most common site. Within the colon, the more common sites are the rectum and, to a lesser degree, the cecum. The incidence of rectal carcinoids has been increasing over the last few decades. The tumors are often quite small, measuring 1 cm on average. However, they may also be of considerable size, particularly in the right side of the colon. The smaller lesions may have a typical mucosal polypoid appearance on barium enema. The larger lesions may be indistinguishable from an adenocarcinoma. Overall survival appears to be greater with the rectal lesions. In general, survival with malignant carcinoids is related to the size of the tumor at the time of diagnosis.

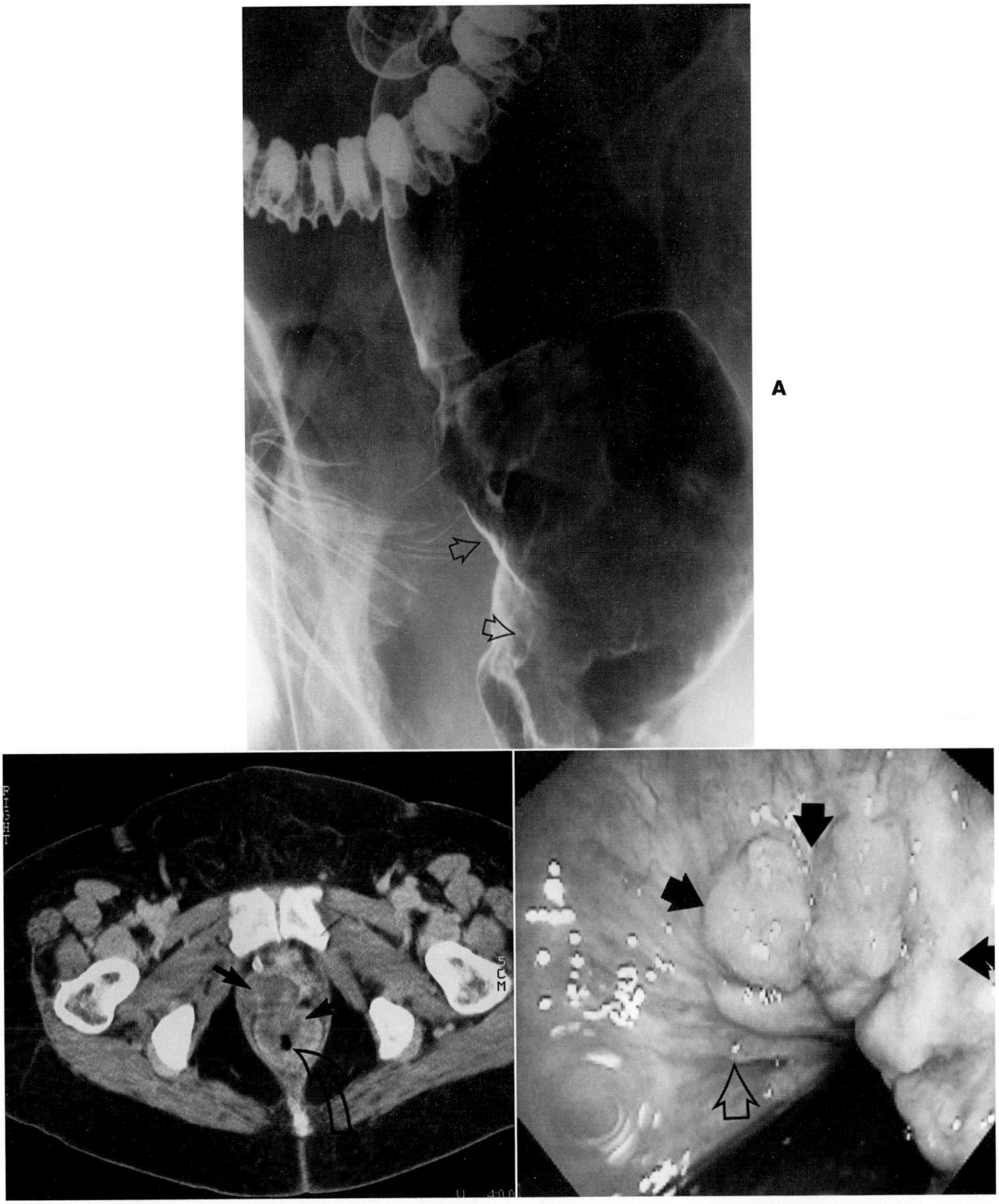

Fig. 7-26   A 71-year-old female presents with low rectal mass with extension into the vagina. **A,** ACBE shows anterior wall nodular rectal mass *(arrows)*. **B,** CT demonstrates rectal mass with anterior extension *(black arrows)*. A rectal lumen is also demonstrated *(open arrow)*. **C,** Retroflexed sigmoidoscope view shows nodular mass *(arrows)* on low anterior rectal wall. Biopsy and resection confirmed a cloacogenic carcinoma. The anterior *(black arrows)* and posterior *(open arrow)* margins are shown.

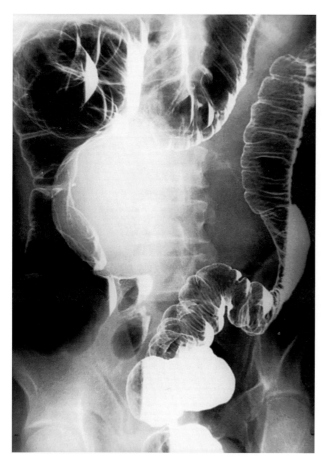

Fig. 7-27 A large leiomyoma is arising from the medial wall of the ascending colon. The lesion is largely exophytic in nature.

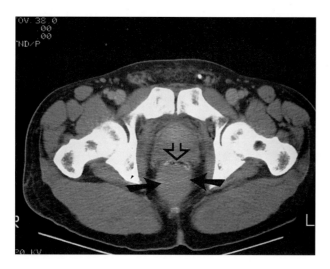

Fig. 7-28 A 54-year-old male presents with rectal mass. CT shows mass in posterior rectal wall *(black arrows)* with some anterior displacement of the rectal lumen *(open arrow)*. Surgical resection revealed stromal cell tumor.

Lymphoma

Lymphoma is a relatively uncommon tumor of the colon and probably represents less than 1% of all malignant neoplasms of the large bowel. The most commonly involved area tends to be the right side of the colon, particularly the cecum. The clinical presentation includes weight loss, weakness, diarrhea, and bleeding. A palpable mass may be discovered if the lesion is sufficiently large. Obstruction is unusual.

The most common radiological presentation is a large, bulky lesion identical in appearance to an adenocarcinoma. Less commonly, it may present as a diffuse nodular or polypoid process. Of interest is the occasional case of Burkitt's lymphoma of the colon, which is seen in the small bowel and colon of children and young adults in North America. This disease is histologically identical to that described by Dennis Burkitt in Uganda during the 1950s that almost exclusively involved children, with the primary site being the mandible. In some parts of Africa, it is the most common malignant neoplasm of childhood. The lesion has been linked to the Epstein-Barr virus. The North American variety of Burkitt's lymphoma more commonly occurs intraabdominally. When colonic involvement is present, it is usually in the ascending region (Fig. 7-29).

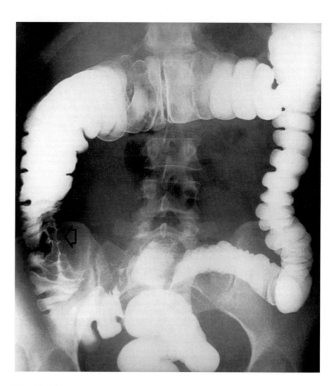

Fig. 7-29 Burkitt's lymphoma involving the ascending colon *(arrow)*.

Colonic Duplication

Colonic duplication is thought to result from intra-uterine vascular insults. They can occur virtually anywhere, from cecum to rectum. The duplication may or may not communicate with the main colonic or rectal lumen. The symptoms depend on the amount of luminal narrowing associated with the mass effect of the duplication. This condition is rare.

Inverted Appendiceal Stump

In a patient with a history of appendectomy, a round, smooth mucosal defect in the cecal tip at the expected orifice of the appendix is almost invariably an inverted appendiceal stump. However, there can be some irregularity associated with the stump, usually as a result of suture granuloma, which may give a suspicious appearance radiologically and result in the necessity of direct visualization (Fig. 7-30). Adenocarcinoma of the appendiceal stump is seen on rare occasion (Fig. 7-31).

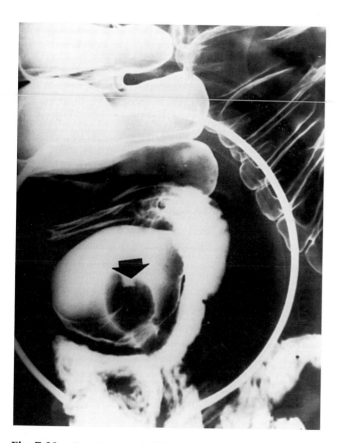

Fig. 7-30   Prominent and slightly irregular polypoid filling defect *(arrow)* at the expected site of the inverted appendiceal stump. Finding represents a variant of normal inverted appendiceal stump, most likely a result of suture granuloma.

Unusual Diverticulum

Under normal circumstances, there is no difficulty in differentiating diverticula from intraluminal filling defects. The so-called unusual diverticulum does occur and can present as a filling defect. This can happen for a couple of reasons. The diverticulum may invert into the lumen, producing a smooth, rounded filling defect (Fig. 7-32). Additionally, the diverticulum may become dis-

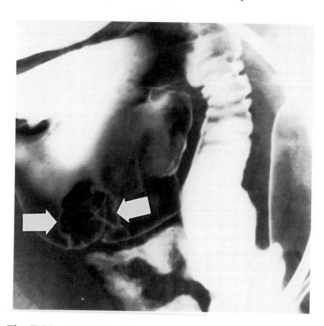

Fig. 7-31   A lobulated filling defect at the cecal tip *(arrows)*. Endoscopic follow-up demonstrated adenocarcinoma arising from the appendiceal stump.

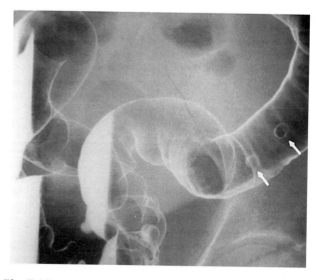

Fig. 7-32   Two small, circular lesions *(arrows)* seen in the proximal sigmoid. Both proved to be diverticula. Note how the barium margin fades toward the center of the more distal lesion, an expected finding with a diverticulum. Note that tangential projection of the upper defect gives a "bowler hat" appearance to this diverticulum.

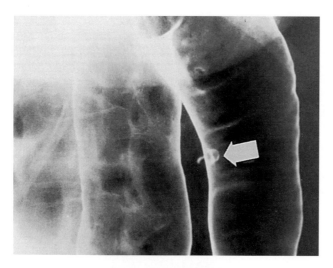

Fig. 7-33 A rounded, smooth filling defect in the splenic flexure *(arrow)* appears to represent a typical polyp. However, a small amount of barium has seeped into the diverticulum and is projected outside the lumen, revealing this polypoid lesion to be a diverticulum.

tended and impacted with stool, some of which may project into the lumen, resulting in a filling defect. During fluoroscopic evaluation, this problem can often be sorted out by the use of compression technique or by rotating the patient in an attempt to profile the diverticulum. Additionally, postevacuation films commonly show some barium within the diverticulum that occurred during evacuation (Fig. 7-33).

Foreign Bodies

Occasionally, medication or vitamin tablets that have traversed the entire small bowel and arrive intact and undissolved in the colon are seen. These are mobile and usually present little difficulty in diagnosis. Metallic foreign bodies in the colon or rectum are not a diagnostic problem. Plastic, glass, latex, and rubber are less obvious but usually apparent.

MULTIPLE FILLING DEFECTS

Hyperplastic Polyps

Hyperplastic polyps of the colon represent the most common type of colonic polyp. The incidence and number of polyps tend to increase with age. Histologically, one finds evidence of epithelial hyperplasia with accompanying elongation and cystic dilatation of the glandular structures. These polyps are also referred to as "metaplastic polyps." They are thought to present no increased risk of malignancy.

Radiologically, the polyps are usually small, measuring from a couple of millimeters to a centimeter, and are almost always sessile. While in themselves the hyperplas-

tic polyps are associated with no particular clinical symptomatology, they do present some difficulty during barium enema because of the inability of the radiologist to distinguish between small adenomatous polyps and hyperplastic polyps. There is also considerable difficulty during colonoscopy in making the differentiation. This and recent observations that suggest that the number of diminutive polyps (less than 5 mm) that are adenomatous is greater than previously thought has led to the assertion that all colorectal polyps should be removed, regardless of size. This position is controversial in the light of widely accepted data that the incidence of carcinoma in adenomatous polyps under 1 cm is less than 1% and is considerably less in polyps under 5 mm in size. Although there is little or no evidence to indicate any malignant potential in hyperplastic polyps, some concern has been expressed regarding the company they keep. There have been reports of increased incidence of both adenomas and carcinomas in patients with multiple hyperplastic polyps of the colon.

Polyposis Syndromes

The various colonic polyposis syndromes are compared in Table 7-1.

Familial polyposis

Familial polyposis represents the most well-known and important of the colonic polyposis syndromes. It is inherited as an autosomal dominant trait with equal distribution among males and females. The frequency of persons with the gene for this disease is somewhere between 1:7000 to 1:8000 in the general population. The first appearance of colonic adenomatous polyps is usually manifested during the teen years. Polyps, although predominantly concentrated within the colon, may also be seen within the stomach, small bowel, and rectum (Fig. 7-34). The large bowel is usually carpeted with several hundred to several thousand small adenomatous polyps.

The disease may be relatively asymptomatic until rectal bleeding occurs (Fig. 7-35). The patients may present in their 20s or 30s with vague abdominal pain or diarrhea, as well as occult or frank rectal bleeding. Because the potential for malignant transformation is so great, frank rectal bleeding may be indicative of the presence of a malignant lesion. Indeed, in two thirds of patients, malignant degeneration has already occurred at the time of diagnosis. If untreated, patients with familial polyposis eventually develop colon cancer, usually during their 30s or 40s.

Radiological examination discloses a colon carpeted with multiple, small polypoid lesions. Distribution may be uniform throughout the large bowel, or it may be more concentrated on the left side. Examination of the stomach and small bowel should also be included as part

Table 7-1 Colonic polyposis syndromes

Syndrome	Type	Inheritance	Other GI sites	Extra-GI manifestations	Cancer risk
Familial polyposis	Adenomatous	Autosomal dominant	Stomach, duodenum, small bowel	Uncommon	High (100%)
Gardner's syndrome*	Adenomatous	Autosomal dominant	Polyps mostly limited to colon	Epidermoids, cysts, fibromas, osteomas	High (100%)
Turcot syndrome	Adenomatous	Autosomal recessive	None	CNS tumors, mostly glioblastomas	High; malignant CNS tumors
Peutz-Jeghers syndrome	Hamartomatous	Autosomal dominant	Small bowel most common, but also stomach, rectum	Perioral pigmentations, GU abnormalities in women	Low (2%-3%); increased risk of breast cancer
Juvenile polyposis	Hamartomatous	Possibly autosomal dominant	Mostly limited to colon, rarely generalized in gut	Increased incidence of congenital malformations, retroperitoneal fibrosis	Low (10%)
Cronkhite-Canada syndrome	Mixed inflammatory/ hamartomatous	Unknown	Stomach, small bowel, rectum	Alopecia, skin pigmentations, onychodystrophy	Low (10%)
Cowden's syndrome (multiple hamartoma syndrome)	Mixed hamartomatous/ fibrosis	Autosomal dominant	Esophagus to rectum	Skin keratoses, oral papillomas, faciotrichilemmomas, thyroid abnormalities	Low; increased risk of breast cancer

CNS, Central nervous system; *GU*, genitourinary.
*May be a variant of familial polyposis.

of the patient's workup to evaluate for the presence of polyps in these sites. Gastric and duodenal polyps can be detected in approximately half of the patients.

Gardner's syndrome

Gardner's syndrome, representing a form of colonic adenomatous polyposis, has been a recognized syndrome since the 1950s and is characterized by extracolonic manifestations such as epidermoid cysts, fibromas, and osteomas of the skull.

It is also inherited by autosomal dominant transmission. It is felt, at this time, that this syndrome most likely represents a variant of familial polyposis. The potential for malignant transformation, as in familial polyposis, is 100% if untreated. Radiological evaluation of the colon discloses numerous colonic polyps. Frequently, the number of polyps is less than is seen in typical familial polyposis. Additionally, some of the polyps may be large and pedunculated. A significant number of these patients also present with symptoms that result from malignant transformation (Fig. 7-36).

Turcot syndrome

This is a rare colonic polyposis condition characterized by adenomatous polyps of the colon, usually larger and in fewer numbers than are seen in Gardner's syndrome or familial polyposis. The syndrome also includes

central nervous system (CNS) tumors, most commonly glioblastoma multiforme and astrocytomas. Despite the high risk of colon cancer, most patients die early as a result of their CNS lesions. The syndrome is thought to be inherited as an autosomal recessive process.

Peutz-Jeghers syndrome

Peutz-Jeghers syndrome is an unusual autosomal dominant inherited disorder consisting of GI polyps, usually of hamartomatous origin, accompanied by mucocutaneous pigment changes of the face and perioral region. The polyps may be asymptomatic or associated with hemorrhage or intermittent small bowel intussusception. The patient may present with iron-deficiency anemia or intermittent cramping and abdominal pain.

The small bowel is the most common site for polyps in the Peutz-Jeghers syndrome, although polyps are seen in the colon and stomach. Polyp size can be variable, from a few millimeters to 2 to 3 cm. The number of polyps can also be variable.

Radiologically, the polyps of this syndrome are indistinguishable from adenomas. The main clinical factor, which raises the level of suspicion, must be the pigmented mucocutaneous lesions that often precede the appearance of the GI symptoms.

Peutz-Jeghers syndrome appears to be associated with a slightly increased risk of GI cancer. However, it is unknown whether the carcinoma arises as part of the hamartomatous process, or spontaneously and coincidentally. At this time, the latter perspective seems to be favored.

Women with this syndrome appear to have an increased risk for developing breast carcinoma. There may also be some slight increase in ovarian cancer in these patients.

Juvenile polyposis

Juvenile polyposis is a disorder thought to be inherited as an autosomal dominant trait. These polyps are hamartomas and may be solitary or multiple, occurring in the colon and rectum of children or young adults.

These polyps can result in GI bleeding, intussusception, and even obstruction. In recent years there has been some increased attention directed at the relationship between this condition and a possible increased risk of carcinoma. However, the polyps are not neoplastic

and no actual malignant degeneration of a polyp composed of hamartomatous elements is known. There may be an increased incidence of adenomatous polyps in these patients.

Associated extracolonic manifestations may include congenital abnormalities and malformations as well as an increased incidence of retroperitoneal fibrosis. Radiologically, the polyps can attain surprisingly large proportions. Quite often they are pedunculated. Occasionally, the larger polyps break free of their stalk, resulting in significant rectal bleeding.

An isolated juvenile polyp, and in some cases, multiple juvenile polyps, can be seen with a negative family history and does not appear to represent the inherited form of juvenile polyposis.

Cronkhite-Canada syndrome

Cronkhite-Canada syndrome was first described in the mid-1950s and is an apparent nonfamilial polyposis

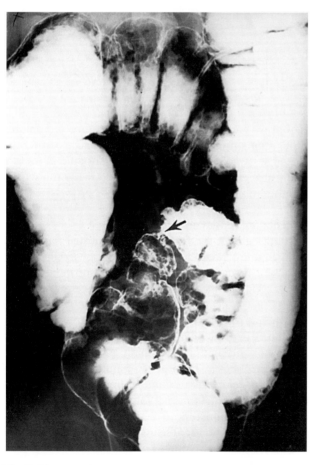

Fig. 7-34 Overhead film from a DCBE reveals numerous polyps throughout the entire length of the colon. An area of stricturing *(arrow)* representing malignant degeneration is demonstrated in the mid-sigmoid in this patient with familial polyposis.

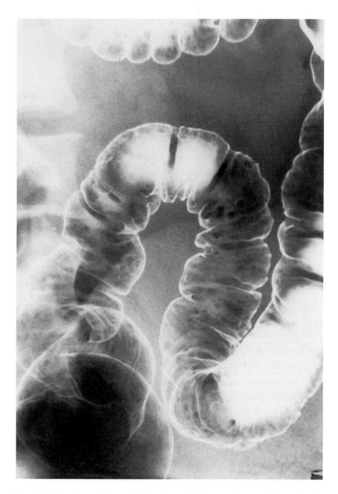

Fig. 7-35 Spot film of the sigmoid in a patient with a family history of familial polyposis. The patient is asymptomatic, and the examination was undertaken because of the family history. Numerous, small sessile polyps are seen throughout the sigmoid and the remainder of the colon.

syndrome. The condition is characterized by GI polyps that can be distributed throughout the gut from stomach to rectum. Associated extragastrointestinal manifestations include alopecia, onychodystrophy, and hyperpigmented lesions of the skin.

The polyps tend to be most numerous in the small bowel, although colonic polyps are not uncommon. Patients are often middle-aged and present with diarrhea relating to an associated protein-losing enteropathy. Although the initial reports considered the polyps to be adenomas, subsequent studies consistently demonstrated a lesion resembling a juvenile polyp with hamartomatous and inflammatory elements. Occasional reports of colon cancer in patients with this condition have raised the question of whether there may be a slightly increased risk.

From a clinical perspective, the chronic diarrhea appears to present more of a threat to the patient's health than the presence of GI polyps does.

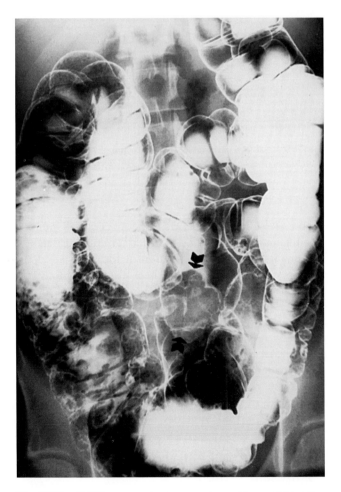

Fig. 7-36 DCBE on a patient presenting with rectal bleeding and a family history of Gardner's syndrome. Multiple polyps of varying sizes are seen throughout the colon. A large, lobulated distal sigmoid mass *(arrows)* is seen and was found to be a polypoid carcinoma.

Cowden's syndrome

Cowden's syndrome is uncommon and is characterized by multiple hamartomatous polyps of the esophagus, stomach, small bowel, and colon. The polyps themselves are not known to be associated with any clinical symptoms. The significant aspect of the syndrome is the extragastrointestinal manifestations, which include skin changes, perioral papillomas, faciotrichilemmomas, thyroid abnormalities (including goiter and cancer), and an increased risk of breast cancer.

Neurofibromatosis

Neurofibromatosis (von Recklinghausen's disease) is a condition in which the most well-known manifestations are multiple subcutaneous neurofibromas. Involvement of the gut with disseminated neurofibromatosis is unusual but does occur. Although involvement of the gut is usually associated with the cutaneous manifestations, the disease may also be confined to the GI tract. Most of the reports of colonic involvement occur in children. They usually present with intussusception or rectal bleeding. There is some slight increased risk of malignant degeneration.

Pseudopolyps

Pseudopolyps are polypoid protrusions into the lumen of a colon exhibiting the changes of severe IBD and are truly named, in that they are not polyps in the typical sense. The pseudopolyp is actually residual edematous mucosa sitting, like an island, on a sea of surrounding ulceration. The denuding of the adjacent mucosa and the swelling of the remaining island of mucosa result in the classic polypoid appearance of the pseudopolyp.

Pseudopolyps may be seen in virtually any IBD involving the colon, although by far the most common is ulcerative colitis. Pseudopolyps are a particularly prominent feature of toxic megacolon.

Postinflammatory Polyps

The appearance of colonic postinflammatory polyps (Box 7-5) is a direct effect of IBD and in particular ulcerative colitis. It may be seen less commonly in Crohn's disease and other inflammatory conditions of the colon.

These polyps are, in fact, composed of normal mucosa. They are often filiform or comma shaped and tend to be mostly found in the distal colon. These projections of normal mucosa into the lumen occur as a result of mucosal healing following severe IBD. They represent what were, during the height of the inflammatory process, pseudopolyps. Once the healing process begins, reepithelialization of the surrounding ulcerated areas occurs. This reepithelialization process

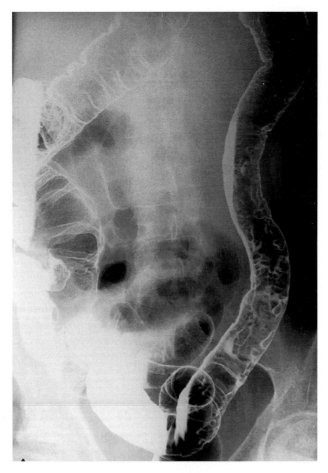

Fig. 7-37 DCBE on a patient with a previous history of ulcerative colitis reveals tubular-appearing left colon with numerous filiform filling defects representing postinflammatory polyposis.

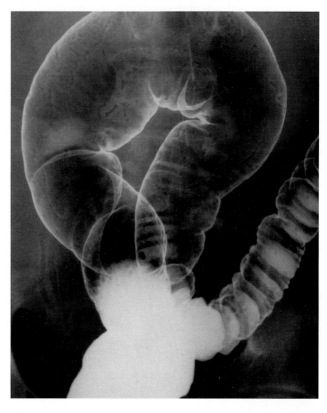

Fig. 7-38 Mucus stranding in the rectum was initially called *filiform polyposis* on ACBE. Sigmoidoscopy was normal.

Box 7-5 Postinflammatory Polyps: How They Come to Be

1. Starts as inflammatory colonic disease (usually ulcerative colitis)
2. Inflammation results in severe ulceration and near denuding of mucosal surface
3. Residual "islands" of edematous mucosa (pseudopolyps are spared)
4. Healing occurs with reepithelialization of the ulcerated surfaces
5. Reepithelialization process surrounds and involves the undermined edges of the pseudopolyps, giving classic appearance of postinflammatory or filiform polyps

---

extends into the undermined base of the pseudopolyp. As a result, when healing is complete, a projection of normal mucosa, usually in a filiform shape and often readily identifiable, is seen (Fig. 7-37). This may be seen on a background of normal colonic mucosa or recurrent disease. Residual fecal debris sometimes closely mimics postinflammatory polyposis, and a careful and detailed examination of the configuration of the "polyps" along with the absence of any evidence of inflammation new or old usually sorts out the problem (Fig. 7-38). Unusual presentations of postinflammatory polyposis include mucosal bridges, which are occasionally seen and represent reepithelialization of a thin strip of viable mucosa that has been totally undermined by ulceration. Additionally, large masses of postinflammatory polyps have been reported, having, in some instances, the appearance of a large villous tumor. These have been called giant postinflammatory polyps.

Lymphoid Hyperplasia/Lymphoid Follicular Prominence

The diagnosis of nodular lymphoid hyperplasia (NLH) presents something of a dilemma. This diagnostic title suggests a disease, whereas the presence of prominent lymphoid follicles throughout the colon is usually a

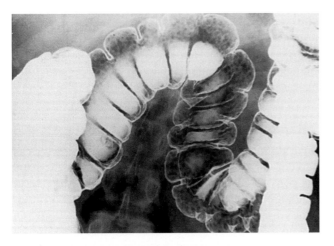

Fig. 7-39   Numerous, tiny filling defects are seen throughout the colon in this adult patient, representing a prominent lymphoid follicular pattern.

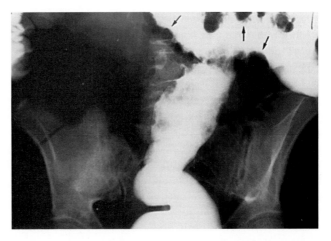

Fig. 7-40   Barium enema reveals numerous marginal nodular filling defects, some of which have the appearance of thumbprinting *(arrows)*. However, the filling defects are air filled and represent pneumatosis coli.

normal finding in children and seen with much more frequency than previously thought in adults.

In most instances, these small lymphoid nodules of the colon are considered a normal variant. They usually measure 1 to 3 mm and are rounded elevations of the mucosa with poor definition of the borders (Fig. 7-39). They tend to occur in areas where lymphoid follicles are most numerous, such as the ileocecal area and rectum. However, they can also be seen distributed throughout the entire colon. When these nodules are larger than 3 mm, the condition is commonly referred to as lymphoid hyperplasia and characterized radiologically by a tiny, central, barium-filled dimple seen on ACBE. This is not a disease but, more likely, the reaction of the lymphoid follicles to an adjacent inflammatory or infectious process, although the process may not always be apparent. The presence of NLH in the small bowel and possibly the colon of patients with hypogammaglobulinemia and associated giardiasis has also been noted. There has been suggestion over the years that lymphoid hyperplasia may represent the earliest changes of IBD or lymphatic disease, although this is quite speculative and has never been proved.

Pneumatosis Cystoides Coli

Pneumatosis coli is manifested by two distinctive patterns. The condition is characterized by air in the bowel wall. The most common form is subserosal cystic blebs (Fig. 7-40). The actual cause is unknown. Speculation has largely centered on coexistent chronic obstructive pulmonary disease in which microruptures of the alveoli occur and air dissects through the vascular-bronchial interstitial pathways to the mediastinum, down the mediastinum into the retroperitoneum, and into the root of the mesentery. Further dissection of air occurs along the leaves of the mesentery until it reaches the peritoneal surface of the bowel. Most of the subserosal cystic air collections are seen in the distal colon, with abrupt termination at the peritoneal reflection off the rectum. The oxygen is largely absorbed and the remaining gas is primarily nitrogen. Another condition that has been associated with this is scleroderma. These patients are almost always asymptomatic and the findings usually incidental. On rare occasion, if a subserosal cyst is sufficiently large, there can be stretching of the overlying mucosa and potential ulceration and bleeding. Additionally, the subserosal blebs on occasion can rupture and the patient can have a benign pneumoperitoneum. Such a finding can often cause confusion in the emergency department.

Another, more ominous form of pneumatosis coli is the presence of linear intramural collections of air. These are not subserosal in location, but usually submucosal. This finding is most frequently associated with underlying acute vascular insults to the bowel, ischemia, and infarction. Air that has percolated into the submucosa as the result of a loss of mucosal integrity is, like food nutrients, taken up in the portal venous system and transported through the mesenteric veins to the portal vein. From there it can be carried into the intrahepatic portal venous system. This can be identified on plain radiographs as tiny, branching, tubular collections of air in the periphery (as opposed to larger air-filled branching structures centrally seen in the biliary tree) of the liver. In most instances, at the time of radiological evaluation, these patients are sufficiently toxic to allow the radiologist to confidently make the diagnosis. However, the findings of air in the bowel wall may precede by several hours the onset of catastrophic decline in the patient's physical status. There may be little more than complaints of abdominal pain in some patients undergoing major bowel infarction who will not survive 24 hours. This may be especially true in older individuals.

A major problem for the radiologist is the occasional discovery of extensive linear submucosal air collections or air within the portal venous system in a relatively asymptomatic patient. This can occur as a benign finding unrelated to bowel wall ischemia or necrosis. Such conditions include GI surgery, pyloric obstruction, peptic ulceration, instrumentation, and mucosal trauma. In these situations, the cause of this condition is related to mechanical and surgical factors rather than bowel necrosis. However, linear pneumatosis on plain film or abdominal CT should always lead to an immediate consultation with the referring clinician.

Metastatic Disease

Metastatic spread of tumor to the colon and rectum can produce a variety of radiological findings and clinical symptomatology. The spread to the colon may occur as a result of seeding through the intraperitoneal pathways, local contiguous spread, or hematogenous dissemination. Tumors that can spread in such a manner and produce multiple and, on rare occasion, solitary filling defects include breast cancer, malignant melanoma, and bronchogenic carcinoma. Radiographic appearances are quite variable and may include well-defined intramural polypoid masses or large, bulky, irregular masses with superficial ulceration. Lesions originating in the ovary and stomach most commonly spread through the intraperitoneal pathways and result in narrowing and stricture. Involvement of the rectum by cervical cancer or prostatic cancer usually results from contiguous invasion.

Colitis Cystica Profunda

Colitis cystica profunda (CCP) is an unusual nonneoplastic condition characterized by the presence of mucus-filled cysts in the submucosa and is usually confined to the rectum or distal sigmoid. The radiographic appearance can be variable, with a classic description of numerous, smooth polypoid lesions that may be indistinguishable from adenomatous polyps. Occasionally the polyps are clustered and irregular, even assuming a masslike configuration that requires differentiation from malignant neoplasm. Clinically, these patients present with rectal bleeding and passage of excessive mucus per rectum.

The etiological basis of the condition is quite confusing. It is felt by some to originate as a primary focal glandular abnormality of the distal large bowel and rectum. Conversely, there is also a fairly convincing argument that this is a variant of the solitary rectal ulcer syndrome. Solitary rectal ulcer syndrome is probably a result of chronic internal rectal prolapse. This causes superficial ulceration, interval episodes of inflammation and healing, and invagination of the glandular structures that become cystic over a period of time.

Kaposi's Sarcoma

For decades, Kaposi's sarcoma has been known as an indolent cutaneous neoplastic disease of older men and was considered uncommon. However, with the advent of acquired immunodeficiency syndrome (AIDS), it has come to the forefront of diagnostic considerations. Of patients with AIDS, 30% to 40% have Kaposi's sarcoma somewhere in the GI tract. Virtually all cases of Kaposi's sarcoma of the gut are associated with AIDS. The lesions can affect the esophagus, stomach, small bowel, or colon. They may predate the cutaneous lesions. Barium enema commonly demonstrates multiple nodular lesions, usually in the distal colon. Infiltrative or irregular masses can also be seen.

These patients may present with GI bleeding as a result of ulceration of the larger nodules. In some instances this may be the presenting complaint before

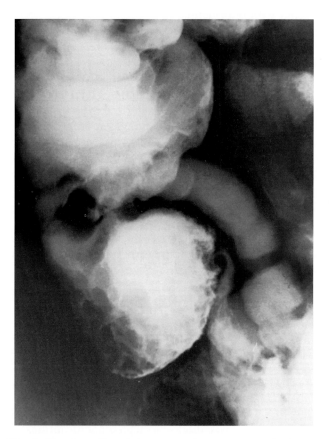

Fig. 7-41 Spot film of the cecum demonstrates multiple mucosal nodules in the cecal tip, giving a somewhat mosaic pattern and representing lymphoma. Other conditions that can give a similar appearance include ischemic changes, Crohn's disease, and *Yersinia* colitis.

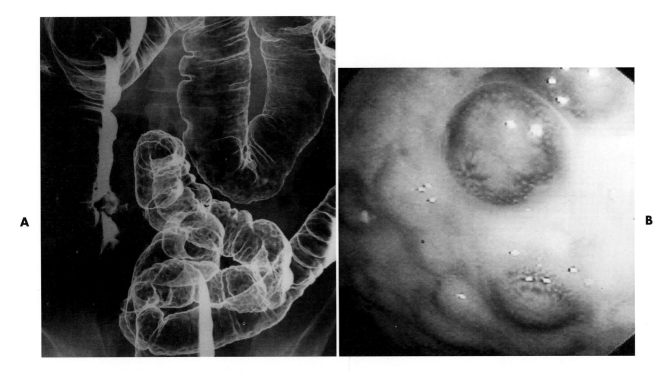

Fig. 7-42 A 53-year-old male presents with Hemoccult-positive stool but is otherwise well. **A,** ACBE reveals multiple colonic polyps. **B,** Colonoscopy reveals multiple atypical-appearing polypoid lesions. Biopsy demonstrated lymphomatous polyposis of the colon, a presentation of colonic lymphoma.

the diagnosis of AIDS is known. The presence of Kaposi's sarcoma within the bowel is indicative of poor prognosis, and few of these patients survive beyond 12 to 18 months following diagnosis.

Colonic Lymphoma

In most instances, lymphoma is indistinguishable from primary adenocarcinoma. However, on occasion this lesion may present as multiple nodular polypoid lesions within the colon, usually on the right side (Fig. 7-41). On rare occasion the appearance is indistinguishable from the more well-known polyposis syndromes (Fig. 7-42).

Colonic Schistosomiasis

Colonic schistosomiasis is a condition rarely encountered in North America, but is occasionally seen in travelers who have visited areas of endemic disease. It presents in the colon as ulcerations associated with polypoid filling defects (Fig. 7-43).

Colonic Varices

Varices are encountered in patients with portal hypertension, most frequently associated with liver cirrhosis. The collateral pathways are usually via the gastroesophageal veins, the mesenteric veins, and occasionally the

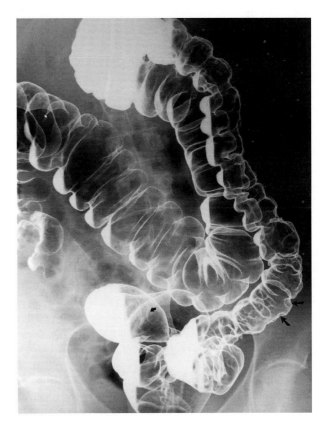

Fig. 7-43 A 46-year-old female presents with abdominal pain and diarrhea following a trip to the Middle East. ACBE shows multiple polypoid lesions in the distal colon *(arrows),* one form of presentation of colonic schistosomiasis.

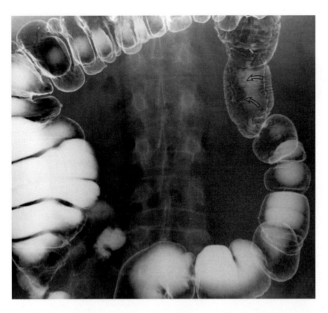

Fig. 7-44   *Colonic varices (arrows) in a patient with portal hypertension and prior colonic surgical resection.*

umbilical veins. It is rare to see colonic varices. They are usually associated pathways that develop as a result of the anastomosis of veins on the visceral surface of the bowel with systemic venous channels in the abdominal wall. This occurs, in almost all cases, in patients with portal hypertension and a history of prior abdominal surgery and resection who develop adhesions between bowel loops, setting the stage for possible abnormal venous collateralizations on the surface of the bowel (Fig. 7-44).

EXTRINSIC DEFECTS

Extrinsic defects affecting the colon may fall within the normal or abnormal category (Box 7-6). In the normal category, one can expect to see impressions from the right lobe of the liver, particularly a Riedel's lobe, where the inferior aspect of the right lobe is somewhat elongated and impresses the ascending colon. A patulous or prominent gallbladder may be seen impressing the superior margin of the proximal transverse colon. Splenic impressions are common, but their presence does not necessarily indicate splenomegaly. Occasionally, individuals with a very prominent sacral promontory demonstrate some posterior impression at the rectosigmoid junction.

Virtually any intraabdominal mass can result in colonic displacement or compression. This ranges from abscesses, the most common of which are due to diverticular, periappendiceal, and pelvic inflammatory disease, to cystic lesions, most commonly of the ovary. Significant cystic disease of the kidney can also impress

Box 7-6   Pushing the Colon Around: Extrinsic Sources of Normal and Abnormal Impressions on the Colon

Liver
Gallbladder
Spleen
Pelvic masses, especially ovarian
Renal disease
Abscesses, especially diverticular or periappendiceal
Mesenteric masses
Small bowel disease

the colon. Intraabdominal tumor masses can compress, displace, or invade the colon.

ULCERATION

Ulcerative Colitis

Of the group of diseases generally known as IBD, ulcerative colitis and Crohn's disease represent the two most important conditions (Table 7-2). Ulcerative colitis is a mucosal disease that involves the colon distally and may progressively advance to affect the proximal colon. The disease, if limited to the rectum at the time of diagnosis, is referred to as ulcerative proctitis.

The cardinal clinical features are diarrhea and rectal bleeding. The severity of the clinical presentation is often dependent upon the amount of large bowel involved. Approximately one third of patients have pancolonic involvement at initial presentation. The disease can present as an acute process, a recurrent process, or a chronic ongoing condition. It is mostly a disease of young people, although it can be seen in any age group. The pathological characteristic of the disease is continuous and concentric superficial involvement of the bowel wall with inflammatory changes, mostly limited to the mucosa. In severe fulminating disease, the extent and depth of disease can significantly increase and become transmural, as in the case of toxic megacolon.

When early active disease is present, the mucosal surface becomes hyperemic, granular, and edematous. Tiny punctate ulcers may also be seen in the acute phase. The haustral pattern is usually diminished but not absent. Progression of disease results in increased ulceration and friability of the mucosal surface. Severe ulceration and denuding of the mucosal surface can occur. As previously mentioned, islands of residual edematous mucosa on this background of ulceration are known as pseudopolyps. Healing can occur with com-

Table 7-2 Inflammatory bowel disease

	Ulcerative colitis	Crohn's disease
Etiology	Unknown	Unknown
Pathology	Superficial mucosal inflammation	Transmural, granulomatous inflammation
Peak age of onset	20-40 years of age	Bimodal, mostly 20-30 years of age, very small secondary peak—60-70 years of age
Male/female ratio	Equal	Equal
Colorectal involvement	100%	65%-70%
Fistula and abscess formation	Rare	Common
Malignant potential	Related to extent and duration of disease, up to 10%-15%	Rare in colon, 2%-5% in small bowel with associated small bowel disease
Rectal involvement	Always, may be limited to rectum initially	Approximately 50% with colonic disease
Disease pattern	Continuous, diffuse ulceration, symmetric involvement of the bowel	Discontinuous, asymmetric skip lesions, asymmetric punctate, linear or branching (cobblestoning) ulceration
Perianal disease	Unusual, can be associated with diarrhea	Common (approximately 50%) with colonic disease
Gastroduodenal disease	No	10%-30%
Major clinical symptoms	Rectal bleeding/diarrhea	Diarrhea, abdominal pain, bleeding less common
Colonic strictures	Yes	Yes (more common)
Pseudopolyp formation	Common	Less common
Toxic megacolon	2%-10%	1%-3%
Extracolonic manifestations		
Arthritis	20%	10%
Skin lesions	Yes	Yes
Liver/biliary	Sclerosing cholangitis 1%-5%	Increased incidence of gallstones
Renal disease	No	Increased incidence of kidney stones
Ophthalmologic disease	4%-5%	Unknown

plete restoration of the normal colonic appearance if the initial insult was not sufficiently severe to cause chronic fibrotic changes.

With more severe disease, there may be distortion of the haustral pattern following healing. Mucosal tags, or postinflammatory polyposis, may be present. With chronic disease, the bowel loses its haustral pattern entirely, assuming a "tubular" appearance. In addition, there is marked foreshortening of the colon. The terminal ileum is usually normal. The condition known as backwash ileitis has been described, resulting from chronic fibrotic changes involving the ileocecal valve and an uninterrupted continuum of the distal ileum and cecum. The terminal ileum appears dilated but is usually not involved in the inflammatory process.

Microscopic changes in the mucosal surface during the initial inflammatory phase reveal not only vascular congestion and leukocytic infiltrates but also inflammatory changes that occur within the crypts of Lieberkühn and resultant microabscesses. Most patients present with mild to moderate disease. However, a small percentage of patients (less than 10%) can initially present with a severe fulminant form of the condition.

Various extracolonic manifestations of ulcerative colitis have been described. Among the most severe is primary sclerosing cholangitis. Although almost half of

patients with ulcerative colitis may have degrees of abnormality of liver function, only a small number have significant hepatobiliary disease, representing approximately 1% to 5% of patients. This includes patients with severe hepatocellular disease and cirrhosis as well as those patients with sclerosing cholangitis.

In about 20% of patients significant periarticular disease is present. Most commonly, this is a monoarticular arthritis involving the lower limbs, usually the ankles or knees. There is also an increased incidence of sacroiliitis and ankylosing spondylitis in patients with ulcerative colitis.

Skin changes are also seen in ulcerative colitis. The most common of these is erythema nodosum, seen in approximately 10% to 15% of patients. Less commonly, pyoderma gangrenosum is seen in patients with severe colonic disease. Other important complications include ocular lesions, such as conjunctivitis, iritis, and episcleritis.

Other recognized but relatively uncommon complications include an increased incidence of thromboembolic disease, growth retardation, and secondary amyloidosis. The potential for the development of colon carcinoma in patients with ulcerative colitis is well known. The risk appears to increase with the extent and duration of disease. A patient with pancolitis and disease over

10 years in duration runs a 10% to 15% risk of developing a malignant lesion, with the risk increasing over time.

The use of the DCBE over the last few decades has greatly enhanced the ability of the radiologist to identify mild early mucosal changes of ulcerative colitis. These findings include mucosal granularity, diminished colonic folds and loss of rectal valves, and the presence of mucosal erosions (Fig. 7-45). In general, the single-contrast study is not very sensitive for the detection of these early changes. Unless there is frank ulceration, they are often missed with single-contrast technique. With more pronounced disease, both techniques can easily demonstrate the diagnostic findings. Frank ulcerations, including the classic "collar button" ulcers, are easily demonstrated on the margins of the bowel using either technique (Fig. 7-46). The "collar button" type of ulceration is indicative of penetration into the submucosa and the undermining of mucosa leading to this classic configuration.

In the chronic phases of ulcerative colitis, there can be colonic foreshortening and narrowing of the lumen. The flexures may virtually disappear.

Fistula formation is extremely uncommon and, if present, should prompt one to reconsider the diagnosis. Following healing or in chronic recurrent disease, postinflammatory polyps may be present.

Crohn's Disease

Crohn's disease is a chronic inflammatory process that, unlike ulcerative colitis, is transmural in nature (see Table 7-2). The cause of the disease remains a mystery. It is largely a disease of young persons, 20 to 30 years of age, although a smaller subset of patients with onset of symptoms beyond 50 years of age is now being identified.

Three primary clinical and anatomical presentations are now recognized. They are small bowel involvement only (30%), distal small bowel and colonic involvement (45%), and colonic involvement only (25%). The pattern of involvement often dictates the clinical presentation. Although diarrhea and abdominal pain tend to be common to all presentations, bowel obstruction and fistula formation are most frequently seen in patients with small bowel involvement. Conversely, rectal bleeding and perianal disease tend to indicate colorectal disease.

The transmural granulomatous type of inflammatory changes is discontinuous within the colon, resulting in the well-known "skip lesions" recognized by pathologists and radiologists. In addition, the pattern of involvement tends to be asymmetric (e.g., one wall of the colon at any given point may be more or less involved than the

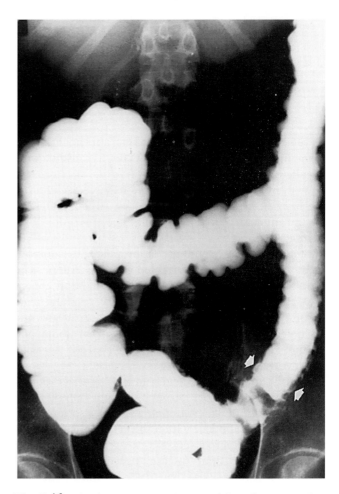

Fig. 7-46 Single-contrast examination of the colon on a patient with bloody diarrhea reveals numerous marginal ulcers *(arrows)* with undermining of mucosa and a "collar button" appearance.

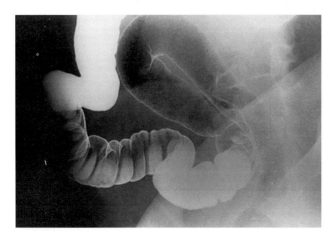

Fig. 7-45 Spot film of the rectosigmoid on a patient with acute ulcerative colitis reveals loss of haustral folds through the affected area, with granularity and tiny, superficial punctate ulcers involving the rectum and distal sigmoid.

opposite wall). This is an important observation, and it contrasts with ulcerative colitis, where involvement is continuous and concentric.

The full-thickness inflammatory disease eventually results in a thickened rigid segment of bowel, with progressive increase in mesenteric fat over the inflamed serosal surface (creeping fat). However, initially the mucosal changes may be little more than aphthoid types of erosions on the mucosal surface. Care should be taken regarding the diagnosis of aphthous ulcers in the colon and rectum, as both a prominent lymphoid pattern and variations of the normal rectal pattern can simulate the appearance (Fig. 7-47). Aphthous ulcers can enlarge, deepen, and extend into long linear ulcerations (Fig. 7-48). Extensive branching linear ulcerations can result in the classic "cobblestone" effect described in the early radiological literature. Penetration of the inflammatory process to the external serosal surface accounts for the high incidence of bowel-to-bowel fistula formation and perforation with abscess formation. These represent the most common complications of Crohn's disease and are rarely seen in ulcerative colitis. Free perforation in Crohn's disease is unusual. There is a slightly increased risk of malignancy as a complication of Crohn's disease. These neoplasms almost always occur in the small bowel in patients with small bowel involvement. Both adenocarcinoma and lymphoma may occur. Colonic malignancy is rare.

Other important complications include toxic megacolon (less common than in ulcerative colitis), enterovaginal, enterovesical, and enteroureteric fistula formation.

In addition, as in ulcerative colitis, there are extra-gastrointestinal manifestations of the disease. Approximately 10% of patients will have peripheral arthritis. Dermatological manifestations include both erythema nodosum and pyoderma gangrenosum.

The radiological evaluation of Crohn's disease begins with the plain film of the abdomen in most patients. Typically, changes include a bowel gas pattern demonstrating thickened irregular folds (Fig. 7-49). The plain film is also of particular benefit in the evaluation for toxic megacolon. Additionally, unusual gas collections may suggest abscess formation.

The radiological evaluation of the patient with non-fulminant disease and no evidence of toxic megacolon or free air should be double-contrast technique. The early superficial aphthous type of erosions will be missed on a single-contrast study. These tiny erosions will be surrounded by apparently normal mucosa.

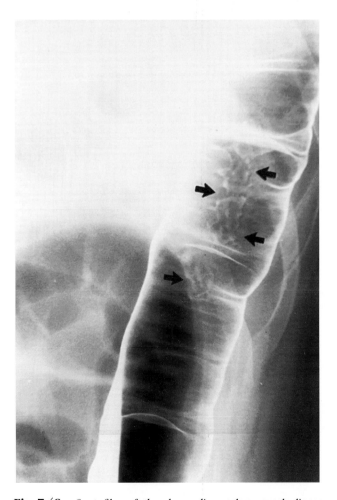

Fig. 7-48   Spot film of the descending colon reveals linear superficial ulceration *(arrows)* typical of early Crohn's disease.

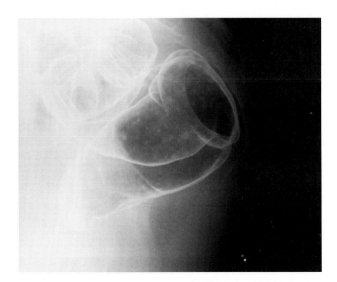

Fig. 7-47   A 35-year-old patient with abdominal pain and bloating. Aphthous ulcers of the rectum diagnosed on the ACBE. Sigmodoscopy was normal. Appearance of rectal mucosa is a normal variant.

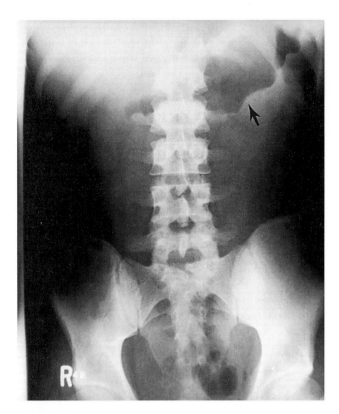

Fig. 7-49 Plain film of the abdomen shows abnormal contours *(arrow)* of the air-filled distal transverse colon in a patient with colonic Crohn's disease. The normal haustral pattern is absent, and narrowing of the mid-transverse colon is seen.

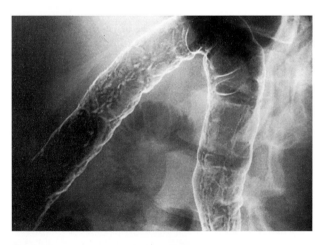

Fig. 7-50 Spot film of the splenic flexure demonstrates eccentric involvement of the flexure with focal areas of more severe involvement (skip lesions). Numerous superficial linear and branching ulcers are seen, particularly in the proximal limb.

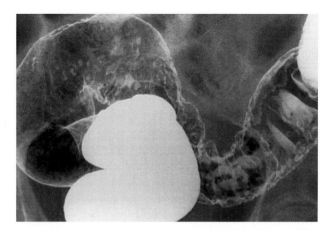

Fig. 7-51 In a patient with severe Crohn's disease, DCBE demonstrates marked involvement of the mid-sigmoid and relative sparing of the distal sigmoid and rectum.

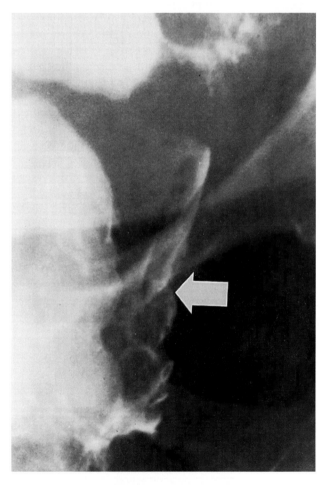

Fig. 7-52 Prominent perirectal sinus tracts *(arrow)* are seen along with rectal involvement in this patient with Crohn's disease.

More severe disease is manifested by deeper and more extensive ulceration, including long linear ulcers (Fig. 7-50). The rectum is histologically involved in over 50% of cases of colonic Crohn's disease but may appear grossly normal on radiological examination. Skip lesions and eccentric involvement of the colon should be identified if present (Fig. 7-51). Fistulas, sinus tracts, and periluminal abscesses may be seen in more advanced disease (Fig. 7-52). The involvement tends to be greater in the proximal portions of the colon. If the disease

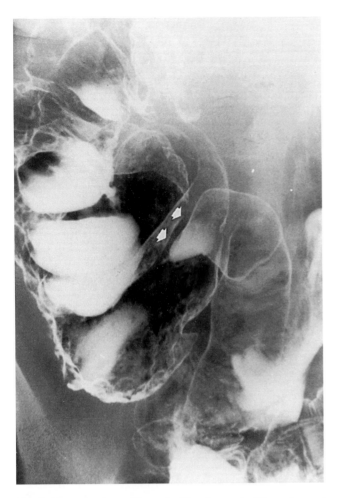

Fig. 7-53   A patient with marked involvement of the colon and particularly the cecal region with Crohn's disease. Note the sparing of the ileocecal valve *(arrows)* and the normal appearance of the terminal ileum.

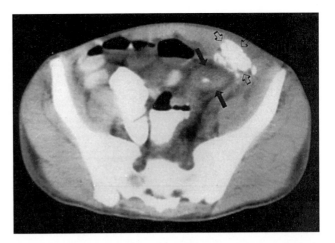

Fig. 7-54   CT image of a patient with known Crohn's disease. Note the marked wall thickening of the descending colon *(arrows)*. A periluminal collection of contrast is also seen *(open arrows)*, representing a pericolic abscess.

involves the ileocecal valve, the valve may be seen as enlarged and rigid. Generally speaking, if the ileocecal valve is involved, this is indicative of terminal ileum involvement (Fig. 7-53).

CT of the involved segments demonstrates the expected thickened, rigid bowel wall. However, CT is especially valuable in the documentation of intraabdominal complications such as abscess formation (Fig. 7-54). It is extremely useful in evaluating right lower quadrant masses, which may be matted, inflamed loops of bowel, but must be differentiated from abscess. CT is also valuable in performing diagnostic aspiration and therapeutic drainage of intraabdominal pus collections.

Ultrasound can demonstrate bowel wall thickening and is very useful in the evaluation of possible abscess formation. Typically, abscesses are seen as sonolucent masses with internal echoes. Radionuclide scintigraphy using indium-labeled leukocytes has also been used in the evaluation of possible Crohn's disease in difficult cases. This tends to be more useful in small bowel than colonic disease.

Viral Colitis

Cytomegalovirus (CMV) colitis is commonly seen in patients suffering from AIDS, as well as other conditions that compromise the immunological system, such as in post-transplant patients with immunosuppression. CMV colitis can have a variety of presentations, from diffuse to focal deep ulcerations. Patients often present with bloody diarrhea (Fig. 7-55).

Barium enema findings can vary from nonspecific, mild, superficial inflammatory changes to dramatic, deep ulcerations. The presence of large, deep ulcers may suggest the possibility of CMV colitis, although biopsy is required for diagnosis.

Bacterial Colitis

A number of bacterial infections of the colon, such as *Shigella, Salmonella, Clostridium,* and *Campylobacter* infections, can result in colonic ulcerations. Most of these are infrequently seen, and few barium enemas are performed for these conditions. The findings tend to be nonspecific. The findings seen in *Campylobacter* colitis have been reported to be identical to those seen in acute ulcerative colitis. *Yersinia* infections of the bowel are generally limited to the distal ileum, although the cecum can be involved. The radiological findings appear to be quite variable, with edema and ulceration the most common findings.

Infectious processes that tend to be limited to the rectum include rectal gonorrhea as well as herpes and *Campylobacter* infections. All of these conditions can present with fold thickening and superficial ulceration.

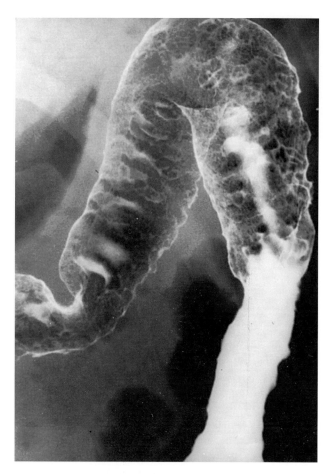

Fig. 7-55   Spot film of the splenic flexure in a patient with AIDS who suffers from severe cytomegalovirus (CMV) colitis. Note the marked ulceration and nodularity of the mucosal surface of the splenic flexure similar to Crohn's disease.

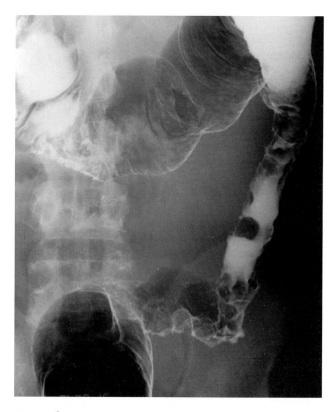

Fig. 7-56   ACBE on a 56-year-old patient who presents with bright red rectal bleeding. ACBE shows segment of left colon with irregular nodular changes consistent with ischemic colitis. Spontaneous healing occurred over several weeks.

Ischemic Colitis

Ischemic colitis is a condition resulting from the deprivation of adequate blood flow to the bowel, usually from the inferior mesenteric artery distribution. Often the condition is more related to hypoperfusion than to occlusive phenomena.

These patients almost uniformly present with bloody diarrhea, occasionally accompanied by lower abdominal pain. The mucosa and submucosa, being most sensitive to the hypoperfusion state, tend to become quickly edematous, hyperemic, and very susceptible to ulceration.

The condition is most frequently encountered in elderly patients, with the disease limited to the colon. Progression of the process to gangrene or to more extensive involvement of the colon, or even the distal small bowel, can also be seen and carries a higher mortality rate. However, most episodes of ischemic colitis run a benign course with over half of the patients recovering with no evident residual problems. Infection of disrupted mucosa can occur in a small percentage of patients, and perforation is uncommon.

The most common finding on either plain film or contrast examination of the colon is marked segmental wall thickening, resulting in the well-known "thumbprinting" sign. Ulceration of the mucosal surface is relatively common (Fig. 7-56). Intramural air can be seen on plain films, barium enema, and CT. The barium enema findings can be easily confused with inflammatory disease of the colon.

Amebiasis

Amebic colitis is the result of colonic parasitic infection by the protozoan *Entamoeba histolytica*. Infection is limited to the colon in most cases although widespread amebiasis can occur. The protozoan is ingested as a cyst in food or water and eventually passes into the small bowel and colon where the cyst dissolves

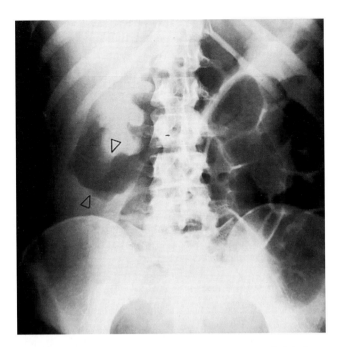

Fig. 7-57   Plain film of the abdomen on a patient with fulminant amebic colitis. Note the narrowing of the proximal transverse colon and the prominent nodularity (thumbprinting) in this region *(arrowheads)*.

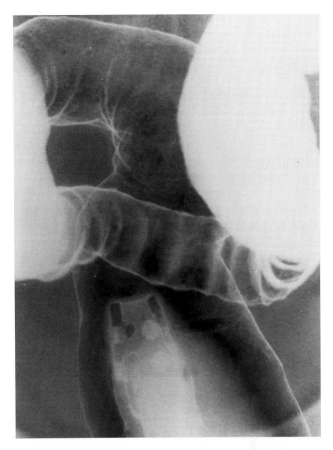

Fig. 7-58   Rectosigmoid spot film from a patient with chronic radiation proctitis and sigmoiditis. There is a general loss of the haustral pattern with a somewhat tubular appearance of the bowel.

and the uninuclear trophozoite form is released. These motile organisms invade the colonic mucosa causing hyperemia and edema. Progression of the infectious process results in mucosal ulcers. The cecum and ascending colon are the areas most commonly affected within the colon. Involvement of the adjacent distal ileum is unusual.

In addition to widespread mucosal inflammation and ulceration, a more localized, masslike form of the process, an ameboma, is occasionally identified. An ameboma is a marked, localized reaction involving extensive granulomatous type of inflammation, thickening of the bowel wall, and narrowing of the lumen. The configuration of an ameboma may look like carcinoma on endoscopic or radiological examination. Fortunately, amebomas are uncommon and are seen in less than 0.5% of cases.

The barium enema often shows severely inflamed spastic bowel with widespread ulceration. In the early stages, superficial discrete ulcers may be identified on ACBE. The disease tends to be more prevalent in the proximal portions of the colon. In severe disease there can be marked edema of the bowel wall, thumbprinting, and even toxic dilatation (Fig. 7-57). The radiological findings are not specific, and any stage of the examination can resemble Crohn's disease or ulcerative colitis. Distinction between amebiasis and inflammatory bowel disease is crucial, as patients with amebiasis who are inadvertently treated with steroids may decline rapidly.

The definitive diagnosis is made by detecting the organisms in the stool or endoscopic aspirate.

A helpful but not specific radiological finding is the conical cecum resulting from diffuse inflammation and spasm of the cecal tip. However, other conditions such as Crohn's disease, tuberculosis, actinomycosis, and even adjacent appendiceal disease can also result in a conical cecum.

Radiation Colitis

Inflammatory changes secondary to radiation are most commonly seen in the rectum and sigmoid colon, usually as a result of radiation therapy for pelvic neoplastic disease. This appears to be most commonly associated with treatment of carcinoma of the cervix. Acute changes are nonspecific and mostly consist of edema and erythema. In more severe radiation damage or chronic radiation damage, the colon tends to lose its haustral pattern and become somewhat tubular (Fig. 7-58). Rectal folds may completely disappear. Frequently, there is widening of the presacral space. Ulceration may be present to varying degrees in both the acute and chronic phases.

Tuberculosis

Tuberculosis involving the GI tract can be either primary or secondary. The primary involvement, usually associated with the ingestion of nonpasteurized milk, is rarely seen in Western countries today. But *Mycobacterium tuberculosis* primarily involving the lungs can secondarily infect the GI tract as a result of swallowed organisms in the sputum. The disease tends to occur around the ileocecal region, possibly because of the abundant lymphoid tissue in that area. Clinical presentation tends to be nonspecific with the most common presenting complaints being abdominal pain, weight loss, fever, and diarrhea. The radiological evaluation may be helpful in identifying an inflammatory mucosal process but is not diagnostic. The radiological appearance can mimic Crohn's disease, including mucosal ulceration, fold thickening, and occasionally stricture. The terminal ileum is commonly involved. In patients with known primary pulmonary tuberculosis, these findings would raise the diagnostic possibility of GI tuberculosis. However, the definitive diagnosis is made by identification of the organism.

The incidence of GI tuberculosis has increased with an increasingly large AIDS population in the community. In addition to *Mycobacterium tuberculosis,* another form of tuberculosis that has been seen with increasing frequency in these patients is *Mycobacterium avium-intracellulare* (MAI). This organism is generally nonpathological. However, in immunoimpaired patients, such as patients with AIDS, MAI infections primarily involving the respiratory tract are seen with increasing frequency. In such patients, this organism may occasionally be found to be the basis of GI infection as well.

Solitary Rectal Ulcer Syndrome

Solitary rectal ulcer syndrome, an unusual and somewhat confusing disorder, was first described in the early 1800s. It is most commonly seen in young or middle-aged adults, and the presenting findings are rectal bleeding and mucous discharge. Many patients also report difficulty passing stool. Ulcers frequently can be identified, although commonly there is more than a solitary ulcer present.

Multiple etiological theories have been suggested. Perhaps the most important is the association of internal rectal prolapse and difficult rectal evacuation. The disease may be associated with or identical to CCP.

Radiologically, inflammatory changes including ulceration can be identified along the anterior rectal wall. The

rectal valves often appear thickened, and a polypoid inflammatory mass may also be identified and may mimic neoplastic disease.

Trauma

Although colorectal trauma may result from a variety of causes, such as gunshot wounds, stabbing, or blunt trauma, the majority of cases are probably iatrogenic. These can occur as a result of the traumatic effect of a barium enema tip on the rectal mucosa or intracolonic instrumentation, such as results from sigmoidoscopy or colonoscopy. Frequently, these instruments may cause mucosal lacerations but infrequently result in serious complications, such as perforation.

Behçet's Disease

Behçet's disease is a condition of unknown etiology characterized by four main clinical findings. These include aphthous ulcers of the mouth, eyes, skin, and genitalia. It tends to be more common in men between the ages of 40 and 50 years. GI involvement occurs in less than half the patients and tends to be a minor manifestation of the condition. However, in a small number of patients, colonic involvement can be severe and significant ulceration may be seen (Fig. 7-59).

The radiological evaluation may be confusing, since the condition can simulate either Crohn's disease or, in some cases, ulcerative colitis. Additionally, because both of these idiopathic IBDs are known to have extracolonic manifestations that involve the eyes and skin, patients with Behçet's disease may carry the diagnosis of IBD for some time.

Diversion Colitis

In patients who have had their fecal stream diverted as the result of a proximal colostomy or ileostomy, a nonspecific inflammation involving the diverted portion of the colon may be seen, representing what has been called "diversion colitis."

The radiological evaluation of the excluded colonic segment will show acute inflammatory changes very similar to mild acute ulcerative colitis. This curious condition usually spontaneously regresses when the ostomy has been taken down and the fecal stream reestablished.

Gonorrheal Proctitis

Gonorrhea is a relatively common sexually transmitted infectious disease that involves the mucous membranes of the urethra, vagina, and cervix. Rectal involvement can occur in women either as a result of infected vaginal discharge and secondary rectal infection, or

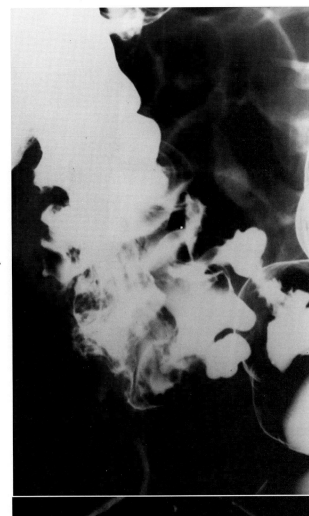

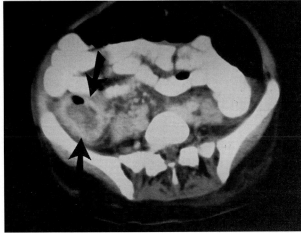

Fig. 7-59 Patient with Behçet's disease with involvement of the right colon. **A,** ACBE shows thickened irregular folds with some areas of ulceration in the cecum. **B,** CT examination shows inflammatory changes in cecal wall *(arrows)*.

primarily as a result of anal intercourse. In men, it always results from direct sexual contact and is seen in the homosexual population. The radiological findings are those of superficial inflammatory changes involving the mucosa of the rectum with fold thickening and areas of

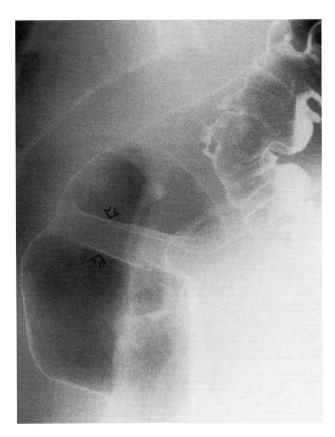

Fig. 7-60 Spot film of the rectum of a patient with known gonorrheal proctitis. Note the thickening of the rectal folds *(arrows)* and the granular appearance of the mucosa.

punctate ulceration (Fig. 7-60). The appearance may be identical to ulcerative proctitis seen early in the development of ulcerative colitis. In addition, other infectious processes such as *Campylobacter* and viral proctitis can give a similar picture.

COLONIC NARROWING

Adenocarcinoma

Although the physical manifestations of colonic adenocarcinoma are numerous, one of the more common is focal irregular narrowing, classically described as the "apple core" configuration or the English equivalent, the "napkin ring" (Fig. 7-61). This lesion involves a short segment of colon, frequently with some degree of proximal dilatation or obstruction, especially in the sigmoid colon.

Annular lesions tend to be relatively uncommon in the rectum, where large bulky polypoid lesions are considerably more frequent (Fig. 7-62). Rectal lesions also occur in a slightly older age group and are associated with a more aggressive course and slightly decreased survival time.

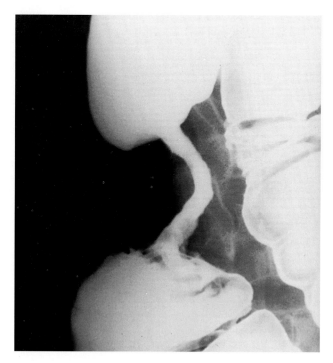

Fig. 7-61 Typical apple core or napkin ring configuration of an annular carcinoma of the colon.

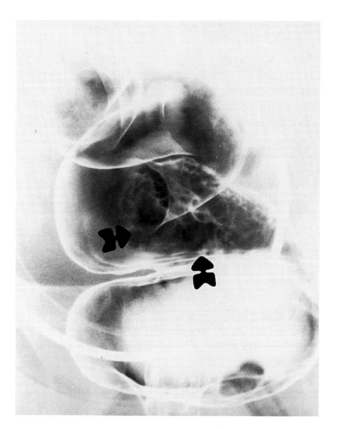

Fig. 7-62 An air-contrast view of rectal carcinoma *(arrows)* demonstrates a large, bulky polypoid lesion with a villous appearance.

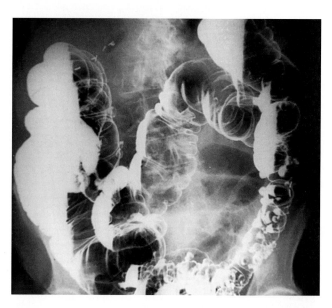

Fig. 7-63 Decubitus view from DCBE demonstrates marked diverticular changes concentrated in the sigmoid region, resulting in considerable distortion of the bowel and difficulty in evaluating the area.

Diverticulitis

Diverticulitis represents one of the two common complications of diverticulosis of the colon (the other being bleeding), and as such, the underlying condition of diverticulosis requires some understanding before this complication can be fully understood.

Diverticular disease of the colon is a condition of twentieth-century industrialized nations and was relatively uncommon before this century. Diverticula can occur anywhere in the colon but are most common in the sigmoid region (Fig. 7-63). These diverticula develop at the site of penetrating blood vessels entering the bowel wall. The mucosa and submucosa of the bowel wall tend to protrude through these natural areas of wall weakness. This anatomical relationship of diverticula to penetrating blood vessels accounts for the high incidence of hemorrhage associated with diverticulum formation.

The etiological origins of diverticulum formation appear to be related to abnormally high intraluminal colonic pressures and abnormally prolonged colonic transit times. Chronic disease results in muscular thickening, and, when severe diverticulosis is present, there can be diffuse narrowing even without the presence of diverticulitis.

The incidence is thought to be slightly more common in women than in men and most definitely increases with age. At age 60, 60% to 70% of patients examined by barium enema have some degree of diverticulum formation. There is also some suggestion that the disease may be occurring in increasingly younger individuals.

As previously mentioned, this condition appears to be most commonly seen in Western industrialized nations and is almost unheard of in Africa and the Far East. This is thought to relate to differences in the fiber content of the diet and to significant differences in colonic transit times. It has also been observed that long-time vegetarians appear to have a decreased incidence of diverticular disease.

It is probably safe to suggest that most patients with uncomplicated diverticulosis are asymptomatic. On the other hand, there is a poorly defined group of patients who experience lower abdominal pain, exacerbated by dietary intake and known under the diagnostic label of irritable bowel syndrome. Whether the so-called irritable bowel syndrome is a manifestation of colonic intraluminal pressure abnormalities leading to diverticulum formation or whether it is a coexisting condition is not absolutely clear, and there is, in fact, difficulty in defining the irritable bowel syndrome. There have been assertions that a correlation exists between the two conditions, although this remains controversial.

Patients who develop complications associated with diverticulosis most frequently develop rectal bleeding. Indeed the most common cause of massive lower GI bleeding is diverticulosis.

Much the same way that appendicitis develops, diverticulitis can occur when a diverticulum becomes occluded by stool, and peridiverticular inflammatory changes associated with microperforations can occur. These can go on to frank pericolic abscess formation (Fig. 7-64). Areas of narrowing may occur as a result of

spasm associated with the inflammation, even in the early changes of diverticulitis without abscess formation. With the presence of abscess formation, the narrowing results from a combination of spasm and mass effect. CT is very useful in the evaluation of diverticulitis, demonstrating thickened edematous bowel wall and pericolic abscesses. The barium enema findings are narrowing and spasm, mass effect, and barium in intramural tracts or pericolic abscess (Fig. 7-65).

Postinflammatory Strictures

A number of inflammatory conditions can cause focal stricturing and narrowing of the colon. They may occur during the acute phase (Figs. 7-66 and 7-67), but commonly are seen as a sequela to chronic disease.

Colonic strictures can be seen in less than 10% of patients with chronic ulcerative colitis (Fig. 7-68). They rarely result in obstructive changes. Additionally, in patients with severe chronic ulcerative colitis, the narrowing may be more diffuse, involving a long segment of the colon (Fig. 7-69).

Because of the transmural inflammatory changes associated with Crohn's disease, areas of focal stricture are slightly more common (Fig. 7-70). The strictures may be asymmetric, reflecting the asymmetric involvement of the bowel at that level.

One of the more common causes of narrowing in the rectum and sigmoid area is radiation colitis. Radiation therapy is usually performed for neoplastic disease of the pelvis. The involved bowel in the radiation port undergoes degrees of vascular injury. Diffuse or focal areas of narrowing are encountered.

Other unusual causes of colonic stricture include amebic, bacterial, and viral colitides.

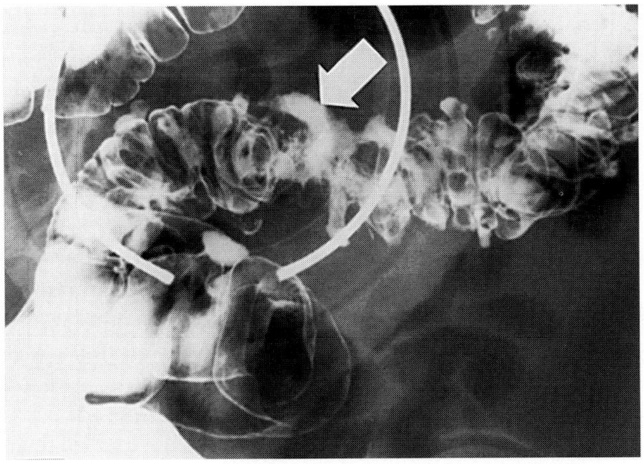

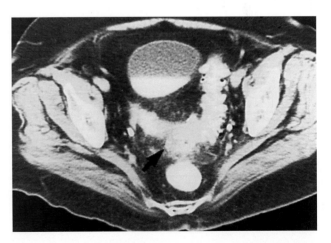

Fig. 7-64   Spot film from DCBE reveals multiple diverticula in the sigmoid region with narrowing and irregularity. A lenticular collection of barium *(arrow)* represents a pericolic abscess secondary to diverticulitis.

Fig. 7-65   CT scan through the pelvis demonstrates a focal area of sigmoid colon where the bowel margin becomes quite blurred *(arrow)*. There is also increased density in the pericolic area and in the surrounding mesenteric fat. These are typical findings of diverticulitis.

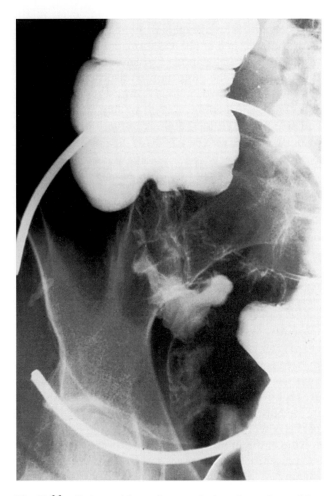

Fig. 7-66   Patient with persistent colonic stricture located just above the ileocecal valve. The mucosa appears to be intact, and this stricture was found to be inflammatory in nature, representing CMV colitis.

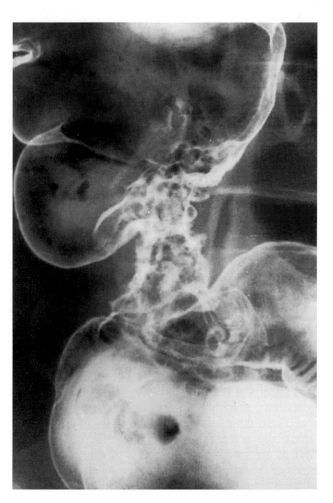

Fig. 7-68   A patient with ulcerative colitis and a well-defined stricture located just above the ileocecal valve, secondary to focal inflammatory changes.

Ischemic Colitis

Over half of patients who experience ischemic colitis undergo complete and spontaneous remission, with return to the normal configuration and appearance of the colon. In a smaller number of patients there is sufficient injury to the mucosa and submucosa that the resultant fibrosis can cause focal luminal narrowing (Fig. 7-71). As with all areas of colonic narrowing, the status of the mucosa in the narrowed segment should be carefully ascertained. In most inflammatory or postinflammatory causes of stricture, a mucosal pattern can be detected, as opposed to the destroyed and replaced mucosa associated with malignant disease.

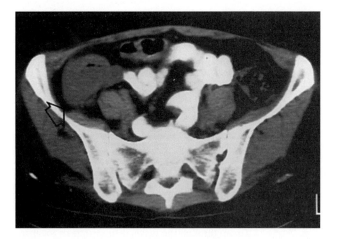

Fig. 7-67   CT scan through the upper pelvis in the same patient as shown in Fig. 7-66. Note the marked thickening of the colonic wall *(arrow)* just above the ileocecal valve.

Adjacent Inflammatory Neoplastic Disease

Processes not originating in the colon can indirectly involve the colon, resulting in luminal narrowing (Fig. 7-72).

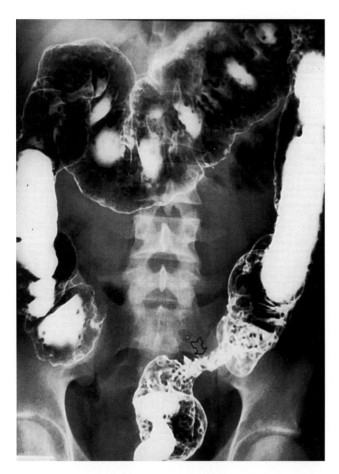

Fig. 7-69   DCBE in a patient with chronic ulcerative colitis. Widespread postinflammatory polyposis is seen along with a strictured segment *(arrow)* in the sigmoid colon.

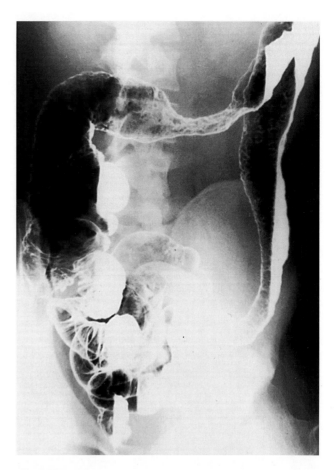

Fig. 7-70   DCBE in a patient with Crohn's disease shows an area of stricturing involving the distal transverse colon.

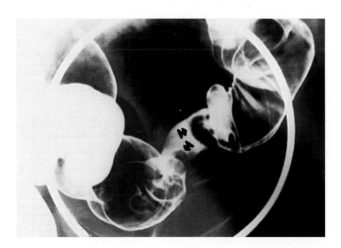

Fig. 7-71   Spot film of the sigmoid colon of a patient with a smooth postischemic stricture. Polypoid filling defects in the stricture *(arrows)* proved to be a polypoid adenocarcinoma arising in the stricture.

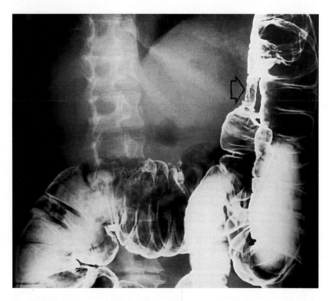

Fig. 7-72   Overhead film demonstrates a fixed area of narrowing *(arrow)* in the ascending limb of the splenic flexure. The mucosa is intact. This area of persistent narrowing is a result of an adjacent pancreatic pseudocyst that involves the colon at that point.

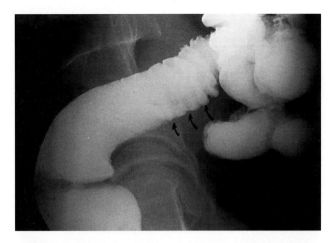

Fig. 7-73   Spot film of the rectum demonstrates some spasm at the rectosigmoid junction and a crenulated appearance along the anterior margin *(arrows)*. This patient had a periappendiceal abscess and pus was discovered in the lower recesses of the pelvis, accounting for these changes.

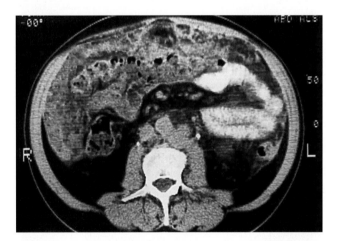

Fig. 7-74   CT of the abdomen discloses widespread infiltration of the mesentery with tumor extending to and involving the transverse colon.

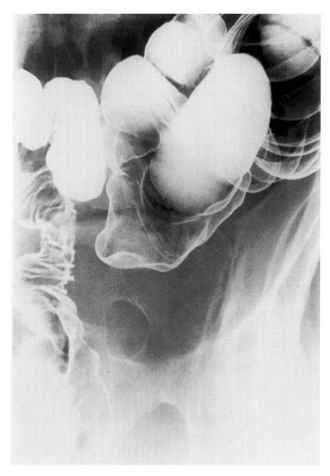

Fig. 7-75   Spot film from DCBE demonstrates a narrowing, spasm, and serrated margins of the sigmoid colon in a patient with widespread ovarian carcinoma involving the serosal surface of the bowel.

In the pelvis, pus or metastatic disease affecting the colon from the serosal side can result in a combination of spasm and infiltration, causing narrowing of the lumen.

Some of the more common inflammatory causes of this condition include periappendiceal abscess and pelvic inflammatory disease (Fig. 7-73).

Secondary neoplastic disease invading this region through the mesenteric pathways and serosal surface is a relatively common occurrence (Fig. 7-74). This results in the spiculated or crenulated margin on the mesenteric side of the bowel commonly seen in this condition. It should also be noted that invasion of the serosal surface of the bowel causes marked spasm of that segment of the bowel (Fig. 7-75). This spasm is among the most painful

types encountered during the course of a barium enema and many times is more uncomfortable than that experienced by patients with acute diverticulitis.

Extension of inflammatory or neoplastic processes through the gastrocolic ligament or the transverse mesocolon can also involve portions of the transverse colon, resulting in eccentric narrowing (Fig. 7-76). These include malignant lesions arising from both the stomach and pancreas. Pancreatitis can result in inflammatory exudates traversing the transverse mesocolon and involving the colon. In addition, there can be moderate to large accumulations of fluid in the lesser sac that may also indirectly involve the transverse colon (Fig. 7-77).

Endometriosis

Endometriosis is the presence of active, functioning endometrial tissue outside of the uterus. In approximately one quarter of the cases, endometriosis involves

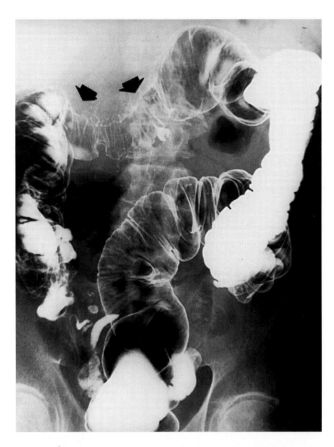

Fig. 7-76   DCBE in a patient presenting with anemia. Extrinsic mass and spiculation seen along the superior margin of the transverse colon *(arrows)* represent metastatic extension of a primary gastric carcinoma down the gastrocolic ligament, investing the transverse colon on its serosal margin.

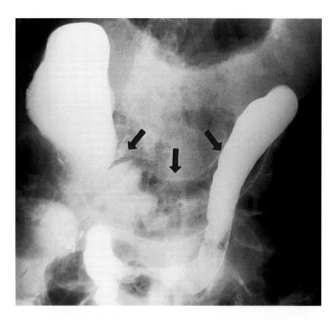

Fig. 7-77   A patient with abscess in the lesser sac. The lesser sac is distended with pus and in turn is impressing and depressing the transverse colon *(arrows)*.

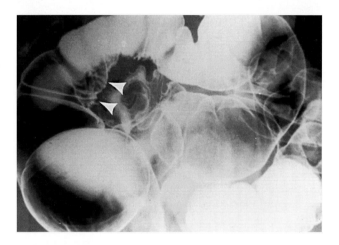

Fig. 7-78   A patient with known endometriosis demonstrates typical findings of serosal involvement at the rectosigmoid junction. The anterior margin of the bowel is crenulated and spiculated at this point with some mass effect *(arrowheads)*.

the bowel. Commonly, the sigmoid and rectosigmoid junctions are involved. However, it can also be seen rarely in the cecum and the terminal ileum.

The patients may be asymptomatic, although complaints of crampy abdominal pain sometimes associated with the menstrual cycle can be elicited. Areas of eccentric luminal narrowing can be seen endoscopically in the sigmoid region. The mucosa may appear distorted but intact. Diagnosis in the proper clinical setting can often be suggested by barium enema. Commonly there is an area of eccentric narrowing with spiculations and nodularity along the affected margin (Fig. 7-78).

Lymphoma

Although lymphoma of the colon can appear as a localized mass lesion with luminal narrowing (Fig. 7-79), it may also be seen as an infiltrating mass lesion in which the lumen of the replaced bowel actually appears widened (aneurysmal dilatation). This appearance is more frequently seen in the small bowel. The colonic

lesions tend to occur with more frequency on the right side and rarely obstruct (Fig. 7-80).

Lymphogranuloma Venereum

Lymphogranuloma venereum (LGV) is a sexually transmitted disease caused by the rickettsial organism, *Chlamydia trachomatis.* Significant inguinal lymphadenopathy is a common finding in this condition. Rectal involvement is also relatively common. When it does occur, it can result in narrowing of the rectum and distal sigmoid associated with marked edematous

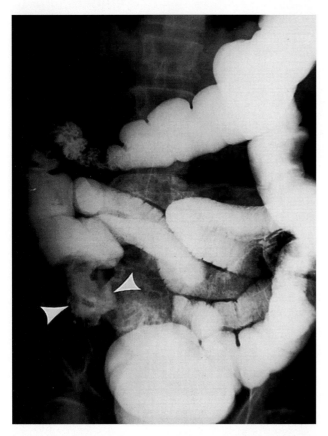

Fig. 7-79 SCBE in a patient with colonic lymphoma demonstrates narrowing and irregularity of the cecum *(arrowheads)*.

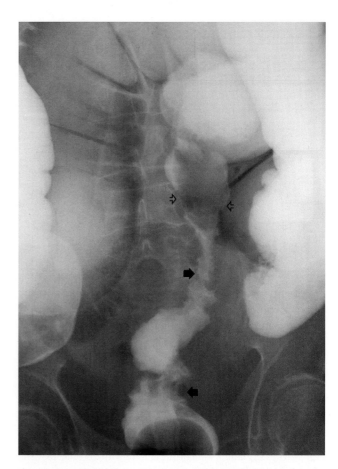

Fig. 7-80 ACBE shows long irregular segment of infiltrated distal colon *(open arrows)* and rectum *(black arrows)*. Resection and pathology revealed colonic lymphoma.

changes and possible ulceration. There may be fistulous tracts communicating to perirectal abscesses or to the perineum.

Actinomycosis

Actinomycosis is an aggressive inflammatory disease that commonly forms multiple sinus tracts. The disease is bacterial in origin, and when it involves the colon or rectum, it is usually associated with luminal mass, narrowing, and sinus or fistulous tracts. The radiological differentiation from colonic malignancy or diverticulitis can be extremely difficult.

Extrinsic Compression

Colonic luminal narrowing can also occur as a result of extrinsic processes compressing the colon. If the processes are inflammatory in nature, the compression accompanied by spasm can result in marked luminal narrowing. Likewise, an adjacent neoplasm with con-

tiguous spread gives a similar appearance. The usual lesions that result in compression of the colon to this degree are pelvic masses compressing the sigmoid region (Fig. 7-81). However, a markedly enlarged spleen can also compress the region of the splenic flexure, while a very enlarged left hepatic lobe can depress and displace the colon (Fig. 7-82).

Carcinoid Tumor

GI carcinoid tumors are most commonly seen in the appendix and the distal small bowel. Colonic involvement is uncommon. When it does occur, the two most frequent sites tend to be the proximal ascending colon and the rectum.

The radiological problems posed by this tumor are multiple. It can be a small polypoid lesion or a large, bulky lesion identical in appearance to colonic carcinoma. Additionally, it may present as an area of focal stricture, which also may be indistinguishable from the common colonic malignancy. Differentiation be-

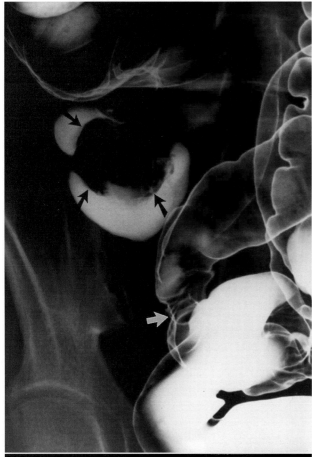

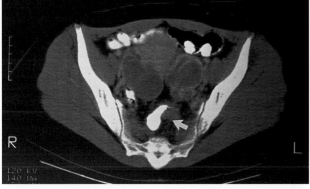

Fig. 7-81 A 46-year-old female with constipation and painful defecation. **A,** ACBE shows tethered narrowing in sigmoid *(white arrow)* and unusual filling defect in cecum *(black arrows).* **B,** CT of the pelvis demonstrates mixed cystic and solid lesion encasing sigmoid *(arrow).* A serosal deposit was also seen on the cecum. Carcinoma of the ovary with serosal spread.

tween benign and malignant lesions is sometimes difficult when there is no evidence of metastatic disease. The presence of malignancy in a focal lesion varies from 10% to 40%. In general, metastatic disease is more frequently associated with carcinoids of the colon than of the small bowel.

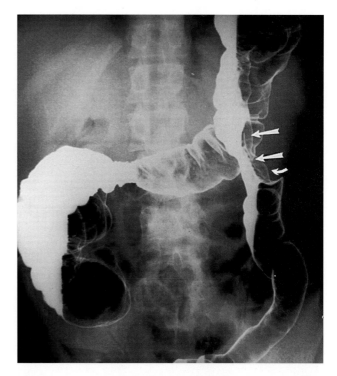

Fig. 7-82 Prominent splenic impression along the descending colon *(arrows)* simulates an intramural colonic lesion, such as a leiomyoma.

MECHANICAL DILATATION

Any condition that compromises the colonic lumen and obstructs the antegrade flow of the fecal stream will result in proximal dilatation. This would include a wide spectrum of lesions, including colonic carcinoma, inflammatory strictures, intussusception, and hernia. On rare occasions, severe ischemic colitis can result in residual narrowing, although obstruction is uncommon. Patients with lymphoma rarely become obstructed. Colonic adhesions are rare but can result in luminal narrowing and proximal dilatation.

Following malignant obstructions and obstruction secondary to inflammatory stricture, volvulus is the third most common cause of colonic obstruction. The two most common forms of colonic volvulus are cecal and sigmoid volvulus. Cecal volvulus is often associated with an abnormally long mesentery of the cecum and ascending colon. This, along with the fact that the amount of retroperitonealization of the ascending colon is quite variable, results in considerable mobility of the right side of the colon, predisposing to volvulus. Commonly, this occurs when the cecum twists on its luminal axis and is displaced upward and to the left of midline (Fig. 7-83). A barium study will often demonstrate the torsion abnormality and the classic beak configuration at the obstructed point.

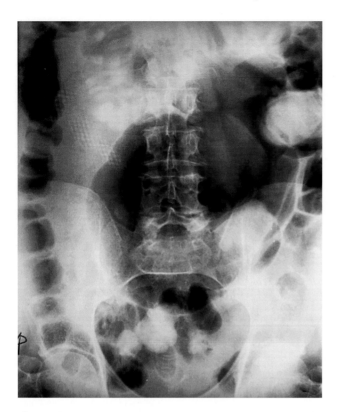

Fig. 7-83 Plain film of the abdomen demonstrates dilated air-filled cecum slightly to the left of midline in a patient with cecal volvulus.

About 10% of cases of cecal volvulus are cecal bascules. This differs from the usual cecal volvulus in that the cecum does not rotate around its luminal axis but instead rotates around a peritoneal band usually located above the cecum. With a cecal bascule, there tends to be less distention of the cecum and less migration of the dilated cecum superiorly and to the left. The origins of the band are unclear, and whether these are congenital or developmental is unknown.

A long, high loop of sigmoid on a mesentery can twist upon itself at the mesenteric base, resulting in a sigmoid volvulus. This is a form of closed-loop obstruction. The hyperinflated sigmoid colon can extend as high as the diaphragm, and the dilated sigmoid loop will have the classic bean-shaped configuration. Again, an SCBE will demonstrate a torsion abnormality at the obstruction point with a beaklike configuration.

Intussusception is relatively uncommon in adults, and, when it does occur, it should be viewed with some suspicion (Fig. 7-84). Most adult intussusceptions have, as their lead point, a neoplastic lesion.

Virtually any type of herniated segment of colon can result in obstruction and proximal dilatation. However, most colonic hernias are asymptomatic. Incidental herniation is commonly seen during barium enema examinations, with portions of the colon in umbilical, inguinal, or femoral hernias. There can be herniation

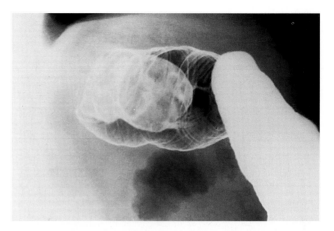

Fig. 7-84 Intussuscepted segment of transverse colon seen on DCBE. A polypoid carcinoma is acting as the lead point of the intussusception.

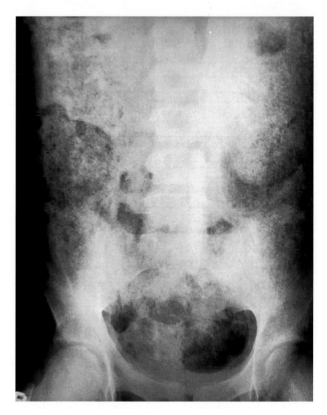

Fig. 7-85 Plain film of a teenage patient with chronic constipation and abdominal distention reveals markedly dilated stool-filled colon.

through incisional defects or through defects in the diaphragm. Herniation of colon through the diaphragm into the pericardial sac in an asymptomatic patient is also possible. Hernias of colon between the lateral muscular layers of the abdominal wall (spigelian hernias) occasionally result in obstruction.

An aganglionic segment of the colon (Hirschsprung's disease) can result in significant dilatation of the proximal colon. This condition is congenital and is more com-

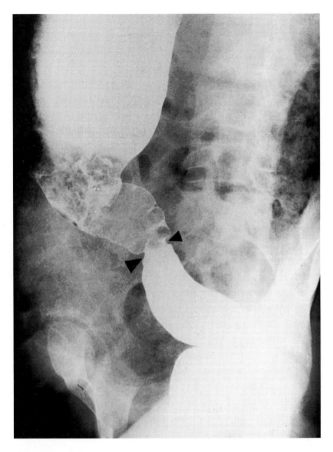

Fig. 7-86   Barium enema (same patient as Fig. 7-85) demonstrates an area of transition in the distal sigmoid, representing the zone of transition *(arrowheads)* from normal to aganglionic colon in a patient with Hirschsprung's disease.

monly seen in male infants. It may not be correctly diagnosed until adolescence or even early adulthood in some individuals. Classically, these patients present with abdominal distention, marked fecal retention, and failure to thrive (Fig. 7-85). Barium enema examination usually demonstrates a normal rectum with normal rectal distention. Above the rectum, there will be an area of transition to grossly dilated colon (Fig. 7-86). The aganglionic segments are almost always focal although they can extend upward for several centimeters, and in very rare instances the entire colon may be involved.

NONMECHANICAL DILATATION

The presence of marked colonic dilatation without obstruction is not uncommon and has been recognized as a frequent finding in mentally retarded patients and particularly in institutionalized patients. This has been referred to as psychogenic megacolon. The exact causes are unknown. There may be some contribution to the situation by the array of anticholinergic medications that many of these patients require.

Additionally, colonic dilatation is a well-recognized complication of the acutely ill, bedridden patient. It is frequently seen in the postoperative patient with prolongation of the postoperative ileus effect. It may also be seen in patients experiencing severe sepsis. Acute passive dilatation of the colon, sometimes called Ogilvie's syndrome, carries with it the risk of perforation of the cecum, where the colon is the most distensible and the wall is the thinnest.

Colonic dilatation can also be seen as a result of underlying systemic conditions such as scleroderma, Chagas' disease, cystic fibrosis, and myotonic dystrophy.

The condition known as idiopathic intestinal pseudoobstruction is thought to represent a neuromuscular disorder of the GI tract involving all parts of the gut. Some of these patients will have colonic distention without acute clinical findings. However, many of these patients will have chronic abdominal complaints, including distention, chronic abdominal pain, and constipation. A plain film of the abdomen will often show marked colonic distention, and without a clinical history the radiologist may be obligated to consider differential considerations that include colonic volvulus or obstruction secondary to inflammatory or neoplastic disease.

DIMINISHED HAUSTRAL PATTERN

A number of conditions, many of which have been previously discussed, can result in a diminished haustral pattern and a tubular appearance of the colon. These include idiopathic inflammatory processes, such as ulcerative colitis and Crohn's disease, as well as bacterial and viral colitides.

In addition, the fold pattern may appear diminished in scleroderma, in which the haustral pattern may assume an asymmetric saccular pattern. Similar changes can be seen in the small bowel. Chronic laxative abuse and resultant cathartic colon also demonstrate a diminished haustral pattern.

Any chronic or healed inflammatory process involving the colon, such as chronic or healed ulcerative colitis or the chronic stages of radiation colitis, can result in diminished or absent haustral pattern.

THICKENED HAUSTRAL FOLDS

A number of conditions can result in varying degrees of thickening of the haustral folds. These can be mild thickening to marked fingerlike indentations of the bowel margin known as thumbprinting. In general, fold thickening and thumbprinting are a result of edema, hemorrhage, or malignancy. Hemorrhage is seen most commonly as a cause of thumbprinting resulting from ischemic colitis. However, thumbprinting resulting from intramural hemorrhage may be entirely indistinguishable from severe inflammation and marked edematous changes such as might be seen in fulminating IBD or toxic megacolon. The clinical history is extremely helpful in sorting out these problems.

Ischemic colitis is a condition seen in the elderly population, with most of the patients being over 70 years of age. The condition relates to an acute reduction of the splanchnic blood flow and is commonly seen in, or distal to, the watershed areas between the inferior mesenteric artery and the superior mesenteric artery circulations. However, more extensive colitis involving longer segments is common.

The exact causes for this diminished blood flow may be multiple. Conditions such as acute hypotensive episodes, underlying vasculitides, or mechanical causes such as herniation or volvulus have been implicated. There is an increased incidence of patients with ischemic colitis who are undergoing hemodialysis. The rectum is rarely involved because of the abundant collateral circulation.

The finding of thumbprinting on either a plain film or during a barium enema examination is most often seen in the transverse or descending portions of the colon and represents intramural hemorrhage. This finding is present in about 20% to 25% of patients. The patients frequently present with painless rectal bleeding. Over half of the cases are transient and reversible. Slightly less than half of the cases develop complications, usually focal stricture, or more seriously, bowel necrosis, which requires surgical intervention. Interestingly, the site of complications is most commonly in the sigmoid colon.

Toxic megacolon (TMC) (Box 7-7) is an acute complication of fulminating inflammatory disease of the colon that involves the entire thickness of the bowel wall (Fig. 7-87). Tissue cohesion is severely impaired, and perforation is a common result. TMC is most frequently seen as a complication of ulcerative colitis, although it occurs with less frequency in Crohn's disease and in bacterial colitis. It has also been reported in pseudomembranous colitis as well as ischemic colitis.

The condition is characterized by a dilated transverse colon with marked thickening and nodularity of the haustral pattern. Multiple nodular filling defects can also be seen profiled and en face, representing pseudopolyps. The reason these changes are mostly seen in the transverse colon is because the transverse colon represents the most anterior portion of the colon in the supine patient. As a result, air gathers in the transverse colon and the findings are most apparent in this region. In fact, toxic megacolon may involve the entire colon and even portions of the distal small bowel. Additionally, it should be remembered that a few cases of toxic megacolon have been reported in which the transverse colon is not significantly dilated. Although radiographically these cases may appear similar to ischemic colitis, the clinical presentation makes differentiation relatively easy. Patients presenting with toxic megacolon are systemically toxic and usually have a history of IBD.

Although the barium enema has been implicated in the development of TMC in patients with IBD, this probably is more of a temporal relationship than cause and effect. However, when presented with plain films of a severely ill patient with findings suggesting TMC,

---

Box 7-7 Characteristics of Toxic Megacolon
Seen in acute fulminating inflammatory bowel disease A full thickness process Breakdown of tissue cohesion Passage of bacteria and bacterial toxins across disrupted mucosal surface Increased incidence of perforation All parts of colon may be affected Dilatation present, but more important radiological signs are thickened folds and prominent thumbprinting.

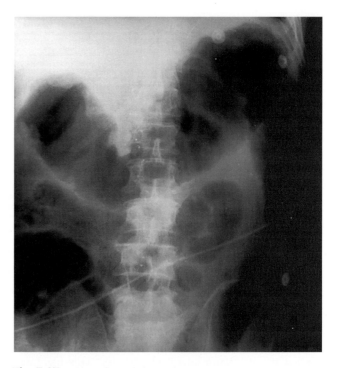

Fig. 7-87   Plain film of the abdomen of a patient with severe inflammatory bowel disease demonstrates dilatation of the colon, particularly in the transverse region, with thickening and nodularity of the folds typical of toxic megacolon.

contrast examination of the colon is contraindicated because of the high risk of perforation.

Pseudomembranous colitis may also present with plain films demonstrating a thickened nodular fold pattern within the colon. This finding occurs as a result of the marked edema and the presence of adherent pseudomembranes along the mucosal surface. This condition, although uncommon, can result in a potentially deadly illness. It has been referred to as antibiotic colitis and is thought to represent a complication of chronic antibiotic therapy. Clinically, the patient often experiences diarrhea with occasional bleeding and abdominal pain. The onset of symptoms is usually within 2 to 3 days following the commencement of antibiotic therapy. Although the condition was initially associated with lincomycin and tetracycline, it is now known that virtually any antibiotic can trigger the disease.

The underlying cause is thought to represent an acute change of the bacterial colonic flora and an overgrowth of the bacterium, *Clostridium difficile,* which is known to produce toxins absorbed across the colonic mucosa. The finding of marked bowel wall and haustral thickening with nodularity and possible thumbprinting in a patient with suspected pseudomembranous colitis should give sufficient warning to the radiologist to avoid doing a barium enema examination. These patients also run an increased risk of perforation.

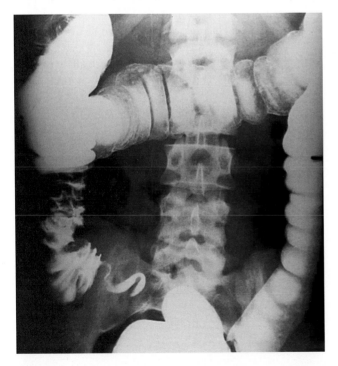

Fig. 7-88 A young patient with leukemia presents with right lower quadrant abdominal pain. Barium enema demonstrates inflammatory and spastic changes involving the cecum and a portion of the ascending colon, representing typhlitis.

Other conditions that may mimic thumbprinting include lymphoma, carcinoma, metastatic extension from the serosal surface, amyloid infiltration of the bowel, and in the cecal region, typhlitis.

Typhlitis, sometimes known as neutropenic enterocolitis, is a condition occasionally encountered in patients undergoing treatment for hematological malignancies, particularly leukemia and lymphoma (Fig. 7-88). The patients are often neutropenic, and changes are most commonly seen in the terminal ileum, cecum, and proximal ascending colon. Marked focal changes of inflammation that can progress to bowel wall necrosis are the manifestations of this condition, and the clinical findings may simulate acute appendicitis.

An interesting condition that, to the inattentive observer, can simulate the appearance of haustral fold thickening and possible thumbprinting is pneumatosis coli. The haustral folds may appear thickened and nodular, but careful attention to the films discloses that this is the result of cystic collections of air in the bowel wall (see Fig. 7-40).

POSITIONAL ABNORMALITIES

Malrotation

Degrees of colonic malrotation can occur and are usually of little clinical significance (Fig. 7-89). These result from the counterclockwise rotation that occurs as the midgut returns from the umbilical sac into the abdominal cavity between 6 and 12 weeks of embryonic life. The amount of rotation may be incomplete, and fixation of the ascending portion of the colon may be either absent or limited. This can cause considerable mobility of the cecum and ascending colon. This condition may potentially predispose to internal torsion abnormalities, such as cecal or transverse colon volvulus. Complete failure of rotation, or nonrotation, is not common. When it does occur, the entire colon is seen on the left side of the abdomen and the small bowel on the right side.

Hernias

Hernias, of both the inguinal and femoral canals, can include segments of colon, most commonly sigmoid. However, the cecum and appendix can also be involved. Internal hernias can involve the colon. These include mesenteric hernias, diaphragmatic hernias, and even herniation through the foramen of Winslow into the lesser sac. Hernias through the diaphragm can occur as a result of traumatic defects in the diaphragm or as a result of congenital defects, such as Morgagni's hernia anteriorly or Bochdalek's hernia of the posterior diaphragm. These herniations may exist for long periods of time with no symptoms. However, strangulation or obstruction of the bowel can occur and result in a surgical emergency.

Herniation of portions of both small bowel and colon through the anterior abdominal wall is relatively common. This includes umbilical hernias and postoperative incisional hernias. Spigelian hernia is an unusual form of ventral hernia in which a defect occurs along the linea semilunaris located in the abdominal wall lateral to the rectus abdominis muscle. The herniated portions of bowel pass through the transverse and internal oblique muscle layers but remain beneath the overlying intact external oblique muscle. As a result, the hernia is difficult to detect clinically and quite frequently there are no symptoms. Occasional, intermittent abdominal pain is reported in some patients. Radiographically, bowel seen on plain film, CT, or barium enema lying laterally to the rectus muscle outside the expected confines of the peritoneal cavity suggests the diagnosis.

MISCELLANEOUS

Presacral Widening

The presacral, retrorectal space normally measures up to 1.5 cm. However, a number of conditions can result in abnormal widening of the presacral space. Most of these conditions involve the rectum itself, and abnormal rectal findings are usually present on the barium enema examination.

The most common cause of presacral widening is inflammatory disease involving the rectum and colon. This is a common finding in ulcerative colitis but can also be seen in Crohn's disease when it involves the rectum (Fig. 7-90). Formation of perirectal fistulous tracts or abscesses in Crohn's disease can result in further widening of the presacral space. Other inflammatory conditions of the rectum, including LGV, radiation proctitis, viral (e.g., CMV) proctitis (Fig. 7-91), and, rarely, ischemic disease can result in increased presacral space size.

Neoplastic disease arising from the colon, such as carcinoma of the rectum, is also an important cause of an enlarged retrorectal space. The most common malignant lesion is adenocarcinoma, which usually results in a large, bulky lesion. However, the mass of the lesion plus the perirectal extension can combine to cause significant widening of the presacral space. Other rare malignancies of the rectum include lymphoma and cloacogenic carcinoma, both of which may produce similar appearances.

Cystic lesions that contribute to presacral widening are dermoid cysts (sacral teratoma), and less commonly, rectal duplications (enteric cysts) (Fig. 7-92).

Lesions arising from the sacrum itself can also contribute to a widened presacral space (Box 7-8). These

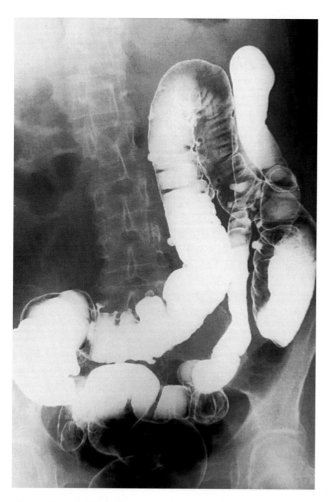

Fig. 7-89 Barium enema in a patient with malrotation demonstrates both flexures on the left side of the abdomen. The cecum is in its expected location.

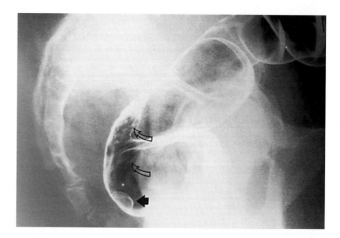

Fig. 7-90 Spot film of the rectum demonstrates inflammatory changes of the rectum *(curved arrows)* associated with widened presacral space. Also note a small adenomatous polyp *(arrow)*.

include infectious processes, such as osteomyelitis of the sacrum, metastatic disease, primary bone tumors, and neurogenic tumors arising from the sacrum. Chordomas are seen in the cervical and sacrococcygeal regions of the spine. These are slow-growing lesions, usually resulting in destructive changes in the sacrum, mass effect with anterior extension and displacement of the rectum, and widening of the presacral space.

Malignant neoplastic lesions arising from structures around the rectum can, by contiguous extension, encircle and deform the rectum and widen the presacral space. This is not common but is occasionally seen in prostatic carcinoma in men and cervical carcinoma in women (Fig. 7-93).

Pelvic abscesses with extension into the pouch of Douglas can result in widening of the presacral space on barium enema examination. Although the abscess itself may not extend beyond the confines of the peritoneal recess into the actual presacral space, the effect of adjacent inflammation presumably results in sufficient edema in the region to separate the rectum and sacral margin. A common example of this is periappendiceal abscess with pus collections in the lower pelvic recesses. Both pelvic inflammatory disease and diverticulitis may have similar effects.

Fistulous Connections and Sinus Tract Formation

Fistulous connections and sinus tract formation are the hallmarks of Crohn's disease. Full-thickness involvement of bowel wall by the disease and extension beyond the wall to the adjacent mesentery and mesenteric fat often result in matting and bonding together of several loops of bowel. Mucosal ulcerations progress, deepen, penetrate, and eventually communicate with the adjacent adherent loops of bowel. This is frequently seen in the right lower quadrant, with fistulous tracts between ileal loops and adjacent ileum, cecum, and ascending colon. These fistulous communications can also extend to the skin, particularly in the postoperative patient. Enteric-colonic fistulous formation does not necessarily present a problem in itself and, in some instances, may actually relieve the potential for obstruction. However,

Box 7-8	Causes of Widened Presacral Space

Inflammatory bowel disease
Pelvic lipomatosis
Sacral lesions
Perirectal lesions (e.g., prostate and cervical cancer)
Pelvic inflammatory diseases

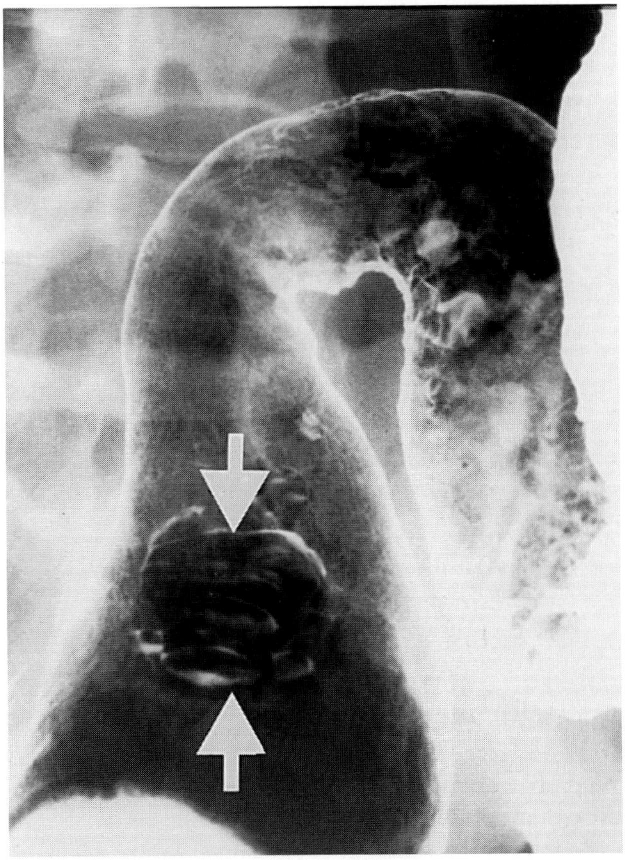

Fig. 7-91   Rectal spot views in a patient with CMV proctitis demonstrate numerous ulcerations, including a huge, superficial ulcer in the rectum *(arrows)*.

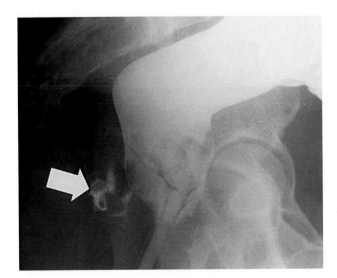

Fig. 7-92   Presacral space is widened secondary to a rectal duplication. There is some communication between the enteric cyst and the bowel lumen, with contrast seen within the duplication *(arrow)*.

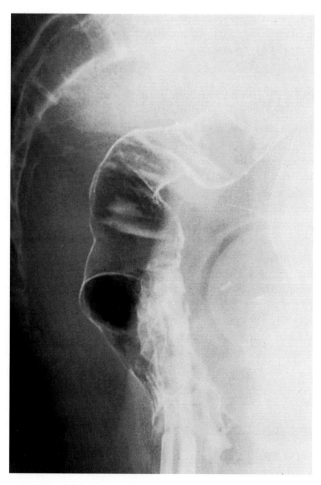

Fig. 7-93 DCBE in a patient with aggressive carcinoma of the cervix. The lesion has invaded the perirectal region with widening of the presacral space.

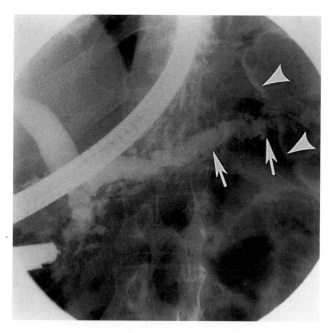

Fig. 7-94 ERCP in a patient with chronic pancreatitis. The pancreatic duct is ectatic and dilated *(arrows)*. There is communication with the splenic flexure of the adjacent colon, and contrast is seen on the colonic mucosa *(arrowheads)*, confirming a pancreaticocolonic fistula.

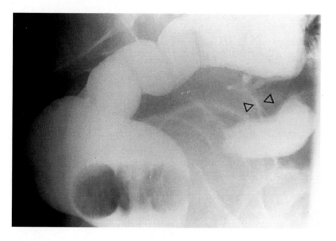

Fig. 7-95 SCBE in a patient with radiation colitis and a narrow fistulous communication *(arrowheads)* to the bladder.

the development of abscess cavities along the tract, the diverting and bypassing of a significant amount of bowel resulting in malnutrition or extension of the fistula to the skin or adjacent organs, can represent serious complications.

Fistulous communications between the stomach and the colon result from either inflammatory or malignant disease arising in the stomach or colon. The large, penetrating benign gastric ulcer (seen in patients on steroids or high doses of aspirin) that communicates with the colon is rarely encountered today. Malignant lesions arising from the greater curvature of the body and fundus of the stomach or the splenic flexure of the colon can form a gastrocolic fistula.

Patients with chronic pancreatitis, on rare occasion, develop a fistulous communication from the pancreatic duct to the colon (Fig. 7-94).

Sinus tracts and fistulous communications are not uncommon in patients with diverticulitis. The fistulous communications are often from colon to bowel loop, particularly adjacent small bowel. However, fistulous

tracts may also develop between the colon and the vagina or the bladder.

On occasion, radiation colitis can result in a fistulous communication between adjacent bowel or other structures, such as the bladder or vagina (Fig. 7-95).

An interesting variation of sinus tract formation is the intramural sinus tract, sometimes referred to as "double-tracking," which is most commonly seen in diverticulitis (Fig. 7-96). However, this can also be seen to a lesser extent in patients with Crohn's disease. Patients with

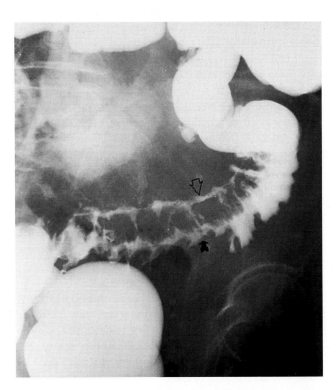

Fig. 7-96   Well-defined example of double-tracking on a barium enema. The narrowed, irregular lumen is seen *(closed arrow)*. Parallel to this is the intramural tract of barium *(open arrow)*.

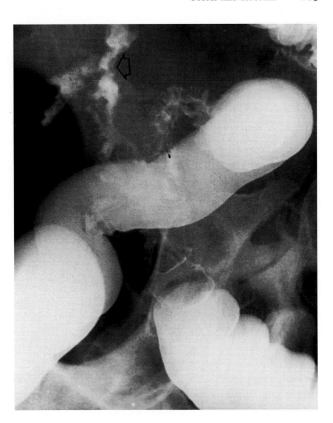

Fig. 7-98   Barium enema in a patient with intraabdominal actinomycosis involving the sigmoid colon, with resultant spasm, narrowing, and development of a branching sinus tract *(arrow)* extending from the affected sigmoid colon.

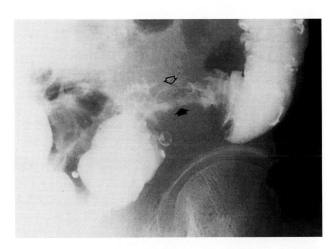

Fig. 7-97   A patient with adenocarcinoma of the sigmoid colon and an apple core type of constricting lesion. Note the narrowed lumen *(closed arrow)* and the adjacent thin, poorly defined periluminal tract *(open arrow)*.

carcinoma of the colon may also have short, irregular intramural sinus tracts (Fig. 7-97).

Actinomycosis with colonic involvement frequently results in sinus or fistulous tracts and communication with adjacent organs or the skin. The blatant disregard of *Actinomyces* for fascial planes is a hallmark of its natural history, and fistulous communications are a common manifestation (Fig. 7-98). Fistula and sinus formation is also a common finding with LGV (Fig. 7-99).

Appendix

The normal appendix originates between the cecal tip and the ileocecal valve. It is a structure of variable length, measuring anywhere from 4 to 12 cm. In a significant number of cases (approximately 25%), the appendix may be retrocecal in position and the tip of the appendix, on occasion, may be located in the right upper quadrant of the abdomen below or at the margin of the liver. Filling of the appendix during a barium enema study occurs in approximately 60% of cases. If a postevacuation film is obtained, one can expect to see additional filling in another 20% to 25% of patients.

The most common condition of the appendix is appendicitis, resulting from occlusion of the appendiceal lumen by a fecalith and development of inflammatory changes within the obstructed appendix. The appendiceal wall becomes thickened, hyperemic, and edematous. Clinical presentation is usually suggestive of the diagnosis. Progression of the inflammatory process can result in perforation with periappendiceal abscess formation or free perforation and generalized peritonitis. On barium enema, spasm at the cecal tip or mass effect from the adjacent abscess may be the expected findings. Incomplete filling of the appendix during barium enema does not exclude appendicitis. However, complete filling and demonstration of the bulbous tip of the appendix do rule out the diagnosis. CT evaluation of the right lower quadrant of the abdomen shows changes of appendicitis from wisps of stranding in the periappendiceal fat-thickened appendiceal wall to frank abscess formation. The CT evaluation is far more sensitive than any other imaging tool currently used.

Crohn's disease of the terminal ileum or cecum may also, by extension, involve the appendix (Fig. 7-100). Isolated appendiceal involvement is extremely rare.

The most common cause of a filling defect at the tip of the cecum is previous appendectomy with an inverted appendiceal stump. Frequently this inverted stump is smooth and in its expected location. On occasion, the stump can appear lobular and require colonoscopy to differentiate it from a neoplasm. Occasionally, a true neoplasm is found arising from the appendiceal stump. There is no reason to suspect that this is any more than coincidental, nor is there evidence to suggest any

increased risk of malignancy at the site of the inverted stump. On occasion, a filling defect at the base of cecum, sometimes with concentric circles arising from the center of the filling defect, can be seen and is the result of appendiceal intussusception. This frequently is asymptomatic and transient, although occasionally it can be associated with acute appendicitis. A similar "coil-spring" appearance can also be seen after appendectomy.

A mucocele of the appendix is another cause of a filling defect at the appendiceal origin. The most widely held etiology for this condition is aseptic obstruction of the appendiceal lumen with mucus accumulation and cyst formation. Most of these lesions are asymptomatic. Occasionally, the mucocele can calcify in its wall. Rupture of an appendiceal mucocele can lead to the condition known as pseudomyxoma peritonei, in which spillage of the mucocele content results in massive accumulations of thick, gelatinous, adhesive type of ascites.

An interesting and rare type of appendiceal mucocele is myxoglobulosis, in which numerous, tiny cohesive translucent globules are mixed with the liquid mucous content of the mucocele. These globules can calcify and, on positional views of the abdomen, may be seen to move within the mucocele.

The most common of appendiceal neoplasms is the carcinoid. The appendix, in fact, represents the most

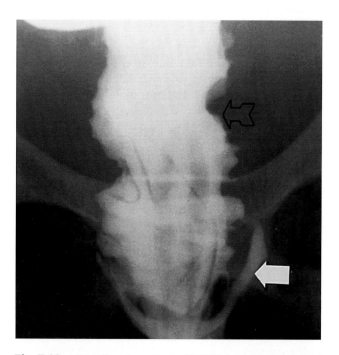

Fig. 7-99 Spot film of a patient with LGV demonstrates marked irregularity and ulceration of the rectal margin *(open arrow)*, as well as prominent bilateral perirectal sinus tracts *(closed arrow)*.

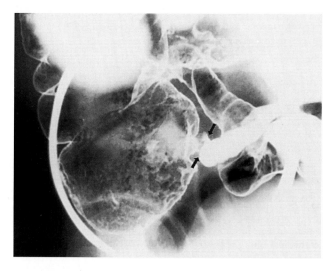

Fig. 7-100 Spot film of the cecum on a patient with Crohn's disease. Inflammatory involvement of the cecum, more severe on its medial aspect around the origin of the appendix, is seen. There is also involvement of the first several centimeters *(arrows)* of the appendix.

common site of carcinoid development within the GI tract. Over 90% of GI carcinoids arise from either the appendix or the distal ileum. These lesions are almost always benign and rarely cause the carcinoid syndrome. The discovery is usually incidental during surgery or autopsy.

Primary malignant neoplasm of the appendix is unusual and is invariably adenocarcinoma. Frequently, this results in gradual luminal obstruction and may present as acute appendicitis. The diagnosis is frequently intraoperative or postoperative.

Ileocecal Valve Enlargement

The appearance of the ileocecal valve can be quite variable, from a small polypoid filling defect on the first transverse fold within the colon to the more typical liplike valvular configuration (Fig. 7-101; Box 7-9). The normal valve may also have a rosette configuration. It is commonly located on the medial side of the cecum, although there can be variation. The valve can be seen on the lateral margin of the cecum in some patients. The size of the normal valve can also be quite variable. The upper limit of normal for the vertical diameter of the valve is probably 3 to 4 cm. Generally speaking, the valve should be measured during full cecal distention. It is not uncommon to see prominence of the valve on a postevacuation film as compared with the distended cecal views (Fig. 7-102). This is because there are degrees of ileal prolapse through the valve when the cecum is collapsed, accentuating the size of the valve.

Reflux of barium across the ileocecal valve into the terminal ileum is a common phenomenon on SCBE, probably occurring in more than 75% of the cases. Fortunately, this is not the case with double-contrast technique, and reflux into the terminal ileum with obscuration of the sigmoid colon occurs with considerably less frequency. The exact reason for this is unclear. It may relate to the smaller amounts and the more viscous nature of the barium used in double-contrast work.

The most common benign neoplastic lesion of the ileocecal valve is the lipoma, which is seen as a rounded, well-circumscribed, smooth mass arising from one of the valvular lips. This should be differentiated from lipomatous valvular infiltration, which is not a neoplastic process (Fig. 7-103). In the latter condition, the valve may appear large and lobulated along both lips. There is also a change of valvular configuration with compression. The diagnosis can be confirmed with CT examination of the cecum, in which the fat density can be seen easily. Both benign adenomas and adenocarcinomas can arise from the ileocecal valve. Like most cecal or right-sided lesions, a valvular malignancy can grow to sizeable proportions before becoming symptomatic, as a result of the fluid nature of the bowel content at this level (Figs. 7-104 and 7-105).

Inflammatory changes involving the terminal ileum and the cecum can also involve the valve. This is particularly the case in Crohn's disease, where involvement of the ileocecal valve frequently indicates involvement of the terminal ileum. *Yersinia,* which involves the distal ileum, may also result in inflammatory changes of the valve.

Box 7-9   When the Valve Looks Big: Ileocecal Valve Enlargement

Normal variation
Valvular lipomatosis
Lipoma of the valve
Adenomatous polyp involving the valve
Carcinoma
Inflammatory changes

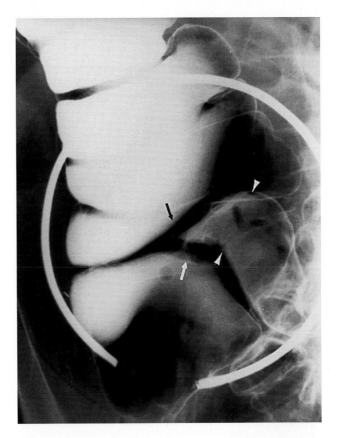

Fig. 7-101   Spot film from a barium enema demonstrates the normal and most common configuration of the ileocecal valve. Note the smooth V-shaped configuration of the valve *(arrows)* and the normal bird's-head configuration of the terminal ileum *(arrowheads)* as it enters the valve.

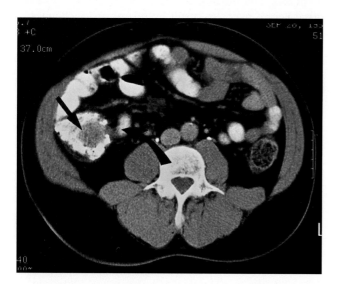

Fig. 7-102 CT study shows filling defect, or *colonic lesion,* in the cecum *(arrow).* Colonoscopy was normal. Finding is pseudo-mass of cecum *(straight arrow)* resulting from some prolapse of valve and distal ileum *(curved arrow)* in undistended cecum. Pseudomasses will disappear with cecal distention.

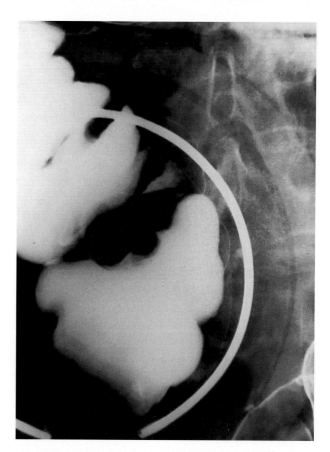

Fig. 7-103 A patient with lipomatous infiltration of the ileocecal valve. The valve is enlarged and nodular. Compression may cause the valve to change shape.

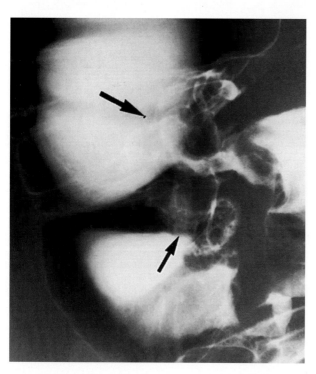

Fig. 7-104 A large polypoid carcinoma arising from the ileocecal valve *(arrows).* Note the narrowing of the lumen of the valve and the adjacent terminal ileum into which the tumor has extended. This patient is not obstructed.

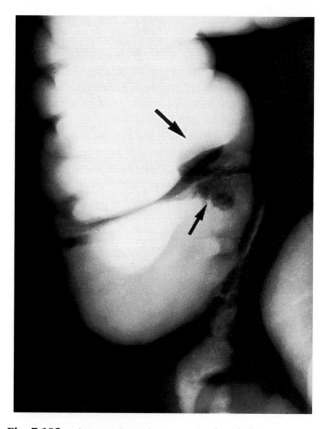

Fig. 7-105 An anemic patient examined with barium enema was found to have a lobulated lesion arising from the ileocecal valve *(arrows),* which proved to be a villous adenoma.

In ulcerative pancolitis, inflammation in the cecal region can result in incompetence of the valve and unimpeded reflux into the terminal ileum. The ileum tends to appear large and distended but is usually not involved in the primary inflammatory process.

Inflammatory conditions that involve the ileocecal region, including tuberculosis, amebiasis, and typhoid fever, can also involve the ileocecal valve.

Defecography

In modern society, the number of patients with complaints of defecation problems is on the rise. It has only been in the last decade that there has been a serious evaluation of this clinical problem. Radiographically, the method that has been used most frequently is that of defecography, which is sometimes called evacuation proctography.

Defecography is the radiographic dynamic assessment of the patient during defecation. Technically, the rectum is filled with a thick, viscous barium material. The material is so thick that it must be injected into the rectum by use of a caulking gun. Also, before this step, the patient ingests thin barium orally to opacify the loops of small bowel. In women, the vagina may also be opacified through use of a radiopaque gel or a tampon soaked with contrast material. The patient is then placed on a radiolucent commode, which is attached to the fluoroscopic table. This commode is commercially available and made of plastic. Radiographs in the lateral projection are obtained. Before the patient defecates, lateral views are obtained with the patient at rest, during straining but without defecation, and with voluntary contracting of the pelvic musculature.

The patient is then asked to defecate, and sequential films or videotape recording of defecation is obtained. Sequential films can be acquired with a 105-mm camera. This can also be acquired digitally, if one has a digital fluoroscopic unit. Some people feel that acquiring the image on videotape is all that is necessary.

There are several measurements that are made from the images. The most commonly used is that of the anorectal angle (Fig. 7-106). The anorectal angle is measured by drawing one line through the anal canal and another along the posterior wall of the rectum. The anorectal angle is created by the contraction of the puborectalis muscle around the anorectal region. At rest this measures about 90 degrees and is rarely greater than 120 degrees. The angle becomes greater on straining and becomes smaller when the patient is asked to squeeze or lift the buttocks. When the patient defecates, this angle becomes quite obtuse and approaches 180 degrees. If this does not occur, it indicates that the puborectalis is failing to relax during defecation, which can have serious consequences.

Another measurement is that of the level of the anorectal junction. It is measured according to its relationship to the ischial tuberosities, which are usually visible on the images. A positive measurement indicates that the anorectal junction is above the inferior aspect of the ischial tuberosity. A negative measurement indicates that the junction is below it. In normal patients, the measurement is slightly positive, but becomes negative during defecation. Normally, this anorectal junction descends a distance of 2 to 4 cm during defecation.

Abnormalities

The most commonly encountered abnormality on defecography is that of the rectocele. This is an outpouching of the rectal wall occurring anteriorly (Fig. 7-107). It is felt to be due to a weakness of the rectovaginal septum. It is such a common finding in women that some feel that only larger rectoceles (larger than 3 cm) should be mentioned, and that smaller rectoceles are probably of little clinical consequence. Sometimes there is also internal rectal prolapse, and the material in the rectocele becomes separated from the rectum and cannot be emptied. In this circumstance, the patient often complains of incomplete evacuation.

Sometimes portions of the small bowel or even the sigmoid colon may descend or herniate into the pouch of Douglas. When this occurs, the small bowel or sigmoid colon may descend between the anterior wall of the rectum and the vagina. When the small bowel does this, it is termed an enterocele (Fig. 7-107) and if it is the sigmoid colon, it is termed a sigmoidocele. In both circumstances, the patient may feel abnormal pressure on the perineum during defecation.

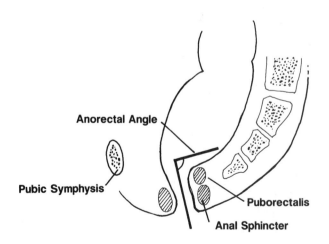

Fig. 7-106   Diagram of the rectum at rest. The anorectal angle is formed by a line drawn through the anal canal and another line drawn along the posterior wall of the rectum. Contraction of the puborectalis muscle is necessary to maintain the angle near 90 degrees. Also, at defecation, the puborectalis relaxes and the anorectal angle becomes more obtuse.

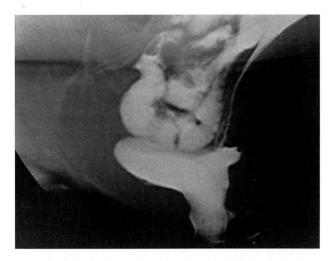

Fig. 7-107   Lateral view during defecation. The large bulge along the anterior wall of the rectum during rectal contraction indicates the presence of a rectocele. The small bowel loops that are opacified by orally ingested barium are descending quite low in the pelvis, indicating an enterocele.

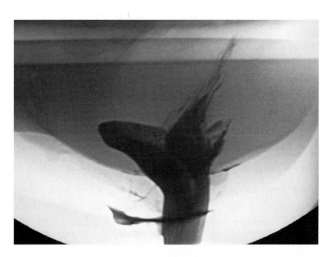

Fig. 7-108   During defecation, a portion of the rectal mucosa invaginates toward the anal canal. Note that a portion of the rectal lumen becomes pinched off anteriorly. This indicates the presence of internal intussusception or prolapse.

Rectal prolapse or intussusception is an invagination of the rectal mucosa toward or even through the anal canal. The invaginated mucosa may just be a portion of the rectal wall (usually anterior) or the entire circumference of the rectum. It starts in the mid to lower rectum near the valves of Houston. This invagination can be seen as a slight ring developing in the lower rectum and is often of little significance. However, it may extend down toward the anal canal and sometimes obstruct defecation (Fig. 7-108). When it is quite severe it can prolapse through the anal canal and can be seen externally (Fig. 7-109). These patients often manually reduce this intussuscepted plug of mucosa in order to continue defecating. With internal rectal prolapse, damage may occur to the mucosa of the rectum, producing ulceration, or the so-called solitary rectal ulcer syndrome. The solitary rectal ulcer syndrome is just a sequela of repeated internal and even external rectal prolapse.

The puborectalis muscle has an important function in maintaining proper rectal function both at rest and during defecation. At rest, the puborectalis maintains an acute angle between the rectum and anus and is felt to be more important in maintaining rectal continence than is the anal sphincter. Patients who are incontinent often have a shallow or obtuse rectal angle at rest because of poor puborectalis contractility. Also, when the patient defecates, the puborectalis must relax and produce straightening of the anorectal angle. If this does not occur, the patient will have a great deal of difficulty defecating, often with resultant pain. This is sometimes called a spastic pelvic floor.

As mentioned previously, the pelvic floor is determined by the relationship of the anorectal junction to the

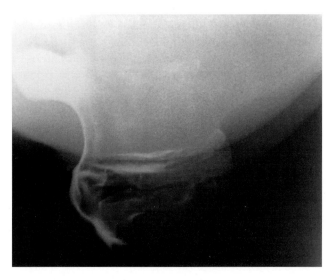

Fig. 7-109   After defecation, a masslike soft tissue density is seen external to the anus. It is coated with barium. This is due to external prolapse of rectal mucosa.

ischial tuberosities. In younger patients the anorectal junction may be above the ischial tuberosities, while in older patients it is at or below the tuberosities. During defecation this descends for a distance of several centimeters, usually 2 to 4 cm. If the descent is 5 cm or greater, it can be considered abnormal. In some individuals this may cause pudendal nerve damage and eventual rectal incontinence. Patients with incontinence often have an exaggerated movement of the pelvic floor on defecation.

On occasion, the posterolateral wall of the rectum may herniate through the pelvic floor musculature, forming a posterolateral pouch. This occurs in people with excessive straining during defecation. It may produce symptoms of a palpable bulge in the buttocks and give symptoms of incomplete evacuation.

SUGGESTED READINGS

Balikian JP, Uthman SM, Khouri NF: Intestinal amoebiasis, *AJR* 122:245-256, 1974.

Balthazar EJ, Megibow AJ, Hulnick D, et al: Carcinoma of the colon: detection and preoperative staging by CT, *AJR* 150:301-306, 1988.

Balthazar EJ, Megibow A, Schinella RA, et al: Limitations in the CT diagnosis of acute diverticulitis: comparison of CT, contrast enema, and pathologic findings in 16 patients, *AJR* 154:281-285, 1990.

Bartram CI: Radiology in the current assessment of ulcerative colitis, *Gastrointest Radiol* 1:383-392, 1977.

Bernstein MA, Feczko PJ, Halpert RD, et al: Distribution of colonic polyps: increased incidence of proximal lesions in older patients, *Radiology* 155:35-38, 1985.

Brady AP, Stevenson GW, Stevenson I: Colorectal cancer overlooked at barium enema examination and colonoscopy: a continuing perceptual problem, *Radiology* 192:373-378, 1994.

Brentall TA, Haggitt RC, Rabinovitch PS, et al: Risk and natural history of colonic neoplasia in patients with primary sclerosing cholangitis and ulcerative colitis, *Gastroenterology* 110:331-338, 1996.

Campbell WL, Wolff M: Retrorectal cysts of developmental origin, *AJR* 117:307-313, 1973.

Cho CK, Morehouse HT, Alterman DD, et al: Sigmoid diverticulitis: diagnostic role of CT—comparison with barium enema studies, *Radiology* 176:111-115, 1990.

Chrispin AR, Fry IK: The presacral space shown by barium enema, *Br J Radiol* 36:319-322, 1963.

Claymon CB: Mass screening for colorectal cancer: are we ready? *JAMA* 261:609, 1989.

deLange EE, Fechner RE, Edge SB, et al: Preoperative staging of rectal carcinoma with MR imaging: surgical and histopathologic correlation, *Radiology* 176:623-628, 1990.

Dworkin B, Winawer SJ, Lighdale CJ: Typhlitis: report of a case with long-term survival and a review of the recent literature, *Dig Dis Sci* 26:1032-1037, 1981.

Feczko PJ, Halpert RD: Reassessing the role of radiology in Hemoccult screening, *AJR* 146:697-701, 1986.

Fishman EK, Kavuru M, Jones B, et al: Pseudomembranous colitis: CT evaluation of 26 cases, *Radiology* 180:57-60, 1991.

Fleischer DE, Goldberg SB, Browning TH, et al: Detection and surveillance of colorectal cancer, *JAMA* 261:580-585, 1989.

Frager DH, Goldman M, Beneventano TC: Computed tomography in Crohn disease, *J Comput Assist Tomogr* 7:819-824, 1983.

Gelfand DW: Decreased risk of subsequent colonic cancer in patients undergoing polypectomy after barium enema: analysis based on data from the preendoscopic era, *AJR* 169:1243-1245, 1997.

Gelfand DW, Wu WC, Ott DJ: The extent of successful colonoscopy: its implication for the radiologists, *Gastrointest Radiol* 4:75-78, 1979.

Glotzer DJ, Glick ME, Goldman H: Proctitis and colitis following diversion of the fecal stream, *Gastroenterology* 80:438-441, 1981.

Golstein SJ, MacKenzie Crooks DJ: Colitis in Behçet's syndrome, *Radiology* 128:321-323, 1978.

Greenall MJ, Levine AW, Nolan DJ: Complications of diverticular disease: a review of the barium enema findings, *Gastrointest Radiol* 8:353-358, 1983.

Greenstein AJ, Janowitz HD, Sachar DB: The extra-intestinal complications of Crohn's disease and ulcerative colitis: a study of 700 patients, *Medicine* 55:401-412, 1976.

Halpert RD: Toxic dilatation of the colon, *Radiol Clin North Am* 25:147-155, 1987.

Henry MM: Pathogenesis and management of fecal incontinence in the adult, *Gastroenterol Clin North Am* 16:35-45, 1987.

Ikenberry S, Lappas JC, Hana MP, et al: Defecography in healthy subjects: comparison of three contrast media, *Radiology* 201:233-239, 1996.

Jackman RJ, Mayo CW: The adenoma-carcinoma sequence in cancer of the colon, *Surg Gynecol Obstet* 93:327-330, 1951.

Johnson CD, Ilstrup DM, Fish NM, et al: Barium enema: detection of colonic lesions in a community population, *AJR* 167:39-44, 1996.

Jones IT, Fazio VW: Colonic volvulus: etiology and management, *Dig Dis* 7:203-209, 1989.

Karasick S, Ehrlich SM, Levin DC, et al: Trends in use of barium enema examination, colonoscopy, and sigmoidoscopy: is use commensurate with risk of disease? *Radiology* 195:777-784, 1995.

Keller CE, Halpert RD, Feczko PJ, et al: Radiologic recognition of colonic diverticula simulating polyps, *AJR* 143:93-97, 1984.

Kelvin FM, Gardiner R, Vas W, et al: Colorectal carcinoma missed on double contrast barium study: a problem in perception, *AJR* 137:307-313, 1981.

Kelvin FM, Maglinte DD, Hornback JA, et al: Pelvic prolapse: assessment with evacuation proctography (defecography), *Radiology* 184:547-551, 1992.

Kelvin FM, Max RJ, Norton GA, et al: Lymphoid follicular pattern of the colon in adults, *AJR* 133:821-825, 1979.

Kelvin FM, Oddson TA, Rice RP, et al: Double contrast barium enema in Crohn's disease and ulcerative colitis, *AJR* 131:207-213, 1978.

Laufer I, Costopoulos L: Early lesions of Crohn's disease, *AJR* 130:307-311, 1978.

Laufer I, Mullens JE, Hamilton J: Correlation of endoscopy and double-contrast radiography in the early stages of ulcerative and granulomatous colitis, *Radiology* 118:1-5, 1976.

Lennard-Jones JE, Morson BC, Ritchie JK, et al: Cancer in colitis: assessment of the individual risk by clinical and histological criteria, *Gastroenterology* 73:1280-1289, 1977.

Maglinte DT, Keller KJ, Miller RE, et al: Colon and rectal carcinoma: spatial distribution and detection, *Radiology* 147:669-672, 1983.

McFarland EG, Brink JA, Loh J, et al: Visualization of colorectal polyps with spiral CT colography: evaluation of processing parameters with perspective volume rendering, *Radiology* 205:701-707, 1997.

Megibow AJ, Balthazar EJ, Kyunghee CC, et al: Bowel obstruction: evaluation with CT, *Radiology* 180:313-318, 1991.

Moon-June C, Ha CS, Allen PK, et al: Primary non-Hodgkin lymphoma of the large bowel, *Radiology* 205:535-539, 1997.

Moss AA: Computed tomography in the staging of gastrointestinal carcinoma, *Radiol Clin North Am* 20:761-780, 1982.

Munyer TP, Montgomery CK, Thoeni RF, et al: Post inflammatory polyposis (PIP) of the colon: the radiologic-pathologic spectrum, *Radiology* 145:607-614, 1982.

Muto T, Bussey HJR, Morson BC: The evolution of cancer of the colon and rectum, *Cancer* 36:2251-2270, 1975.

Ott DJ, Donati DL, Kerr RM, et al: Defecography: results in 55 patients and impact on clinical management, *Abdom Imaging* 19:349-358, 1994.

Ott DJ, Gelfand DW: How to improve the efficacy of the barium enema examination, *AJR* 160:491-495, 1993.

Ott DJ, Gelfand DW, Wu WC, et al: Sensitivity of double-contrast barium enema: emphasis on polyp detection, *AJR* 135:327-330, 1980.

Peskin GW, Orloff MJ: A clinical study of 25 patients with carcinoid tumors of the rectum, *Surg Gynecol Obstet* 109:673-682, 1959.

Pradel JA, Adel JF, Taourel P, et al: Acute colonic diverticulitis: prospective comparative evaluation with US and CT, *Radiology* 205:503-512, 1997.

Rifkin MD, Ehrlich SM, Marks G: Staging of rectal carcinoma: prospective comparison of endorectal US and CT, *Radiology* 170:319-322, 1989.

Rose CP, Stevenson GW, Somers S, et al: Inaccuracy of radiographic measurements of colon polyps, *J Can Assoc Radiol* 32:21-23, 1981.

Rubesin SE, Levine MS, Bezzi M, et al: Rectal involvement by prostatic carcinoma: barium enema findings, *AJR* 152:53-57, 1989.

Sauerbrei E, Castelli M: Hypogammaglobulinemia and nodular lymphoid hyperplasia of the gut, *J Can Assoc Radiol* 30:62-63, 1979.

Schuffler MD, Rohrmann CA, Templeton FE: The radiologic manifestation of idiopathic intestinal pseudoobstruction, *AJR* 127:729-736, 1976.

Stanley RJ, Melson GL, Tedesco FJ: The spectrum of radiographic findings in antibiotic-related pseudomembranous colitis, *Radiology* 111:519-524, 1974.

Thoeni RF, Petras A: Detection of rectal and rectosigmoid lesions by double-contrast barium enema examination and sigmoidoscopy, *Radiology* 142:59-62, 1982.

Van Fleet RH, Shabot MJ, Halpert RD: Adenocarcinoma of the appendiceal stump, *South Med J* 83:1351-1353, 1990.

Vogl TJ, Pegios W, Mack MG, et al: Accuracy of staging rectal tumors with contrast-enhanced transrectal MR imaging, *AJR* 168:1427-1434, 1997.

Yang XM, Paranen K, Farin P, et al: Defecography, *Acta Radiol* 36:460-468, 1995.

Miscellaneous Conditions

HERNIAS

A hernia can be described as the protrusion of an organ through an opening or aperture that can exist normally or be due to congenital, developmental, or acquired causes. Within the abdominal cavity, we tend to consider hernias only when portions of bowel protrude abnormally through some opening, because the large majority of hernias are manifested through the symptoms of bowel obstruction, ischemia, or related complications. Only a small portion of hernias are discovered incidentally. With the increasing use of cross-sectional imaging, it is common to encounter asymptomatic hernias. It also must be stressed that hernias can contain omentum rather than bowel; even

solid viscera can be within a hernia, which also can produce symptoms.

Diaphragmatic Hernias

Esophageal hiatus
Of the diaphragmatic hernias, those through the esophageal hiatus are by far the most common. These types of hernias are extensively discussed in Chapter 1.

Foramen of Bochdalek
During development, the posterolateral portion of the diaphragm is the last portion of the diaphragm to fuse during fetal development. This typically occurs during the eighth week of gestation by fusion of the pleuroperitoneal membrane. If this membrane fails to close before the intestines return to the abdominal cavity, a herniation of intestinal loops can result through what is called the foramen of Bochdalek. When significant portions of the intestines herniate into the hemithorax, they usually do so on the left side. If sufficiently large, herniation will interfere with lung development, resulting in pulmonary hypoplasia on the affected side. Some of these defects can be apparent in utero by ultrasound or detected in the neonate because of respiratory distress. When the hernia is quite small and contains only portions of retroperitoneal structures, it is unlikely to produce symptoms; hernias are usually discovered by chance in adulthood (Fig. 8-1). These defects are situated posterolaterally and sometimes detected on chest radiographs as a small protrusion of the posterior aspect of the diaphragm. They are typically encountered on the left side because the liver on the right side will block passage of material through the hernia unless the material is fairly large.

Foramen of Morgagni
The foramen of Morgagni is a retrosternal or parasternal hernia produced by small clefts between the muscle

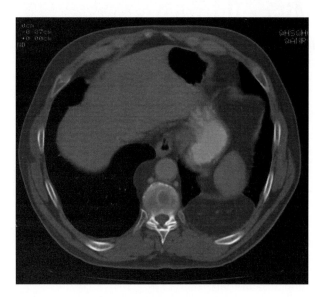

Fig. 8-1   Computed tomography of the lower chest demonstrates intraabdominal fat herniated through the foramen of Bochdalek into the left posterior costophrenic angle.

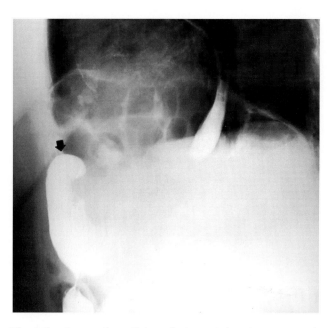

Fig. 8-2   Loop of small bowel *(arrow)* herniates anteriorly through the foramen of Morgagni.

fibers of diaphragm that arise from the sternum and the costal cartilages. A triangular portion of diaphragm can exist that does not contain any muscle and through which the internal mammary vessels can pass. Unlike the Bochdalek hernia, the Morgagni hernia is more frequently seen on the right side because the presence of the heart on the left side tends to block its development. The Morgagni hernia also typically does not become apparent until adulthood even though it is a developmental defect. That is because additional mechanisms, such as increased intraabdominal pressure, obesity, and related conditions, must be present for the abdominal contents to herniate through the defect. The hernia sac also frequently contains omentum, and only the largest Morgagni hernias contain portions of bowel (often stomach). The majority of Morgagni hernias are asymptomatic and identified only as masses in the right cardiophrenic region that contain fat or portions of bowel (Fig. 8-2). They can even extend, although rarely, into the pericardial sac. As previously stated, the vast majority are asymptomatic, although those containing portions of bowel have been known to produce bowel ischemia; surgical intervention is usually considered in those patients.

Acquired

Traumatic diaphragmatic hernias are an increasingly diagnosed entity, as the result of both high-speed motor accidents and penetrating trauma. Despite the increased incidence, less than half are diagnosed at the time of injury, which can cause significant morbidity and mortality.

The mechanism of injury in blunt trauma is due to a rapid increase in intraabdominal pressure at the time of the trauma, with transmission of the pressure to all portions of the abdominal cavity. Because the diaphragm is relatively weaker than other portions of the abdominal cavity, it is the most likely to tear as the result of a sudden increase in intraabdominal pressure. These traumatic diaphragmatic tears are more frequent on the left side because of several reasons. First, the liver to some extent protects the right diaphragm from the increase in pressure, and next, the left hemidiaphragm is relatively weaker than the right. In penetrating trauma, the diaphragmatic defect occurs at the site of injury and no special predilection exists for site. These defects may be overlooked initially because of the seriousness of other injuries the patient may have received.

Although the diaphragmatic defect can occur with the injury, the actual herniation of abdominal contents can be delayed for varying lengths of time, which gives rise to the patient's symptoms. The gradual herniation of intraabdominal contents is due to both the negative intrathoracic pressure generated by respiration and the intermittent waves of intraabdominal pressure generated by everyday activities. Thus, at the time of injury, a hernia may not be present, but the patient may return several years later with herniation of abdominal contents into the lower chest (Fig. 8-3). Because of the gradual development of the "delayed" herniations, the patient's symptoms can be vague; some nonspecific abdominal or lower chest pain is typical. Eventually, this can culminate in ischemia of the herniated structures, and surgical repair is warranted once the diaphragmatic tear is

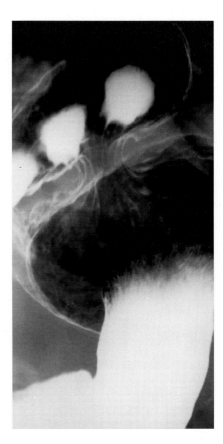

Fig. 8-3 Upper gastrointestinal examination shows the fundus of the stomach herniating through the central portion of the diaphragm and not the esophageal hiatus because of a posttraumatic diaphragmatic injury with delayed herniation of abdominal contents.

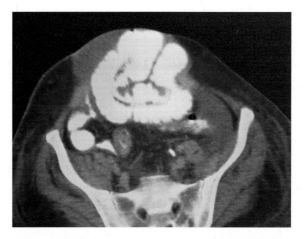

Fig. 8-4 Computed tomography of the lower abdomen shows an incisional hernia containing loops of small bowel located in the midline of the lower abdomen.

discovered. As with the other diaphragmatic hernias, omentum, bowel, and even solid viscera can herniate into the lower chest.

Anterior Abdominal Wall Hernias

Acquired hernias

The majority of hernias through the anterior abdominal wall are iatrogenic, the result of previous surgical intervention in the abdominal wall. Although hernias develop in only a small percentage (5% or less) of surgical patients, that number becomes enormous when one considers that several million abdominal surgeries are performed in any given year. The development of laparoscopic techniques will not have much effect on the development of hernias. In fact, many cases of hernias through the laparoscopic holes left in the abdominal wall have been encountered.

Most iatrogenic hernias develop in the first few months after the surgical procedure. This shows failure of complete healing of the fascial layers of the abdominal wall, with weakness of the underlying muscular layer as a result of the procedure. Many of these hernias are the

result not of poor surgical technique, but rather obesity or other predisposing conditions that hinder the healing process. However, with laparoscopic techniques the defects through the abdominal wall are not closed with a multilayer technique and inherent weaknesses in the wall are produced. Although the openings are quite small, omentum or loops of bowel can herniate into these openings before they have a chance to close.

Postprocedural abdominal hernias often become apparent within 1 year of the surgical procedure, although some remain silent for many years (Fig. 8-4). With the increasing use of cross-sectional techniques, asymptomatic occult herniations are commonly found in the abdominal wall. As with other hernias, the symptoms depend on the size of the hernia and the abdominal contents that are herniated. Smaller hernias are more likely to incarcerate loops of bowel and lead to strangulation and ischemia; thus the size of the hernia has no direct relationship to the severity of the clinical condition. A very small hernia may contain only half the wall of the bowel, a so-called Richter hernia (Fig. 8-5). These typically do not obstruct, but they can be associated with nonspecific abdominal symptoms.

A small number of acquired abdominal wall hernias result from penetrating trauma or other causes of abdominal wall injury with resultant injury to the layers of the abdominal wall and development of weaknesses. This is encountered primarily with severe penetrating injuries to the abdominal wall, and underlying conditions such as obesity often exist as well.

Ventral hernias

Ventral hernias occur in the anterior or lateral abdominal wall. Most of these occur in the midline, through a defect in the aponeurosis that forms the linea alba. Those located superior to the umbilicus are called *epigastric*, whereas those inferior to the umbilicus are called *hypogastric*. The superiorly located ventral hernias are much more common than those located inferior to the umbilicus. Mediolateral ventral hernias are the most infrequently encountered. Preceding surgery or other trauma can often predispose to their development.

Umbilical hernias

Defects in the abdominal wall adjacent to the umbilicus are frequent occurrences, especially in infants. Many of those encountered in neonates spontaneously disappear with time. Some of these infantile umbilical hernias contain loops of bowel and fail to close, necessitating surgery in some instances. It should be noted that omphaloceles are not true umbilical hernias in that the bowel never returns to an intraabdominal location during development. A second peak of umbilical hernias typically occurs in middle age and is associated with multiple pregnancies, obesity, ascites, or other conditions with increased intraabdominal pressure. These hernias can become large and contain omentum and loops of bowel. Surgery is often necessary if the bowel becomes incarcerated within the hernia sac.

Spigelian hernias

An uncommon hernia of the anterior abdominal wall is the so-called spigelian hernia, named after the physician who first described this entity. This is the result of a weakness of the linea semilunaris, which is the fibrous sheath of tissue between the rectus abdominis muscles and the transverse and oblique abdominal muscles of the lateral abdominal wall. A weakness may exist along this aponeurosis that allows portions of bowel to herniate into the anterior abdominal wall. Typically, the loops of bowel dissect laterally through the abdominal wall and are visible as they project beyond the lateral confines of the abdomen (Figs. 8-6 and 8-7).

Lumbar hernias

A rare flank herniation is the lumbar hernia. Superior and inferior lumbar spaces exist, called the Grynfeltt-Lesshaft and Petit triangles, respectively. The inferior lumbar space of Petit has as its inferior border the top of

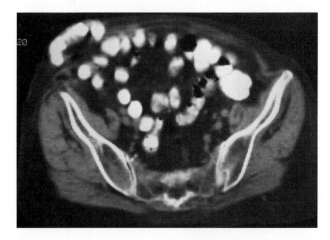

Fig. 8-6   A loop of small bowel in the right anterior, lateral abdomen is herniating through the linea semilunaris. This is a spigelian hernia.

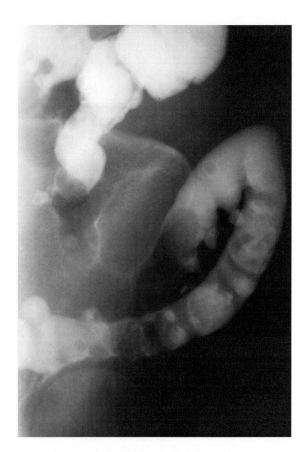

Fig. 8-7   Barium enema demonstrates the sigmoid colon herniating through a spigelian hernia in the left flank.

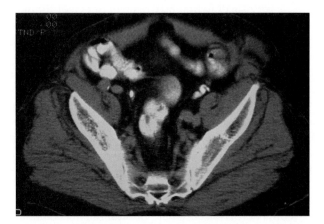

Fig. 8-5   A loop of small bowel partially enters a hernia along the left flank. Only one wall of the bowel is involved, a so-called Richter hernia. (Courtesy of Duane Mezwa, M.D.)

the iliac crest, and these hernias are encountered in that location (Fig. 8-8). The superior lumbar space of Grynfeltt-Lesshaft has as its superior border the twelfth rib. These hernias can contain retroperitoneal structures or sometimes loops of bowel, and they are best demonstrated by computed tomography (CT) examination. For some reason, they are typically seen on the left side and are thought to be more common among middle-aged men.

Pelvic Hernias

Inguinal hernias

The most common type of abdominal hernia by far is the inguinal hernia. This accounts for the vast majority of detected hernias, and its repair is one of the most common surgical procedures.

The most common type is the indirect inguinal hernia, which develops from the embryological formation of the pelvic structures. During movement of the testis into the scrotum, a peritoneal extension called the processus vaginalis accompanies the testis. In females, it follows the round ligament. This peritoneal communication is usually closed in utero; however, it may persist in up to one third of infants and a somewhat smaller number of adults. The persistence of the processus vaginalis allows the subsequent development of an indirect inguinal hernia in certain circumstances. When the processus vaginalis persists, abdominal contents can slide into the scrotum and less frequently into the labia majora. Loops of bowel, omentum, and even bladder or ureters have been known to extend into these inguinal hernias. Obstruction, incarceration, and strangulation are known complications of this type of hernia.

Conversely, the direct inguinal hernia is actually a direct protrusion through the lower abdominal wall in a weak area medial to the epigastric vessels. These hernias

are short, do not extend into the scrotum, and are usually asymptomatic because of the nature of the hernia sac. They are much more common in men and are rarely seen in women or children.

Femoral hernial

The femoral hernia is a much more common complication in women and is rarely seen in children and men (Fig. 8-9). These hernias begin lateral to the pelvic tubercle and below the inguinal ligament. Omentum or loops of bowel can protrude through the hernia, and these hernias are much more prone to incarceration or strangulation than are inguinal hernias. Although femoral hernias can be difficult to diagnose, barium studies show a loop of bowel projecting over the femoral head much more lateral than what is seen with an inguinal hernia.

Sciatic hernias

Sciatic hernia is an uncommon hernia that protrudes through the sciatic foramen (Fig. 8-10). This is actually the greater sciatic notch that has this complication and is the pathway for the sciatic nerve, gluteal vessels and nerves, and pyriformis muscle into the buttocks. This rare hernia often contains the distal ureter and sometimes a loop of bowel. Because of this, it is more frequently diagnosed on intravenous urography. CT may show a loop of bowel extending lateral behind the acetabulum and hip joint.

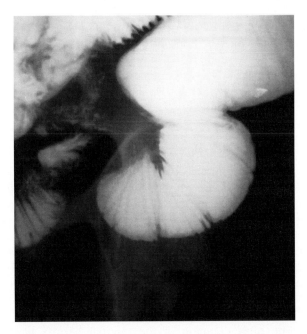

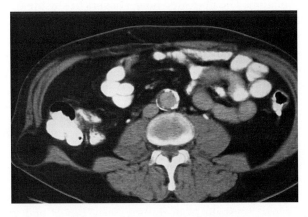

Fig. 8-8   A portion of retroperitoneal fat is herniating through Petit's triangle along the right posterior flank, producing a lumbar hernia. (Courtesy of Duane Mezwa, M.D.)

Fig. 8-9   A loop of small bowel projects over the femoral head in a femoral hernia. Note the constriction of the lumen. Femoral hernias produce obstructive changes more frequently than do inguinal hernias.

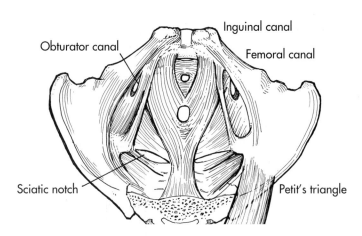

Fig. 8-10   Diagram of the pelvic inlet. Hernias of the pelvis occur through preexisting openings or spaces in the pelvic structures.

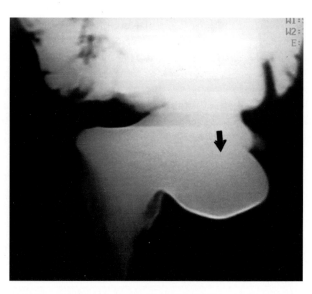

Fig. 8-11   During a barium enema, the left portion of the rectum *(arrow)* herniates through the pelvic floor into a perineal hernia.

Obturator hernias

An obscure pelvic hernia is the obturator hernia. The obturator nerve and vessels course through what is known as the obturator foramen. A CT scan may demonstrate a loop of bowel between the pectineus and obturator muscles; otherwise, this hernia is extremely difficult to diagnose. Obturator hernias are seen predominantly in women and in a much older age group. For some unknown reason, they are more common on the right side.

Perineal hernias are defects in the floor of the pelvis through which a portion of bowel or rectum can herniate. These are found more frequently among older women (Fig. 8-11). Weakness of the pelvic floor musculature, along with multiple births and even surgical procedures, is thought to predispose perineal hernias.

Internal Hernias

An internal hernia occurs when an abdominal structure passes through an opening or defect within the abdominal cavity and moves into another compartment of the abdomen. The structure itself does not lead out of the abdominal cavity but rather takes up residence in another portion of the abdomen where it should not be. The openings within the abdominal cavity can be naturally occurring or congenital or acquired defects.

Paraduodenal hernias

The most common of the internal hernias is the paraduodenal hernia, more commonly found in men. Two types of paraduodenal hernias exist, with the left paraduodenal hernia more common than the right.

The left paraduodenal hernia involves the fossa of Landzert and occurs just lateral to the fourth portion of the duodenum. Small bowel loops pass into the left upper quadrant behind the fourth portion of the duodenum and transverse mesocolon. These loops of bowel can become fixed in that location and produce symptoms such as recurrent pain and distention. Ischemia is the most serious complication of this hernia. Barium studies can show a fixed portion of small bowel in a confined clump in the left upper quadrant. CT can show similar findings and demonstrate distortion of the mesentery and displacement of mesenteric vessels.

The right paraduodenal hernia occurs through the fossa of Waldeyer. This orifice is behind the superior mesenteric artery and inferior to the third portion of the duodenum. The herniated bowel occurs below the right side of the transverse mesocolon. On barium studies a rounded clump of small bowel loops can be seen lateral to the descending duodenum (Fig. 8-12). Again, stretching of the mesentery and vessels occurs, and this can be seen with angiography or CT (Fig. 8-13).

Foramen of Winslow hernias

The foramen of Winslow is the orifice by which contents of the lesser sac communicate with the rest of the peritoneum. This is a relatively rare hernia and can be dependent on the size of the foramen and the mobility of the bowel. Herniation through the foramen of Winslow is usually done by the small bowel and less commonly by the gallbladder, kidney, or even large bowel. Barium studies can demonstrate loops of bowel protruding into the lesser sac.

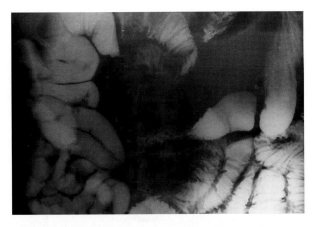

Fig. 8-12   In this patient with a right paraduodenal hernia, the duodenum is displaced to the left and there is a fixed loop of small bowel in the right upper quadrant.

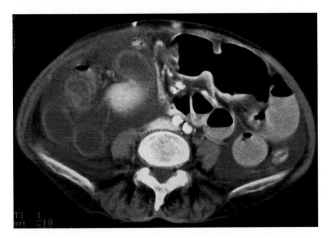

Fig. 8-13   Computed tomography demonstrates dilated bowel loops in the right upper quadrant. Incarcerated bowel loops are shown in a right paraduodenal hernia with resultant obstruction.

Transmesenteric hernias

Transmesenteric hernias occur through defects in the mesentery of the small bowel. This type of hernia is more frequently encountered in the pediatric population and may result from congenital defects within the mesentery. In these children the defects are thought to be the sequelae of previous vascular insults to the mesentery and bowel, which are frequent associated occurrences. In adults the mesenteric defects are typically associated with previous surgical procedures. Because loops of small bowel are usually herniated through these defects, a high incidence of obstruction or strangulation exists with transmesenteric hernias.

Other hernias

There are several other intraabdominal hernias, although they are all considered rare. Pericecal hernias occur when loops of bowel herniate beneath the cecum and become trapped in the right paracolic gutter.

Internal hernias also have been described in the region of the mesentery of the sigmoid colon. Whenever surgical intervention occurs, particularly with bowel anastomoses, hernias can develop in mesenteric defects or can occur adjacent to stoma or bowel anastomoses. All of these types of hernias can produce symptoms of closed-loop obstruction or strangulation.

PNEUMOPERITONEUM

Free intraperitoneal air is a significant radiographic finding within the abdominal cavity. Its presence can indicate serious abdominal pathology. At the same time, it can also be encountered frequently in the hospitalized patient and may just be iatrogenic. Determining the presence of a pneumoperitoneum and its etiology is of utmost importance.

The detection of free intraperitoneal air can be difficult and can be easily overlooked. A general rule of thumb is that free intraperitoneal air rises to the most superior portion of the abdominal cavity. However, its movement is not rapid and can take 10 to 20 minutes to percolate to the highest portion of the abdominal cavity when the patient changes position. Similarly, free intraperitoneal air is best detected by a horizontal beam radiograph. Typically, this is done in the upright position but it can also be done using cross-table views with the beam in a horizontal position. Also, it can be detected best when the center of the x-ray beam is aligned with the position of the free intraperitoneal air. In some circumstances, such as in an upright abdominal film, the angle of the beam at the edge of the film is too oblique to separate two adjacent structures separated by a small portion of air. In ideal conditions, as little as 1 ml of intraperitoneal air can be detected on radiographs.

Radiographic Signs

A variety of signs have been described for the detection of free intraperitoneal air (Box 8-1). Of all the signs described, the one most easily detected and most definitive in diagnosis is when free intraperitoneal air is located beneath the hemidiaphragm. Air in this position can be detected even when it is only a few milliliters. This is best seen on the right side because the liver offers a distinct outline between the free air and the soft tissues. On the left side, free air can be difficult to discern from the air in the stomach or splenic flexure. The free air occasionally can cross the midline, producing the cupola sign. Also, subdiaphragmatic air is best seen on the chest radiograph because of the difference in radiographic technique and because the central portion of the radiographic beam is somewhat more closely aligned to the diaphragms compared with what is normally depicted on abdominal upright radiographs.

A corollary position for detecting air in this position is the left side down decubitus film with a cross-table radiographic beam. This detects air between the liver and right lower ribs, which also offers a sharp demarcation because of their radiographic densities. This may have to be used when the patient is too sick to be placed in a true upright position. The free air on the decubitus view occasionally can be detected near the edge of the iliac bone because that may be the highest portion of the abdominal cavity in some individuals in the decubitus position.

In the supine position, air accumulating in the abdomen can give rise to an area of increased lucency over the liver (Fig. 8-14). This can be subtle and is often

detected when the margin of the free air produces a rather sharp border.

Rigler's sign is produced when both sides of the bowel wall become outlined by air. Under normal circumstances only the inner wall of the bowel may be defined by air. However, when free intraperitoneal air exists, both sides of the bowel wall may become visible, hence the term the "double-wall" sign (Fig. 8-15). This is typically seen on supine radiographs and unfortunately requires a substantial amount of air within the abdomen to be detected with confidence.

Associated with the Rigler's sign are triangular or rhomboidal collections of air. Air in this configuration is actually rare within the abdomen. It occurs when free intraperitoneal air becomes trapped in the potential space between adjacent loops of bowel and its margins take on a triangular or rectangular shape. Also, on a cross-table supine view of the abdomen, which can be obtained in seriously ill or traumatized patients, the free intraperitoneal air seen anteriorly has a triangular shape. Its superior margin is the anterior abdominal wall, and the two lower margins are produced by adjacent loops of bowel. This sign also can be evident by CT in detecting small quantities of free intraperitoneal air.

As free intraperitoneal air collects over the liver on the supine radiograph, it outlines the edges of the falciform ligament (Fig. 8-15). These are not usually visible on radiographs; however, it is a common location for free intraperitoneal air to collect and makes the falciform ligament readily visible. Also, air can collect in Morison's

---

Box 8-1   Signs of Pneumoperitoneum

Subdiaphragmatic air
Perihepatic air (lucency over liver)
Rigler's (double-wall) sign
Triangle or rhomboid sign
Visualization of falciform ligament
Morison's pouch air
Football or dome sign
Scrotal air
Visualization of lateral umbilical ligaments

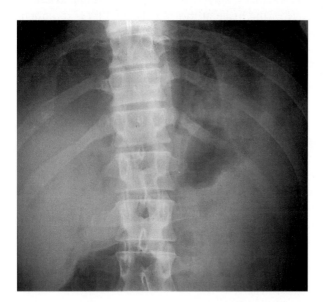

Fig. 8-14   An area of lucency exists over the upper abdomen and crosses the midline in this supine radiograph of the abdomen. This is a result of free intraperitoneal air.

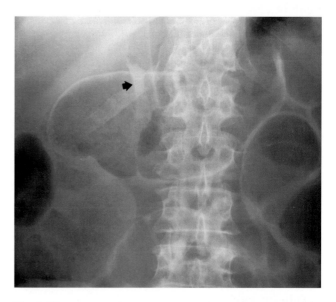

Fig. 8-15   Massive free intraperitoneal air is present in this supine abdomen film. Both sides of the bowel are evident in the right upper quadrant. The arrow indicates the falciform ligament. Rhomboidal air collections in the midabdomen also indicate free air.

pouch, which is inferior to the liver and above the right kidney. The free edge of the liver can become visible with air in this location.

A number of signs are more frequently seen in the pediatric/neonatal age group. One of these is the football sign, named for the large amount of free air that forms an oval "football" shape within a young child, as shown on the supine radiograph. Also, air within the scrotum is more typically seen in the younger patient and rarely encountered in the adult. The lateral umbilical ligaments in the lower abdomen form an inverted-V. They can be seen on the supine radiograph when large amounts of free intraperitoneal air are present. Again, this is more typically seen in children.

There are a number of conditions that can mimic free intraperitoneal air and can lead to a false-positive diagnosis. The most common of these are loops of bowel interposed beneath the diaphragm and liver or other abdominal structures (Chilaiditi syndrome). Also, a band of curvilinear atelectasis in the lung bases can be mistaken for the diaphragm and lead to a false diagnosis. The same can be said for a subpulmonic pneumothorax on a supine chest radiograph, which can lead to a false diagnosis of pneumoperitoneum. When loops of bowel are dilated in the abdomen, it can appear that both sides of the bowel wall are evident, producing a pseudo-Rigler's sign. Pneumatosis intestinalis also can mimic a Rigler's sign.

Causes

A variety of conditions can lead to a pneumoperitoneum (Box 8-2). It must be emphasized that a pneumoperitoneum does not equate to a surgical condition, and numerous "benign" conditions can produce free intraperitoneal air.

By far the most common cause of spontaneous free intraperitoneal air is the result of a perforated hollow viscus. Peptic ulcer disease, of either the stomach or the duodenum, is the most likely cause. Diverticulitis actually causes free air in relatively few patients. Usually, the inflammatory condition walls off the perforation and does not lead to free air. However, patients who have renal failure or are immunosuppressed tend to have a higher incidence of free air when they develop diverticulitis. Appendicitis also rarely produces free air, and bowel obstruction infrequently leads to free intraperitoneal air. Several inflammatory conditions can produce free intraperitoneal air; the best known is toxic megacolon, which can result from a variety of causes. Often the site of perforation is not detectable and simply may be the result of loss of integrity of the bowel wall.

The next most common cause of free intraperitoneal air is iatrogenic. Most free intraperitoneal air encountered in hospitalized patients is the result of some type of invasive procedure or diagnostic test. The rate at which free air becomes absorbed after surgery/laparoscopy depends on the amount of air introduced and the presence of peritoneal problems. Obesity also can delay its absorption. It is believed that the peritoneal cavity can absorb about 100 ml of air per day. This amount may be diminished in the presence of peritoneal inflammation. Typically, most air introduced during a procedure is gone in a few days and rarely takes longer than a week to be reabsorbed. Some reports indicate air remaining up to 3 weeks, but this is rare. CT is much more sensitive in detecting small amounts of free intraperitoneal air. CT often shows tiny amounts of free air a week or more after surgery, and this should not be considered significant. However, an increase in the amount of intraperitoneal air can signal the possibility of a surgical complication such as anastomotic breakdown.

Free intraperitoneal air may be introduced through the female reproductive tract from gynecologic procedures or sexual intercourse. Rarely, it even can occur in certain traumatic conditions.

In certain thoracic conditions, particularly pneumothorax or pneumomediastinum, air can enter the peritoneal cavity. A number of potential pathways exist for the dissection of air from the chest into the peritoneal cavity. This possibility increases with increased intrathoracic pressure from assisted ventilation or other causes. Air in the peritoneal cavity has no effect on the clinical status of the patient and does not require alteration of therapy.

Box 8-2 Conditions Producing Pneumoperitoneum

PERFORATED VISCUS

Peptic ulcer disease
Penetrating trauma
Diverticulitis
Bowel obstruction
Appendicitis

INFLAMMATORY CONDITIONS

Toxic megacolon
Tuberculosis
Peritoneal inflammation

IATROGENIC CAUSES

Postsurgery
Postlaparoscopy
Endoscopy
Peritoneal dialysis

GYNECOLOGIC CAUSES

INTRATHORACIC CAUSES

PNEUMATOSIS INTESTINALIS

In patients with pneumatosis of the bowel wall, the subserosal collections of air can rupture, with resultant pneumoperitoneum. This is not a serious consequence, however, and produces no significant complications. There are many "benign" causes of pneumatosis that have associated pneumoperitoneums. When pneumoperitoneum exists over a period, this is called a "balanced" pneumoperitoneum.

For patients with suspected perforation, the radiologist is often requested to assist in the preoperative evaluation. The last situation a surgeon wants is to operate and be unable to identify the site of perforation. For patients with spontaneous pneumoperitoneum, the simplest method is to inject a substance through a nasogastric tube and obtain radiographs. This could be either air- or water-soluble contrast material, although the latter is preferred. Since upper intestinal tract perforation is more common, it can frequently be identified with this method. In patients who are postoperative or have extensive abdominal problems, CT is probably the best modality for evaluating for underlying bowel or abdominal pathology. Rarely, water-soluble enemas can be used in suspected colonic perforation. This typically should be done in patients who have had recent bowel cleansing, such as postcolonoscopy or postsurgical patients. If a perforation is detected, the bowel contents will be flushed into the peritoneal cavity with this procedure. A water-soluble contrast material must always be used in suspected abdominal perforation.

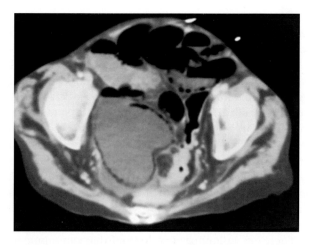

Fig. 8-16   Computed tomography demonstrates pneumatosis of the bowel. In the posterior pelvis, the linear air is seen in the dependent portion of the cecum. Bubbles of air are also seen in a loop of bowel in the left anterior pelvis as a result of pneumatosis.

PNEUMATOSIS

Gas within the bowel wall (pneumatosis) is an uncommon diagnostic finding for the radiologist. Although first described on abdominal radiographs, it is now appreciated as more easily and reliably diagnosed by CT. Its radiographic appearance, by either plain abdominal radiographs or CT, can be either linear or bubbly, or even a combination of both (Fig. 8-16). The distribution of the air can be variable and is not always related to the underlying pathologic condition producing the pneumatosis.

Pathology

On pathologic examination, pneumatosis of the bowel is found in the subserosal layer of the gut. It can be found less commonly in the submucosal layer and rarely in the muscularis propria. The pneumatosis typically forms bubbles or blebs that can range from a few millimeters to greater than a centimeter. They are found more commonly along the mesenteric side of the bowel but also can occur circumferentially around the bowel and even in the mesentery itself. The cysts do not communicate with the lumen and contain gas that is typically under pressure. On histological examination, the cysts have a defined lining with multinucleated giant cells. Initially these were thought to represent dilated lymphatics, but this is no longer accepted. A mild inflammatory reaction is thought to occur around these cysts, and often an associated mild inflammatory change is evident in the mucosa and submucosa of the affected bowel.

Analysis of the gas within the cysts shows a high concentration (approaching 50%) of hydrogen, compared with intestinal gas with a composition of 14% hydrogen. This high level of hydrogen suggests that the gas is probably bacterial in origin and not due to the passage of intestinal gas into the bowel wall. Also, pulmonary gas does not have such a high hydrogen concentration.

Etiology

Several theories exist regarding the etiology of pneumatosis. Given the numerous causes of pneumatosis, it may vary according to the underlying condition. Evidence suggests that intramural gas in pneumatosis is bacterial in origin, based on its high hydrogen content. Also, breath hydrogen levels are typically elevated in patients with pneumatosis, indicating increased activity of anaerobic, gas-producing bacteria. Two methods of treatment of pneumatosis—hyperbaric oxygen and antimicrobial therapy—diminish anaerobic bacteria growth. Bacteria also would account for the mild inflammatory changes that are frequently encountered in portions of the bowel affected by pneumatosis. However, for bacteria to flourish in the intestinal wall, other factors must come into play, including loss of integrity of the mucosa of the bowel and diminished oxygen levels in the bowel.

Many believe that some type of mucosal disruption must occur in all forms of pneumatosis for bacteria to gain access into the bowel wall. This can occur simply from ulceration of the mucosa, as seen in many conditions, or from the depletion of the Peyer's patches in patients undergoing steroid therapy. Once the anaerobic bacteria gain access to the bowel wall, a low oxygen level, caused by ischemia or a variety of other conditions, assists in the growth of these organisms. The development of pneumatosis in patients with underlying pulmonary disease was thought to result from direct dissection of air along lymphatic channels into the bowel. This could never be proved, and it is now thought that the development of pneumatosis is a combination of low oxygen levels from the pulmonary disease and steroids or other medications the patient may be taking. Other theories have been proposed, but in effect they all lead to a condition that promotes anaerobic bacterial growth and possible loss of integrity of the bowel mucosa.

Associated Conditions

As seen in Box 8-3, numerous conditions from clinically innocuous to immediately life threatening can produce pneumatosis. The radiologist cannot differentiate the etiology based on the radiographic appearance (e.g., linear gas is not of greater significance than bubbly gas collections). Also, the distribution of the gas may not relate to the underlying cause of the condition except in certain circumstances (e.g., air in gastric wall). The presence of a pneumoperitoneum (so-called balanced pneumoperitoneum) can be encountered in both innocuous and life-threatening causes of pneumatosis. The finding of pneumatosis must be coupled with the patient's underlying clinical state to determine the significance of the pneumatosis. Idiopathic pneumatosis of an unknown cause is rarely encountered nowadays.

Most radiologists immediately consider a serious vascular insult to the bowel when encountering pneumatosis, and this is warranted because a significant proportion of cases of pneumatosis are due to ischemic bowel disease (Fig. 8-17). Ischemia produces the two changes necessary for pneumatosis: loss of integrity of the mucosa and lowered oxygen levels. Most bowel ischemia is not due to occluded vessels, and pneumatosis does not imply vascular obstruction. Other findings that may support ischemia as an underlying etiology include the appearance of portal venous gas, which is seen predominantly with bowel ischemia and a few other conditions (Fig. 8-18). Surprisingly, many patients with portal venous gas survive if aggressively treated.

Numerous inflammatory or infectious conditions of the bowel cause the development of pneumatosis. Pneumatosis has been seen with both Crohn's disease

Box 8-3 Conditions Associated with Pneumatosis

VASCULAR CONDITIONS

Ischemia

INFLAMMATION OR INFECTION

Diabetes
Necrotizing enterocolitis
Typhlitis (neutropenic colitis)
Crohn's disease
Ulcerative colitis
Infectious or parasitic agents
Peptic ulcer disease

PULMONARY DISEASE

Asthma
Chronic obstructive pulmonary disease
Cystic fibrosis

COLLAGEN VASCULAR DISEASE

Scleroderma and mixed connective tissue disease
Systemic lupus erythematosus

BOWEL OBSTRUCTION

DRUGS

Steroids
Chemotherapy

TRAUMA

Surgery
Postendoscopy
Penetrating injuries

OTHER CONDITIONS

Idiopathic cause
Whipple's disease
Posttransplantation

and ulcerative colitis, although admittedly this complication is rare. A unique situation exists in patients with diabetes, in whom a condition known as emphysematous gastritis develops (Fig. 8-19). This is not the result of ischemia but rather an infection of the gastric wall, usually by hemolytic streptococci. Emphysematous gastritis is a grave complication with a high mortality rate. Pneumatosis has also been reported in patients with infections or parasitic infestations of the gut.

In debilitated infants, necrotizing enterocolitis is a serious complication. It is typically encountered in premature infants. It is thought that bacteria invade through the bowel lumen because of the diminished resistance of the infant. This leads to necrosis of the mucosa and eventually the bowel wall, with resultant septicemia.

Also seen in children, and some adults, is typhlitis, or neutropenic colitis. This is a necrotizing infection of the ascending colon and to some extent the terminal ileum. It was first described in children undergoing treatment for leukemia. It is now seen as a complication not only of leukemia, but also of lymphoma, aplastic anemia, acquired immunodeficiency syndrome (AIDS), and im-munosuppressive therapy as in transplant patients. It still is more frequently encountered in children but can be seen in adults.

One of the initial descriptions of pneumatosis was of a condition in patients with significant underlying pulmonary disease (Fig. 8-20). It was thought that the gas developed because of rupture of alveoli with dissec-

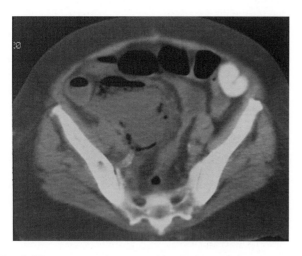

Fig. 8-17   Computed tomography is highly sensitive in demon-strating pneumatosis. Air that remains in the dependent portion of the bowel, as in this patient with ischemia, is suggestive of pneumatosis.

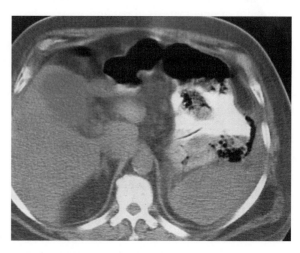

Fig. 8-19   Bubbly and linear air collections are seen in the stomach wall in this diabetic patient with emphysematous gastritis.

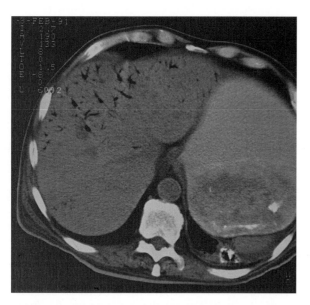

Fig. 8-18   Linear air collections rising to the anterior portion of the liver are compatible with air in the portal venous system. Air in the biliary system is more centrally located.

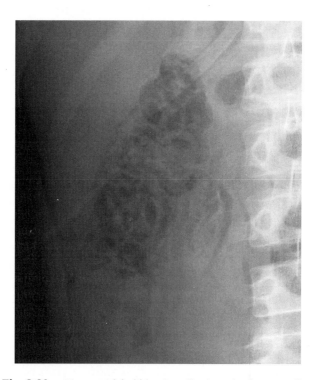

Fig. 8-20   Linear and bubbly air collections in the ascending colon are present in this patient with pulmonary disease. The pneumatosis was believed to be due to underlying asthma.

tion of air along tissue planes, along the mediastinum, and down into the mesentery and gut. This theory could never be substantiated, no other evidence exists to support this as a hypothesis, and it is no longer thought to be valid. Instead, many now believe that pneumatosis is due to low oxygen levels in bowel promoting the growth of anaerobic bacteria. Many patients with this condition are taking steroids, which depletes the Peyer's patches and reduces resistance to infection. Pneumatosis is not unusual in severe asthma. It can be seen less frequently in severe chronic obstructive pulmonary disease and even cystic fibrosis.

Pneumatosis is known to develop in patients with collagen vascular disease. This can be seen in scleroderma or mixed connective tissue disease (Fig. 8-21) and is due to a combination of factors. These patients are often taking steroids. Also, they frequently have underlying pulmonary disease. Furthermore, their small bowel transit tends to be altered, leading to bacterial overgrowth, which increases the probability that pneumatosis will occur.

Bowel obstruction has been known to produce pneumatosis but this is rare considering the number of patients encountered with bowel obstruction. It is usually a result of progressive bowel dilatation, which leads to ischemic changes in the bowel, along with disruption of the mucosa. Increased intraluminal pres-

sure also can play a small part in its development. Pneumatosis has also been described in patients with gastric outlet obstruction, but this typically develops some distance from the site of obstruction.

When encountering a patient with pneumatosis, the physician needs any clinical information concerning procedures or medications. As already stated, many patients with pneumatosis are on steroid therapy. The cause for the pneumatosis is twofold: depletion of Peyer's patches disrupting the integrity of the mucosa and the reduced ability to fight infection. The physician should also ask about chemotherapeutic drugs (Fig. 8-22). Pneumatosis can develop in transplant patients on immunosuppressive therapy, which often includes steroids. Pneumatosis is rarely encountered in postsurgical or postendoscopic patients. Considering the millions of patients undergoing these procedures, the occurrence of pneumatosis is rare. This may be the one circumstance in which the pneumatosis is related to direct injury to the mucosa with dissection of intraluminal gas.

Numerous other conditions have been associated with pneumatosis. The idiopathic or unknown is frequently listed as a cause. However, with increasing awareness of the underlying mechanism of its pneumatosis, its etiology can typically be determined.

Treatment for pneumatosis can be directed at the underlying etiology, such as ischemia. When pneumatosis has a more innocuous cause, no treatment is usually required. However, some patients experience pain, bloating, and discomfort with the condition. These patients can be treated with hyperbaric oxygen, although this treatment is not readily available. Some antibiotics also have been known to reduce or eliminate pneumatosis.

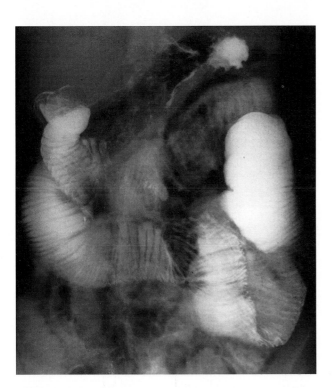

Fig. 8-21 Air is present in the wall of the jejunum in the left upper quadrant. The patient has severe scleroderma and associated pulmonary disease.

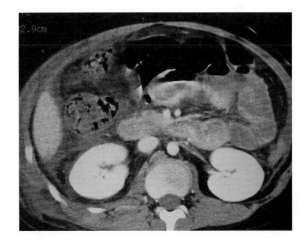

Fig. 8-22 Pneumatosis is evident in the ascending colon, and associated pericolonic inflammatory changes also exist, indicating inflammation and probable impending bowel necrosis.

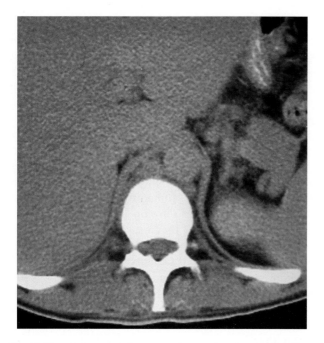

Fig. 8-23   Enlarged nodes are evident in the retrocrural region. Typically, any lymph nodes in this region measure only a few millimeters.

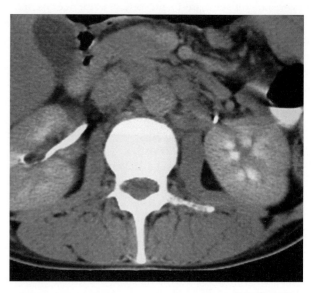

Fig. 8-24   Several soft tissue densities in the periaortic region are evident. This is due to mildly enlarged lymph nodes, which exceed 10 mm in diameter.

LYMPHADENOPATHY

The presence of enlarged lymph nodes in the abdomen is used for the staging of many abdominal and extraabdominal malignancies. However, a number of benign diseases can also produce abdominal adenopathy. Over 200 lymph nodes exist within the abdomen and pelvis. Additionally, the sole criterion of CT in the evaluation of lymph nodes is their size (Figs. 8-23 to 8-25). Unfortunately, significant disease can exist in normal-sized lymph nodes, and enlarged lymph nodes can be of little significance. Thus the potential for both false-positive and false-negative diagnoses exists when lymph nodes are evaluated by just their size. The size of the lymph nodes is determined by measuring across their short axis, and normal size varies according to their position in the abdomen, as listed in Box 8-4.

Internal architecture or characteristics are extremely difficult to determine by CT. However, the CT attenuation of the lymph nodes, particularly in enlarged nodes, may be determined to be different than normal (e.g., soft-tissue density). If the CT attenuation is greater than normal, the disease processes are likely benign (Box 8-5).

On occasion, the lymph nodes may be lower in attenuation than expected (Fig. 8-26). This is best identified when the lymph nodes are enlarged. The causes of

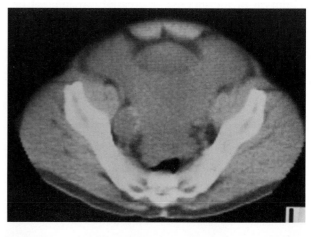

Fig. 8-25   Enlarged lymph node is seen on the right side of the pelvis. Ascites is also present.

low-density lymph nodes in the abdomen are listed in Box 8-6.

In the vast majority of cases, enlarged lymph nodes detected are associated with malignancy. CT is still the primary modality used in staging of abdominal malignancies as well as lymphoma. CT can be performed to evaluate for possible adenopathy from extraabdominal tumors that have spread to the abdomen. However, a small percentage of lymphadenopathies are actually due to benign processes rather than malignancy. The radiolo-

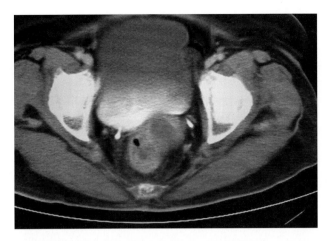

Fig. 8-26 A low-density area is seen on the left side of the rectum. The rectal wall is thickened. This was due to an infiltrating mucinous carcinoma of the rectum with a single large low-density lymph node adjacent to the rectum found at resection.

Box 8-4	Criteria for Enlarged Abdominal Lymph Nodes	
Retrocrural and porta hepatis nodes		6 mm
Retroperitoneal and mesenteric nodes		10 mm
Pelvic nodes		15 mm

Box 8-5   Causes of Calcified Lymph Nodes

Postinflammation—tuberculosis
Treated lymphoma
Teratosarcoma
Mucinous carcinoma

Box 8-6   Causes of Low-Density Lymph Nodes

Nonseminomatous testicular tumors
Whipple's disease
Mycobacterium infection
    M. tuberculosis
    M. avium-intracellulare
Epidermoid genitourinary tumors
Lymphoma and mucinous tumors (rarely)

gist must be aware of this because the presence of lymphadenopathy does not signify that the disease process is malignant. Also, previously treated malignancies that produce adenopathy (e.g., lymphoma) sometimes leave residual enlarged lymph nodes, which is

Box 8-7   Causes of Benign Abdominal Lymphadenopathy

Granulomatous infections
    Tuberculosis
    Sarcoid
Other abdominal infections
Crohn's disease
Sprue
Whipple's disease
Previously treated malignancies

thought to be due to fibrosis. The causes of benign abdominal adenopathy are listed in Box 8-7.

HUMAN IMMUNODEFICIENCY VIRUS INFECTION

The occurrence of human immunodeficiency virus (HIV) infection and AIDS has been one of the major medical stories in the latter part of the twentieth century. HIV can be transmitted through sexual intercourse and through exposure to blood and other body fluids. Although the initial impact of AIDS was seen in young men, the incidence of disease among women and children has grown at an alarming rate, and this disease is now evident in all segments of our society and worldwide in its distribution. Its ubiquitous nature is important for the radiologist, because the patient can have a variety of symptoms, often related to the gastrointestinal (GI) tract. The radiologist must be aware of the changes produced by AIDS and its associated infections and neoplasms, because he or she may be the first to have the opportunity to make the diagnosis.

AIDS actually represents the advanced stages of a viral infection. Because of the selective loss of helper T-cells in the victims' immune systems, it was initially thought that the disease was the result of a retrovirus. The AIDS virus was initially called HTLV-III, or lymphadenopathy virus. By convention, it is now called HIV, of which several types have been described. Infection by this viral agent is termed HIV infection, of which AIDS is just a latter segment of the stages of infection. HIV belongs to the subfamily of retroviruses termed lentivirus, named for their slow course of infection. It is a single-stranded RNA virus surrounded by a lipid envelope. When the virus enters the target cells, it is translated into DNA and incorporated into the host nucleus. HIV attaches itself not only to helper T-cells, but also to macrophages, monocytes, certain glial cells, and crypt cells in the intestinal epithelium.

Clinical Features

The hallmark of retroviruses is their prolonged course of infection within the host organism. Initially, the infection can be asymptomatic or present as a viral-like illness. Initially the patient can suffer viral-like symptoms of fever, pharyngitis, gastrointestinal upset, and even neurologic symptoms. This occurs as the HIV virus attaches itself to the various target cells. The time from initial exposure to acute illness can be anywhere from days to a few months. During this initial phase the patient often seroconverts to an HIV-positive state. There are two major clinical tests for HIV infection. One is the seropositive conversion, which usually occurs within 12 weeks of exposure, and the other is the peripheral lymphocyte level. Both helper T-cells (CD4) and suppressor T-cells (CD8) can be measured. Since helper T-cells are destroyed by HIV infection, their level is diminished. Correspondingly, there may be an increase in suppressor T-cells, resulting in an inversion of the CD4/CD8 ratio.

GI symptoms such as diarrhea, nausea and vomiting, anorexia, and even GI ulceration can occur, prompting GI evaluation. During this initial phase, radiographic evaluation can demonstrate subtle abnormalities (Box 8-8). The HIV virus may cause discrete ulceration in the esophagus (Fig. 8-27). Nodular fold thickening can be present in the intestinal tract. Finally, CT can demonstrate mild hepatosplenomegaly, and prominent lymph nodes can be evident in various portions of the abdomen, although they are not necessarily enlarged.

The second phase, that of a relatively asymptomatic carrier, can last up to a decade. In some patients HIV infection never develops into the clinical state considered AIDS, and there have been some reports of eventual seronegative reconversion. The next phase of disease is indicated by the presence of adenopathy for several months. The phase commonly considered AIDS occurs when any of a number of complications occur. There can be the development of secondary infections with *Can-*

dida or other opportunistic organisms. Neoplastic conditions such as lymphoma or Kaposi's sarcoma can also occur. Neurologic symptoms and diffuse constitutional symptoms such as weight loss and fever are also indicative of this final stage.

GI symptoms develop in the vast majority of patients who reach the category of AIDS. Radiologists are frequently called on to evaluate the complications of this disease. Since much of the disease processes can be confined to the superficial mucosal layer of bowel, barium studies still have an important role in the diagnosis of abnormalities. CT is the preferred method of evaluating the abdomen for more severe complications such as adenopathy, malignancy, or abscess. Ultrasound can also be used, particularly in evaluating the liver and biliary system. In using these modalities, the radiologist must still consider certain principles:

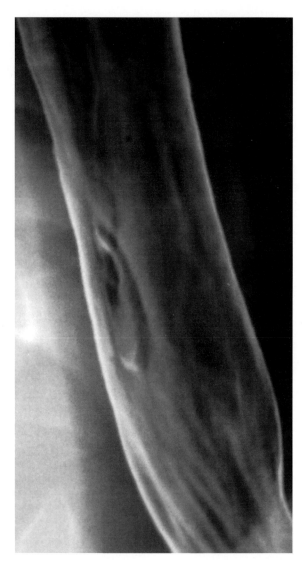

Fig. 8-27   Large oval ulcer in the lower esophagus is due to viral esophagitis in this AIDS patient.

Box 8-8   Possible Gastrointestinal Abnormalities During Initial Human Immunodeficiency Virus Infection

Focal esophageal ulceration
Nodular fold thickening in the small bowel
Mild hepatosplenomegaly
Multiple lymph nodes, nonenlarged or borderline
   enlarged

1. Infections are often multifocal and involve separate segments of the GI tract.
2. Multiple organisms may be involved simultaneously, either in the same segment of bowel or in separate portions of bowel.
3. The GI tract has only a limited number of changes that occur, predominantly fold thickening and ulceration. It is difficult to distinguish the exact organism by the radiographic appearance.
4. Weak association exists between symptoms and radiographic findings.
5. Infections and neoplasms can occur together.

Associated Infections

A variety of pathogens can be isolated from the GI tract in AIDS patients (Box 8-9). This constellation of organisms is more extensive than that seen in other immunosuppressed patients such as transplant recipients.

Of the viral infections, cytomegalovirus (CMV) is the most commonly encountered in AIDS patients. It is found in the immunocompetent, but it has considerable clinical impact once the immune system is compromised and contributes significantly to the morbidity in these patients. It can involve all segments of the intestinal tract. In the esophagus it can produce large, flat ulcers. In the upper GI tract the changes include fold thickening and ulceration. CMV commonly produces colitis with superficial ulceration similar to ulcerative colitis, but with more focal distribution.

Herpes simplex is a common cause of esophagitis in AIDS patients. It typically manifests as small, discrete ulcers against a background of normal mucosa (Fig. 8-27). The ulceration can be diffuse in severe instances. As mentioned previously, HIV can cause a primary infection of the intestinal mucosa. It is one of the causes of large, flat ulcers in the esophagus. It can also manifest in the small bowel where it produces diffusely thickened folds.

Candida albicans is the most common symptom-producing mucosal infection in patients with AIDS, ultimately affecting all patients with advanced disease. It most commonly involves the oropharynx. In the esophagus it produces either diffuse ulceration with pseudomembranes or discrete plaques, causing dysphagia (Fig. 8-28). Motility can also be impaired. AIDS is one of the few conditions in which *Candida* can also affect other portions of the GI tract and has been known to produce ulceration in the stomach and even the rectum. Other rare fungal infections such as histoplasmosis also can involve the GI tract, but their occurrences are rare.

A variety of protozoa exist as enteric pathogens in HIV patients. *Cryptosporidium* is the most common. It is a coccidial protozoan that produces a debilitating watery diarrhea. Infection is predominantly of the small bowel, producing thickened folds, dilatation, and increased secretions. It also can involve the biliary system, causing an ascending cholangitis and significant liver dysfunction (Fig. 8-29). *Isospora belli* is another coccidial protozoan, and it produces changes similar to those of cryptosporidiosis. These two are clinically indistinguishable.

Giardia lamblia is a flagellated protozoan that occurs naturally in small epidemics in the immunocompetent, usually related to infected water. However, it has been well described as a pathogen in the immunosuppressed and occasionally involves AIDS patients. It has a predilection for the proximal small bowel, producing diarrhea because of malabsorption. Radiographic examination shows thickened, irregular folds with evidence of fluid or increased secretions in the bowel.

Entamoeba histolytica is an amoeba that can infect both normal patients and the immunosuppressed. It produces inflammatory changes in the distal small bowel and the colon. This inflammation can be diffuse or focal with changes of stricturing and even masses. It can be mistaken for Crohn's disease.

The *Mycobacterium* group of bacteria includes the most common pathogens in AIDS patients. *M. tuberculosis* of the GI tract typically occurs after a pulmonary infection. It can involve the small bowel distally, where it can produce severe stricturing and even fistula or perforation, and the adjacent ascending colon, where it

---

Box 8-9 Opportunistic Infections of the Gastrointestinal Tract in Acquired Immunodeficiency Syndrome

VIRAL

Herpes
Cytomegalovirus
Human immunodeficiency virus

FUNGAL

Candida
Histoplasmosis

PROTOZOAN

Cryptosporidiosis
Isosporiasis
Giardiasis
Amebiasis

BACTERIAL

Mycobacterium tuberculosis
Mycobacterium avium-intracellulare
Salmonella
Campylobacter
Shigella
Yersinia

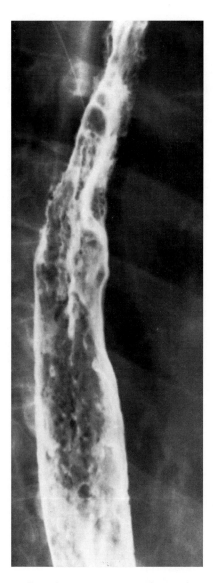

Fig. 8-28 Diffuse shaggy ulceration of the esophagus as a result of *Candida* infection.

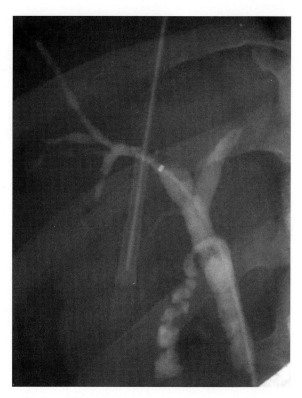

Fig. 8-29 There is attenuation of the intrahepatic biliary system with some beading of the smaller branches. This patient with AIDS has cryptosporidiosis of the biliary system.

can produce wall thickening and ulceration. It can also involve the esophagus, although this is rare. *M. avium-intracellulare* is an atypical mycobacterium that involves the small bowel, usually through infected water, and invades only the immunosuppressed. In the small bowel it produces enteritis with diarrhea, fever, and wasting. On radiographic examination, the folds are thickened in a regular fashion (Fig. 8-30). Some think that the changes can mimic Whipple's disease. Both mycobacteria are known to cause lymphadenopathy, and this can be seen as low-density lymph nodes by CT examination. The adenopathy can be in the mesentery or in the retroperitoneum.

A variety of other bacteria can infect AIDS patients. These include both *Salmonella* and *Shigella,* which can produce severe enteritis and colitis. *Campylobacter* can also produce colitis. All of these agents are indistinguishable on radiographic examination, usually producing either diffuse or patchy areas of superficial ulceration. *Yersinia enterocolitica* typically involves the distal small bowel and to a lesser extent the colon.

Associated Neoplasms

The development of neoplasms is a well-recognized complication in immunosuppressed patients, both AIDS patients and transplant recipients. The development of tumors in young men first prompted the recognition of AIDS. As AIDS patients continue to have a longer survival, more secondary neoplasms will likely become associated with HIV infection (Box 8-10).

Kaposi's sarcoma is a skin sarcoma composed of endothelium-lined vascular channels, spindle-shaped cells, and varying degrees of inflammatory infiltrate. Until the AIDS epidemic it was considered a rare neoplasm usually found among elderly men. Interestingly, the incidence of Kaposi's sarcoma in AIDS is more frequent in the homosexual AIDS population than in those who have acquired AIDS through drug use or other causes. The incidence of Kaposi's sarcoma in AIDS patients appears to be decreasing. Kaposi's sarcoma in the AIDS population is much more aggressive than the neoplasm that has

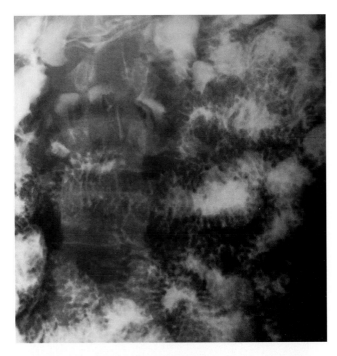

Fig. 8-30 Markedly thickened small bowel folds are demonstrated along with segmentation of the barium. This AIDS patient has an opportunistic infection of the small bowel. It usually is not possible to determine the type of infection by the radiographic appearance.

Box 8-10   Neoplasms Associated with Acquired Immunodeficiency Syndrome

Kaposi's sarcoma
Lymphoma
Anal carcinoma
Esophageal or oropharyngeal carcinoma

---

been classically described. One form produces diffuse skin lesions along with visceral involvement, and another form has marked lymph node involvement with little cutaneous disease.

Involvement of the GI tract is one of the most common manifestations of Kaposi's sarcoma. Lesions can occur throughout the GI tract, from the mouth to the rectum. One major form is that of a discrete nodule or mass projecting into the bowel lumen, sometimes with central ulceration, producing a so-called bull's-eye lesion; it also can be a superficial spreading lesion, appearing as thickened folds, similar to what can be seen with hemorrhage into the bowel wall. Kaposi's sarcoma occasionally produces massive adenopathy (Fig. 8-31), which can be low density, similar to mycobacterial

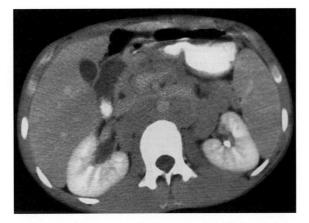

Fig. 8-31 Extensive retroperitoneal adenopathy is present in this patient with AIDS-related Kaposi's sarcoma. (Courtesy of Duane Mezwa, M.D.)

infection of the gut. It is well known that Kaposi's sarcoma of the abdomen, either gut or adenopathy, can appear before any cutaneous lesions are visible. Liver metastases also have been described, appearing as low-density lesions.

Lymphoma encountered in AIDS patients is a non-Hodgkin's lymphoma, usually B-cell type. It is distinctive in AIDS in that it is highly aggressive, has a high-grade histological subtype, and has a high proportion of extranodal involvement such as the central nervous system or gastrointestinal tract (Fig. 8-32). Some speculation exists on a link to the Epstein-Barr virus. The radiographic appearance of lymphoma is variable and similar to what can be seen in immunocompetent patients. Lesions of the bowel can have the appearance of mucosal fold thickening, discrete nodules or masses, or infiltrating neoplasms with mucosal destruction. Besides the bowel lesions, associated adenopathy often occurs, and CT is the examination of choice in patients with suspected lymphoma. Unfortunately, the presence of adenopathy can be seen in a variety of benign conditions with AIDS and is not an indicator of neoplasm. CT-guided biopsy can be necessary to obtain tissue for differentiation.

Scattered reports show that other neoplasms develop in AIDS patients. One of the more common is squamous cell carcinoma of the anus. Its development may be related to a viral oncogenic stimulus. This tumor is best evaluated clinically, although CT has limited use for staging. Some reports also indicate squamous cell carcinoma of the oropharynx and esophagus. Again, these lesions can be induced by viral infections, which are prevalent in those locations. As HIV patients survive longer, the possibility of further intestinal malignancies must be considered.

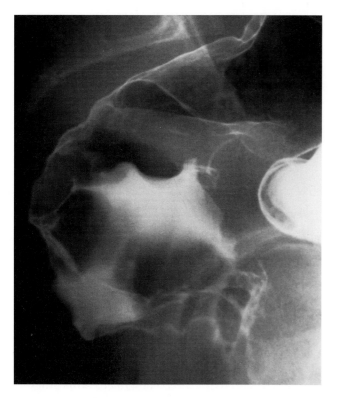

Fig. 8-32 Double-contrast colon examination demonstrates marked mucosal destruction in the rectum. This is secondary to infiltrating lymphoma of the bowel in this AIDS patient.

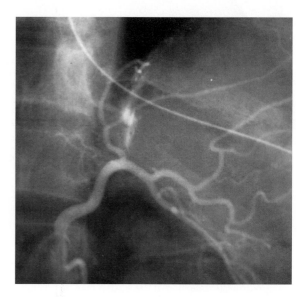

Fig. 8-33 Selective injection of the left gastric artery shows a small area of extravasation near the gastroesophageal junction of the stomach. This is a result of a Mallory-Weiss tear.

GASTROINTESTINAL HEMORRHAGE

Acute GI hemorrhage is a major clinical problem resulting in substantial morbidity and mortality. The prompt diagnosis of the site and possible etiology of the bleeding is important, and it is an area in which the radiologist can serve an important interventional role. Acute hemorrhage for this discussion involves patients with a loss of blood sufficient to produce dizziness, which usually requires a loss of at least 2 units of blood, or shock, which begins after the loss of 3 to 4 units of blood. Of course, this can vary among individuals.

Localization of the site of bleeding is crucial in the initial stages. Hematemesis, or the vomiting of blood (either bright red or "coffee-ground" color), is associated with lesions proximal to the ligament of Treitz (Fig. 8-33). Melena, or black tarry stools, is also more commonly associated with upper GI bleeding and less commonly with the small bowel or proximal colon. Hematochezia, the passage of red or maroon blood through the rectum, typically is seen with colonic hemorrhage and less frequently with bleeding from the small bowel or upper GI tract.

Box 8-11 Common Causes of Gastrointestinal Hemorrhage

UPPER GASTROINTESTINAL TRACT

Ulcers (gastric or duodenal)
Gastritis
Varices
Mallory-Weiss tear
Neoplasm (primary or secondary)
Vascular anomalies
Esophagitis

LOWER GASTROINTESTINAL TRACT

Diverticula
Vascular anomalies
Neoplasm
Inflammatory bowel disease
Hemorrhoids
Ischemia

A myriad of disorders can cause GI bleeding, but the most common are listed in Box 8-11. The frequency with which these are encountered depends on the demographics of the clinical population at a particular hospital.

Box 8-12 Diagnostic Procedures in Gastrointestinal Hemorrhage

Endoscopy
Angiography
Nuclear scintigraphy
  Tagged red blood cells
  Sulfur colloid
Barium studies

Box 8-13 Sensitivity of Modalities in Detecting Gastrointestinal Bleeding

Endoscopy	Variable
Angiography	0.5 ml/min
Tagged red blood cells	0.05-0.2 ml/min
Sulfur colloid	<0.1 ml/min

A sufficient knowledge of the patient's medical and surgical history is important in establishing a prompt diagnosis, but this is not always feasible in an emergency situation.

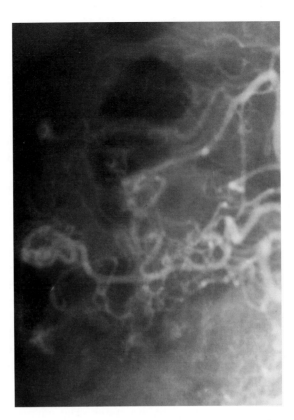

Fig. 8-34   Angiodysplasia of the cecum is demonstrated angiographically in this patient with lower gastrointestinal bleeding.

Diagnostic Imaging

Several diagnostic modalities exist for establishing of the site and etiology of the bleeding point (Boxes 8-12 and 8-13).

Whenever possible, endoscopy should be considered the primary diagnostic tool for the evaluation of acute hemorrhage. Its advantages include accurate diagnosis as to the bleeding site, delineation of the cause of the hemorrhage, and possible therapeutic intervention. Diagnosis is relatively independent of the rate of bleeding. The accuracy of endoscopy for upper GI hemorrhage can approach 90% or higher for some endoscopists. Accuracy is typically lower in lower GI hemorrhage because measurement is somewhat impeded by blood and stool. Also, small bowel hemorrhage cannot be visualized—only inferred—with endoscopic procedures. An advantage of endoscopy is that an accurate delineation of the cause and severity of the bleeding can be obtained. A bleeding malignant ulcer can be differentiated from gastritis, potentially causing a significant change in management. Also, arterial bleeding, including the visualization of the bleeding vessel, can be differentiated from slower venous bleeding, again changing management. Bleeding at multiple sites, which is not an unusual occurrence, can be identified. Finally, therapeutic attempts to control the bleeding can be used with variable success by the endoscopist. Usually this consists of using lasers or injecting sclerotherapeutic agents.

Angiography is another modality best performed on patients who are having a brisk, acute bleeding episode. Diagnostic accuracy depends somewhat on the site of the bleeding and its underlying etiology. Most important for angiography, however, are the rate and nature of the bleeding. For angiography to be successful, it is generally considered that the rate of bleeding should exceed 0.5 ml per minute. Also, the bleeding must occur over the few seconds that the arterial injection occurs. If bleeding is intermittent, which is common, it may not be demonstrated unless it is sufficiently active at the time of injection. Some find angiography the most advantageous technique, perhaps better than endoscopy, in massive lower GI hemorrhage (Figs. 8-34 and 8-35).

Another advantage of angiography is the potential for therapeutic intervention. The two major tools of the angiographer are vasopressin infusion and embolotherapy. Vasopressin is a vasoconstrictor that, when given intraarterially, diminishes blood flow and causes bowel wall contraction. Although its use is complex, usually doses of 0.2 to 0.4 unit per minute decrease or stop arterial bleeding. This rate of infusion is diminished over a period of hours as long as bleeding has stopped. Complications include ischemia or infarction of the bowel, thrombosis, peripheral ischemia, elevated blood pressure, arrhythmias, and fluid imbalance.

Embolotherapy consists of the placement of temporary or permanent material intraarterially through the catheter. Embolotherapy is performed when vasopressin or other measures cannot control the bleeding. It can also be the initial choice if unusual lesions such as arteriovenous malformations or large tumors are encountered. The risks of embolization include infarction of that segment or adjacent segments of bowel. The material can also be displaced or migrate to other parts of the body, causing secondary complications. Finally, if embolization is too proximal, bleeding can continue as other collateral channels open up to the bleeding site.

Radionuclide scintigraphy is one of the most sensitive methods for detecting GI hemorrhage. With this technique Tc-99m isotope is attached to either red blood cells (RBCs) or sulfur colloid. There are certain advantages with each type. Tagging of RBCs is best done in vitro but is more difficult. The tagged RBCs will stay within circulation for hours, and scanning can be done both immediately and with a delay of up to 24 hours. When an active site of bleeding exists, the tagged RBCs will be seen as an area of increased radioactivity in the bowel, distinct from the vascular structures. The amount of bleeding that can be identified is usually 0.1 to 0.2 ml per minute, and on delayed images amounts as low as 0.05 ml per minute can be detected. Usually at least 5 ml of blood must extravasate to be visualized. The major advantage is that intermittent bleeding can be identified, since the isotope remains within the blood for many hours. Difficulty arises in that the exact origin of the bleeding may not be determined on delayed images because of bowel peristalsis. Artifact from excretion of unbound Tc-99m can also be encountered, yielding false positive results.

The other radionuclide is Tc-99m sulfur colloid. After injection of the material, it actively circulates for a matter of minutes before it becomes bound within the liver, spleen, and bone marrow. By 15 minutes a substantial amount of tracer has been cleared from the blood. Active bleeding during this interval will be seen as a focal area of activity within the abdomen. A major advantage is that minute amounts of bleeding, 0.1 ml per minute or even less, can be detected. Also, smaller amounts of bleeding can be seen since the background activity diminishes, thus providing better contrast. Unfortunately, for the bleeding to be visualized, it must be active during the 10 to 15 minutes of maximum circulation of the isotope. Also, activity in the liver and spleen can obscure bleeding points.

The use of barium is rarely indicated for acute hemorrhage. Even if barium studies demonstrate a pathologic condition such as a tumor, this still does not confirm that the bleeding is from that point or possibly from an ulcer or diverticulum. A barium study never identifies the actual site of bleeding; it only demonstrates gross pathology. Finally, residual barium within the gastrointestinal tract can interfere with other modalities such as angiography or endoscopy if those have to be performed after a barium study. Barium probably never should be introduced into someone with acute bleeding.

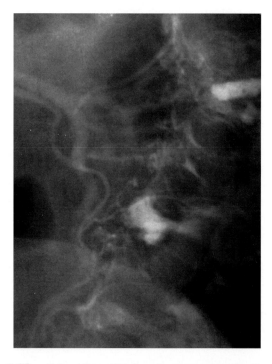

Fig. 8-35 At least three bleeding sites are seen in the descending colon because of diverticula. Multiple areas of simultaneous bleeding are unusual.

SUGGESTED READINGS

Baker SR: Imaging of pneumoperitoneum, *Abd Imag* 21:413-422, 1996.

Bunker SR, Lull RJ, Tanasescu DE, et al: Scintigraphy of gastrointestinal hemorrhage: superiority of 99mTc red blood cells over 99mTc sulfur colloid, *AJR* 143:543-548, 1984.

Caudill JL, Rose BS: The role of computed tomography in the evaluation of pneumatosis intestinalis, *J Clin Gastroenterol* 9:223-226, 1987.

DeMeo JH, Fulcher AS, Austin RF: Anatomic CT demonstration of the peritoneal spaces, ligaments and mesenteries: normal and pathologic processes, *Radiographics* 15:755-770, 1995.

Deutch SJ, Sandler MA, Alpern MB: Abdominal lymphadenopathy in benign diseases: CT detection, *Radiology* 163:335-338, 1987.

Earls JP, Dachman AH, Colon E, et al: Prevalence and duration of post-operative pneumoperitoneum, *AJR* 161:781-785, 1993.

Einstein DM, Singer AA, Chilcote WA, et al: Abdominal lymphadenopathy: spectrum of CT findings, *Radiographics* 11:457-472, 1991.

Feczko PJ, Mezwa DG, Farah MC, et al: Clinical significance of pneumatosis of the bowel wall, *Radiographics* 12:1069-1078, 1992.

Galandiuk S, Fazio VW: Pneumatosis cystoides intestinalis: a review of the literature, *Dis Colon Rectum* 29:358-363, 1986.

Gomes AS, Lois JF, McCoy RD: Angiographic treatment of gastrointestinal hemorrhage: comparison of vasopressin infusion and embolization, *AJR* 255:497-500, 1986.

Gostout CJ, Wang KK, Ahlquist DA, et al: Acute gastrointestinal hemorrhage, *J Clin Gastroenterol* 14:260-267, 1992.

Harrison LA, Keesling CA, Martin NL, et al: Abdominal wall hernias: review of herniography and correlation with cross-sectional imaging, *Radiographics* 15:315-332, 1995.

Jeffrey RB, Nyberg DA, Bottles K, et al: Abdominal CT in acquired immunodeficiency syndrome, *AJR* 146:7-13, 1986.

Lecklitner ML, Hughes JJ: Pitfalls of gastrointestinal bleeding studies with 99mTc-labeled RBCs, *Semin Nucl Med* 16:151-154, 1986.

Lee GM, Cohen AJ: CT imaging of abdominal hernias, *AJR* 161:1209-1213, 1993.

Marshall JB: Acute gastrointestinal bleeding, *Postgrad Med* 87:63-70, 1990.

Miller PA, Mezwa DG, Feczko PJ, et al: Imaging of abdominal hernias, *Radiographics* 15:333-347, 1995.

Murray JG, Evans SJ, Jeffrey PB, et al: Cytomegalovirus colitis in AIDS: CT features, *AJR* 165:67-71, 1995.

Nyberg DA, Federle MP: AIDS-related Kaposi sarcoma and lymphoma, *Semin Roentgenol* 22:54-65, 1987.

Panicek, DM, Benson CB, Gottlieb RH, et al: The diaphragm: anatomic, pathologic, and radiologic considerations, *Radiographics* 8:385-425, 1988.

Pantongrag-Brown L, Nelson AM, Brown AE, et al: Gastrointestinal manifestations of acquired immunodeficiency syndrome: radiologic-pathologic correlations, *Radiographics* 15:1155-1178, 1995.

Radin R: HIV infection: analysis in 259 consecutive patients with abnormal abdominal CT findings, *Radiology* 197:712-719, 1995.

Redvanly RD, Silverstein JE: Intra-abdominal manifestations of AIDS, *Radiol Clin North Am* 35:1083, 1997.

Scheidler J, Stabler A, Kleber G, et al: Computed tomography in pneumatosis intestinalis: differential diagnosis and therapeutic consequences, *Abdom Imag* 20:253-258, 1995.

Shackleton KL, Stewart ET, Taylor AJ: Traumatic diaphragmatic injuries: spectrum of radiographic findings, *Radiographics* 18:49-59, 1998.

Solomon JA, Levine MS, O'Brien C, et al: HIV colitis: clinical and radiographic findings, *AJR* 168:681-687, 1997.

Wall SD, Ominsky S, Altman DF, et al: Multifocal abnormalities of the gastrointestinal tract in AIDS, *AJR* 146:1-5, 1986.

Wechsler RJ, Kurtz AB, Needleman L, et al: Cross-sectional imaging of abdominal wall hernias, *AJR* 153:517-521, 1989.

Wood BJ, Kumar PN, Cooper C, et al: Pneumatosis intestinalis in adults with AIDS: clinical significance and imaging findings, *AJR* 165:1387-1391, 1995.

Zarvan NP, Lee FT, Yandow DR, et al: Abdominal hernias: CT findings, *AJR* 164:1391-1399, 1995.

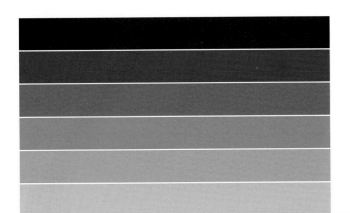

Index